# The Neurological Manifestations of Pediatric Infectious Diseases and Immunodeficiency Syndromes

# Infectious Disease™

**Series Editor:** ***Vassil St. Georgiev***

National Institude of Allergy and Infectious Disease

National Institutes of Health

---

**National Institue of Allergy and Infectious Diseases, NIH: Volume 1: Frontiers in Research,** edited by ***Vassil St. Geogiev, PhD***, 2008

**The Neurological Manifestations of Pediatric Infectious Diseases and Immunodeficiency Syndromes,** edited by ***Leslie L. Barton, MD and Neil R. Friedman, MBChB,*** 2008

**Diagnosis and Treatment of Human Mycoses,** edited by ***Duane R. Hospenthal, MD, PhD, and Michael G. Rinaldi, PhD***, 2007

**Foodborne Diseases,** edited by ***Shabbir Simjee, PhD***, 2007

**Reverse Transcriptase Inhibitors in HIV/AIDS Therapy,** edited by ***Gail Skowron, MD and Richard Ogden, PhD,*** 2006

**Vaccine Adjuvants:** *Immunological and Clinical Principles*, edited by ***Charles J. Hackett, PhD and Donald A. Harn, Jr., PhD***, 2006

**Congenital and Perinatal Infections:** *A Concise Guide to Diagnosis*, edited by ***Cecelia Hutto, MD***, 2006

**Drug Interactions in Infectious Diseases:** *Second Edition*, edited by ***Stephen C. Piscitelli, PharmD and Keith A. Rodvold, PharmD***, 2005

**Biological Weapons Defense:** *Infectious Disease and Counterbioterrorism*, edited by ***Luther E. Lindler, PhD, Frank J. Lebeda, PhD, and George W. Korch, PhD***, 2005

**Microbial Genomes**, edited by ***Claire M. Fraser, PhD, Timothy D. Read, PhD, and Karen E. Nelson, PhD***, 2004

**Management of Multiple Drug-Resistant Infections**, edited by ***Stephen H. Gillespie, MD***, 2004

**Aging, Immunity, and Infection**, by ***Joseph F. Albright, PhD, and Julia W. Albright, PhD***, 2003

**Handbook of Cytokines and Chemokines in Infectious Diseases**, edited by ***Malak Kotb, PhD and Thierry Calandra, MD, PhD***, 2003

**Opportunistic Infections:** *Treatment and Prophylaxis,* by ***Vassil St. Georgiev, PhD***, 2003

*Innate Immunity*, edited by ***R. Alan B. Ezekowitz, MBChB, DPhil, FAAP*** and ***Jules A. Hoffmann***, PhD, 2003

**Pathogen Genomics:** *Impact on Human Health,* edited by ***Karen Joy Shaw, PhD***, 2002

**Immunotherapy for Infectious Diseases**, edited by ***Jeffrey M. Jacobson, MD***, 2002

**Retroviral Immunology:** *Immune Response and Restoration,* edited by ***Giuseppe Pantaleo, MD and Bruce D. Walker, MD***, 2001

# The Neurological Manifestations of Pediatric Infectious Diseases and Immunodeficiency Syndromes

Leslie L. Barton, MD
Professor of Pediatrics and Director, Pediatric Residency Program,
Codirector, Pediatric/Emergency Medicine Residency Program,
University of Arizona College of Medicine, Tucson, AZ

Neil R. Friedman, MBChB
Staff Physician, Neurological Institute
Director, Pediatric Neurology Residency Program,
Cleveland Clinic, Cleveland, OH

Foreword by

Joseph J. Volpe, MD
Bronson Crothers Distinguished Professor of Neurology
Harvard Medical School
Boston, MA

Humana Press

Leslie L. Barton, MD
Professor of Pediatrics and Director
Pediatric Residency Program
Codirector, Pediatric/Emergency Medicine
Residency Program
University of Arizona College of Medicine
Tucson, AZ 85724
llb@peds.arizona.edu

Neil R. Friedman, MBChB
Staff Physician, Neurological Institute
Director, Pediatric Neurology Residency Program
Cleveland Clinic, Cleveland, OH
friedmn@ccf.org

ISBN: 978-1-58829-967-3 e-ISBN: 978-1-59745-391-2

Library of Congress Control Number: 2007933722



Printed on acid-free paper.

9 8 7 6 5 4 3 2 1

springer.com

*We dedicate this work to those who have:*

- *Enabled and encouraged us—our spouses, William Holmes (LLB) and Joanne Friedman (NRF), our children, our grandchildren (LLB), our parents and Johanna Grimes (LLB)*
- *Inspired us—our students, housestaff, and teachers*
- *Endured us—our colleagues*

# Foreword

A major portion of all of acute child neurology involves the neurological complications of infectious diseases. However, none of the currently available excellent texts on infectious disease focus specifically on the neurological aspects. Drs. Neil R. Friedman and Leslie L. Barton have filled this important void with a superb, multi-authored text, addressing directly "the neurological manifestations of pediatric infectious diseases and immunodeficiency syndromes."

The book is organized logically according to the responsible microorganisms and addresses sequentially a broad spectrum of viruses, bacteria, fungi, rickettsiae, spirochetes, mycobacteriae, and parasites, as well as cat-scratch disease and human immunodeficiency virus (HIV) infection. The chapters are consistently similar in organization and begin with an introduction that provides a synopsis and perspective. The substance of the chapters follows in sections devoted to epidemiology, pathogenesis, clinical manifestations, diagnosis, treatment, and references. The discussions of epidemiology are particularly informative and current. The sections on pathogenesis include valuable neuropathology and critical distinctions among disorders caused by primary infection by the microorganism and those related to parainfectious and postinfectious immunological phenomena. The sections on clinical manifestations emphasize the neurological features and often are subdivided into specific neurological syndromes. Results of modern brain imaging are illustrated, and tables highlight neurological and other features. Sections on diagnosis are especially valuable and emphasize the value of polymerase chain reaction (PCR) and related means of identifying microbial nucleic acids and proteins. The discussions of treatment are especially current and valuable. The citations are up-to-date and reflect a broad spectrum of both the neurological and infectious disease literature.

This text is very well balanced. It is comprehensive yet readable. It emphasizes neurological aspects, yet includes detailed and current infectious disease aspects. The balance undoubtedly reflects particularly the expertise of the two editors, one a child neurologist (Dr. Neil R. Friedman), and the other, an infectious disease expert (Dr. Leslie L. Barton).

The editors are to be congratulated for the superb organization of the text and their important personal contributions, the assembling of an outstanding group of authors, and the orchestration of a consistent and clear message throughout the text. It should prove useful to anyone involved in the evaluation and care of sick children.

Joseph J. Volpe, M.D.
Bronson Crothers Distinguished
Professor of Neurology
Harvard Medical School
Boston, MA

# Preface

Infectious diseases and immunodeficiencies remain the leading causes of morbidity and mortality in the world's children today (World Health Organization [WHO], 2006). The WHO estimates that nearly one third of the global deaths in 2005 were attributable to communicable diseases, an acknowledged underestimate. Despite the optimism engendered by the development of antimicrobial therapy and vaccines, and improvements in sanitation—especially in developed countries—infections both prevail (e.g., malaria) and emerge (e.g., human immunodeficiency virus/acquired immunodeficiency syndrome). Infectious diseases respect neither geographic nor medical specialty boundaries.

Pediatricians and all who care for children are faced virtually on a daily basis with classic and unusual presentations of infectious diseases and immunodeficiencies in their patients. The neurological consequences of infectious diseases and immunodeficiency syndromes have, however, not been previously compiled in a readily accessible volume.

Our goal is to provide a succinct authoritative, up-to-date, evidence-based, practical, and accessible reference. This book is written for physicians-in-training, primary care physicians, and subspecialists. We aim to alert practitioners to the neurological manifestations of infectious disease entities and, conversely, to alert physicians who encounter a neurological process to the possibility of an underlying infectious disease or immunodeficiency syndrome.

All chapters provide a general description of the disease or disorder, its epidemiology, etiology, clinical synopsis, neurological manifestations, diagnosis, differential diagnosis, and therapy. We have endeavored to enhance the volume's usefulness by maintaining a structured format, at the same time offering refreshing and diverse expositions by an international group of authors. Although we attempted to minimize duplication, some repetition was unavoidable.

The editors are grateful to these expert contributors, to our teachers and to our mentors, and to the many individuals who helped bring this text to fruition.

Leslie L. Barton, M.D.
Neil R. Friedman, M.B.Ch.B

# Contents

# Contributors

Motasem A. Abuelreish, M.D.
Pediatric Infectious Diseases Consultant, King Hussein Cancer Center; Pediatric Residency Program Director, Specialty Hospital, Amman, Jordan

Lemuel Aigbivbalu, M.D.
Pediatric Infectious Diseases and Immunology, University of Florida College of Medicine, Jacksonville, FL

Ana M. Alvarez, M.D.
Assistant Professor of Pediatrics, University of Florida College of Medicine, Jacksonville, FL

Leslie L. Barton, M.D.
Professor of Pediatrics, Director Pediatric Residency Program, Codirector, Pediatric/Emergency Medicine Residency Program, University of Arizona College of Medicine, Tucson, AZ

Daniel J. Bonthius, M.D., Ph.D.
Associate Professor, Department of Pediatrics, Division of Child Neurology, University of Iowa College of Medicine, Iowa City, IA

Nancy E. Bonthius, Pharm.D.
Clinical Assistant Professor, Division of Clinical and Administrative Pharmacy, University of Iowa College of Medicine, Iowa City, IA

Kimberley C. Brown, Pharm.D.
Assistant Professor of Pediatrics, University of Florida College of Medicine, Jacksonville, FL

Megan Connick, M.D.
Staff Physician, Christian Hospital, St. Louis, MO

Hannah Klein de Licona
Neuroscience Program, University of Iowa College of Medicine,
Iowa City, IA

Sean P. Elliott, M.D.
Associate Professor of Clinical Pediatrics, University of Arizona College of Medicine, Tucson, AZ

Allan D. Friedman, M.D., M.P.H.
Professor and Chair, Division of General Pediatrics, Department of Pediatrics, Virginia Commonwealth University School of Medicine, Richmond, VA

Neil R. Friedman, M.B.Ch.B.
Staff Physician, Neurological Institute, Director, Pediatric Neurology Residency Program, Cleveland Clinic, Cleveland, OH

Patrick J. Gavin, M.B., M.R.C.P.I.D.(A.B.M.M.)
Consultant Pediatric Infectious Diseases, Rainbow Clinic, Our Lady's Hospital for Sick Children, Crumlin, Dublin, Ireland

C. Diane Halstead, Ph.D.
Professor of Pediatrics, University of Florida College of Medicine, Jacksonville; Pathology Associates, P.A./Baptist Health, Jacksonville, FL

Lisa D. Inge, Pharm.D.
University of Florida College of Pharmacy, Jacksonville, FL

Bahri Karacay, Ph.D.
Adjunct Assistant Professor, Department of Pediatrics, University of Iowa College of Medicine, Iowa City, IA

Abeer Khayat, M.D.
Chief of Pediatrics, American Hospital of Dubai, Dubai, United Arab Emirates

Andrew M. Margileth, M.D., F.A.A.P., F.A.C.P.
Professor of Pediatrics, University of Florida College of Medicine, Jacksonville, FL

Sean O. McKenna, M.D.
Assistant Professor, Division of General Pediatrics, Department of Pediatrics, Virginia Commonwealth University School of Medicine, Richmond, VA

Ayesha Mirza, M.D.
Assistant Professor of Pediatrics, Division of Infectious Diseases and Immunology, University of Florida College of Medicine, Jacksonville, FL

Manikum Moodley, M.B.Ch.B.
Staff Physician, Neurological Institute, Cleveland Clinic, Cleveland, OH

Jason G. Newland, M.D., F.A.A.P.
Assistant Professor of Pediatrics, University of Missouri–Kansas City; Section of Infectious Disease, Children's Mercy Hospital, Kansas City, MO

Mobeen H. Rathore, M.D., C.P.E., F.A.A.P.
Professor of Pediatrics and Associate Chairman, Chief Division of Pediatric Infectious Diseases and Immunology, University of Florida College of Medicine and Wolfson Children's Hospital, Director Rainbow Center for Women, Adolescents, Children and Families, Jacksonville, FL

José R. Romero, M.D., F.A.A.P.
Professor of Pediatrics, Pathology, and Microbiology, Director, Section of Pediatric Infectious Diseases, University of Nebraska Medical Center, Omaha, NE

Barbara Stechenberg, M.D.
Vice Chairman and Director, Pediatric Infectious Diseases, Baystate Children's Hospital; Professor of Pediatrics, Tufts University School of Medicine, Springfield, MA

Meera Varman, M.D., F.A.A.P.
Assistant Professor of Pediatrics, Creighton University School of Medicine, Omaha, NE

# Section I
# Viruses

# Chapter 1
# Herpes Viruses

**Sean P. Elliott, M.D.**

## Herpes Simplex Virus

### *Introduction*

Herpes simplex virus (HSV) is a ubiquitous virus that infects most humans and is responsible for a broad spectrum of disease, ranging from asymptomatic infection to fatal, sporadic viral encephalitis. HSV occupies a prominent place in the differential diagnosis of infectious neurological disease and has led to large modifications in the diagnostic and interventional approach to acute encephalitis and neonatal infection.

### *Epidemiology*

HSV is highly infectious, but requires close interpersonal contact for transmission. Such transmission can occur via saliva or direct apposition of infected with uninfected mucous membranes. HSV-1 typically is associated with gingivostomatitis, pharyngitis, and encephalitis in children and adults. HSV-2 primarily is associated with genital herpes. Both can cause neonatal disease, acquired either transplacentally or via exposure to cervical secretions. Age-linked seroprevalence data differ for HSV-1 and HSV-2, reflecting patterns expected for a sexually transmitted disease (HSV-2) compared with a mostly nonsexually transmitted disease (HSV-1). HSV-1 seroprevalence increases in a linear fashion with increasing age, reaching at least 40% by age 15 years and 60 to 90% in older adults; HSV-2 seroprevalence is very low in those younger than 15 years, but increases precipitously during the sexually active years and plateaus after age 40 years [1]. The seroprevalence of HSV-2 continues to increase in the United States, recently reaching 20.8% overall, with high-risk groups demonstrating 46 to 77% [1, 2]. Asymptomatic shedding of HSV is common: patients with known recurrent genital disease shed HSV up to 10% of the time that they are lesion free [3]. Not surprisingly, the incidence of neonatal HSV infection has shown a similar increase, rising from 2.6 per 100,000 live births to 11 to 28.2 per 100,000 live births [4, 5]. Preventive measures and planned cesarean delivery may eventually halt or reverse this trend [6].

L.L. Barton and N.R. Friedman (eds.), *The Neurological Manifestations of Pediatric Infectious Diseases and Immunodeficiency Syndromes.*

## *Pathogenesis*

HSV is the fastest growing member of the *Herpesviridae* family of DNA viruses, existing in humans in two serotypes, HSV-1 and HSV-2, which share approximately 50% nucleotide homology. HSV is highly neurotropic and can establish latent infections with periodic reactivation. Initial infection and viral replication occur at the site of entry, typically skin or mucous membranes. Cellular response to injury precipitates local inflammation with formation of vesicles in the affected areas. After resolution of primary infection, HSV remains latent in sensory ganglia. The route of transmission to the brain in encephalitis is less well understood. Neonates with disseminated HSV disease likely experience viremia with secondary diffuse encephalitis resulting in generalized encephalomalacia [7, 8]. Neonates, children, and adults with primary encephalitis may experience retrograde axonal transport via the trigeminal ganglia or nerve after HSV reactivation or new infection, resulting in distinctive, localized inflammation in the mediotemporal and orbitofrontal lobes [9,10].

## *Clinical Manifestations*

### Perinatal Disease

Neonates are especially vulnerable to HSV infections, acquired most often via vertical transmission in the peripartum period and less frequently in utero or via postpartum exposure. Prevention of HSV transmission is difficult because 70 to 80% of infected infants are born to mothers with asymptomatic HSV infection [11]. Risk for neonatal infection is much higher in those babies born to mothers with primary infection (33%) than those born to mothers with reactivated disease (3%) [12]. Additional risk factors include maternal antibody status, duration of ruptured membranes, and placement of a scalp monitor [13]. Neonatal infection may be classified into four syndromes: intrauterine disease; skin, eye, and mouth (SEM) disease; disseminated disease; and encephalitis. Demographics and characteristics of infants with neonatal HSV disease are listed in Table 1.1, compiled from National Institute of Allergy and Infectious Diseases (NIAID) Collaborative Antiviral Study Group Data [14,15].

### Intrauterine Disease

True congenital HSV infection acquired in utero is rare. Infants are born with congenital malformations and evidence of HSV infection detected at or shortly after delivery. One series of such infants found the clinical manifestations to include skin lesions, chorioretinitis, microcephaly, hydranencephaly, and microphthalmia, with all infants demonstrating at least two malformations in combination.

**Table 1.1** Demographic and clinical characteristics of infants enrolled in a National Institute of Allergy and Infectious Diseases (NIAID) collaborative antiviral study [14,15]

| | Disease classification | | |
|---|---|---|---|
| | Disseminated | CNS | SEM |
| No. of infants | 93 (32%) | 95 (33%) | 102 (35%) |
| Clinical findings | | | |
| Skin lesions | 72 (77%) | 60 (63%) | 86 (84%) |
| Brain involvement | 69 (74%) | 95 (100%) | 0 (0%) |
| Pneumonia | 46 (49%) | 4 (4%) | 3 (3%) |
| Mortality at 1 yr[a] | 56 (60%) | 13 (14%) | 0 (0%) |
| Neurological impairment of survivors (affected/total) | | | |
| Total | 15/34 (44%) | 45/81 (56%) | 10/93 (11%) |
| Adenine arabinoside | 13/26 (50%) | 25/51 (49%) | 3/34 (9%) |
| Acyclovir | 1/6 (17%) | 18/27 (67%) | 4/51 (8%) |
| Placebo | 1/2 (50%) | 2/3 (67%) | 3/8 (38%) |

[a]Regardless of therapy.

All survivors developed significant neurological sequelae, including hearing and vision defects, mental retardation, severe developmental delay, and complex seizure disorders [16]. The triad of skin vesicles/scarring, eye damage, and microcephaly/hydranencephaly suggests the diagnosis. Central nervous system (CNS) damage is caused by intrauterine encephalitis. Other data indicates a higher risk of spontaneous abortion for women with genital HSV infections, suggesting the majority of fetuses infected in utero are not viable [17,18].

## Skin, Eye, and Mouth Disease

SEM disease typically presents in the first or second week of life, with discrete, vesicular skin lesions present on any part of the body. Clusters of vesicles also occur, especially on traumatized skin, such as scalp monitor sites, or on the presenting part of the body. SEM disease is not associated initially with significant neurological disease. However, if left untreated, 35 to 40% of patients with SEM disease may develop neurological disease [13]. Recurrences occur in 90% of patients and may be associated with CNS involvement. Moreover, 20 to 30% of infants who experience more than three recurrences in the first 6 months of life develop evidence of neurological impairment [11,15], including cognitive defects, spastic quadriplegia, microcephaly, and blindness [13]. Risk for neurological sequelae seems to be even higher with HSV-2 infections than HSV-1 infections [11]. Although the safety of oral suppressive acyclovir therapy has been established [19], evaluation of its efficacy in preventing such recurrences and neurological sequelae is ongoing. Thus, infants with both primary and recurrent SEM disease deserve evaluation for CNS involvement and initial, aggressive treatment with antiviral agents.

### Disseminated Disease

Infants with disseminated HSV disease develop symptoms in the first week of life, although diagnosis occurs more commonly in the second week of life. Disseminated HSV disease carries the worst prognosis. Any organ may be affected, but the lungs, liver, adrenal glands, and brain are the most common targets. Encephalitis occurs in 60 to 70% of infants, most likely as a result of hematogenous spread to the brain, causing multiple areas of cortical hemorrhagic necrosis [15]. Signs and symptoms of disseminated disease include irritability, lethargy, seizures, respiratory distress, jaundice, bleeding diathesis, and shock. Unfortunately, at least 20% of infants with disseminated disease will not demonstrate skin vesicles [13], thus complicating initial diagnosis. Without treatment, mortality exceeds 80%. Even with timely initiation of antiviral agents, mortality remains high (50–60%) [11].

### Neonatal Encephalitis

Primary neonatal HSV encephalitis usually presents in the second to third week of life. Typical signs and symptoms include focal, multifocal, or generalized seizures; lethargy; irritability; poor feeding; temperature instability; apnea; bradycardia; and cranial nerve abnormalities [15]. Only 60% will develop skin lesions during their disease course [11]. Typical cerebrospinal fluid (CSF) findings include pleocytosis and mild reduction of glucose. Although initial CSF protein concentrations may be normal or only slightly elevated, most infants usually demonstrate progressive increases up to more than 1000 mg/dL. The hemorrhagic nature of HSV encephalitis may result in apparent bloody CSF, making differentiation from a traumatic lumbar puncture difficult. Electroencephalography (EEG) and neuroimaging demonstrate abnormalities in 85% and 74%, respectively, of patients with HSV CNS disease [14]. Untreated neonatal HSV encephalitis carries a 50% mortality. With prompt initiation of antiviral therapy, mortality drops to 15 to 18% [8,11]. Antiviral therapy has no significant impact on neurological sequelae in survivors: 50 to 66% will develop neurological impairment such as psychomotor retardation, microcephaly, hydranencephaly, spasticity, blindness, chorioretinitis, or learning disabilities [8,11,15]. Neuroimaging typically demonstrates progression of focal parenchymal lesions into multicystic cerebral degeneration [20].

### Sporadic Encephalitis

HSV is the most common cause of sporadic, acquired, focal encephalitis in the United States, occurring in approximately 1 in 250,000 to 500,000 people annually [8]. A bimodal age distribution exists, with more than 80% of cases found in patients younger than 20 years or older than 50 years of age and, unlike most other causes of viral encephalitis, cases occur throughout the year [10]. HSV-1 is the cause of 93 to 96% of cases, more often as a result of recurrent or reactivated (70%) disease than primary (30%) infection [21].

HSV encephalitis may have an acute or subacute onset. Most patients develop signs of localized lesions in the temporal lobes, often taking the form of personality changes, hallucinations, or bizarre behavior. Fever, headache, and alterations in consciousness also are prominent early symptoms, followed by seizures, hemiparesis, dysphasia, and superior quadrant visual field defects (Table 1.2). Without treatment, most patients progress from stupor to coma to death very rapidly [9].

The CSF frequently demonstrates pleocytosis ranging from 50 to 2000 white blood cells/mm$^3$, with a lymphoid predominance. Red blood cells may be seen in 75 to 85% of cases, reflecting the hemorrhagic, necrotic nature of HSV encephalitis. Five to 25% of patients have hypoglycorrhachia, and 80 to 88% have elevated protein levels, beginning at a median of 80 mg/dL and rising dramatically as the disease progresses. CSF findings in early disease may be subtle, with mild pleocytosis and neutrophil predominance, normal glucose, and minimally elevated protein levels [9,22]. EEG (Fig. 1.1) may show unilateral or bilateral periodic focal spikes against a background of slow (flattened) activity (periodic lateralized epileptiform discharges [PLEDS]), which typically has been associated with HSV encephalitis [22]. PLEDS is not, however, pathognomonic for this, and may be associated with other neurological conditions. Magnetic resonance imaging (MRI) scanning is more sensitive than computed tomographic (CT) scanning for early detection of HSV encephalitis [23]. Findings include hyperintensity on T2-weighted images of temporal areas and gadolinium enhancement (Fig. 1.2)

Without appropriate antiviral treatment, the mortality of HSV encephalitis exceeds 70% [8]. Use of acyclovir reduces the mortality rate to 19%, although this may be negatively influenced by increased patient age and lower initial level of consciousness [9]. A poor therapeutic outcome is uniform in those patients with an initial Glasgow Coma Score of 6 or less [8]. Even with treatment, patients who survive HSV encephalitis may have severe sequelae, including major motor and sensory deficits, aphasia, and an amnestic syndrome (Korsakoff's psychosis) [9].

**Table 1.2** Historical and clinical findings in HSV encephalitis [8–10,22]

| Historical findings | | Clinical findings at presentation | |
|---|---|---|---|
| Alteration of consciousness | 97% | Fever | 92% |
| Fever | 90% | Personality changes | 85% |
| Headache | 81% | Dysphasia | 76% |
| Persistent seizures | 67% | Autonomic dysfunction | 60% |
| Personality change | 71% | Ataxia | 40% |
| Vomiting | 46% | Seizures | 38% |
| Hemiparesis | 33% | Focal | 28% |
| Memory loss | 24% | Generalized | 10% |
| | | Cranial nerve defects | 32% |
| | | Visual field loss | 14% |
| | | Papilledema | 14% |

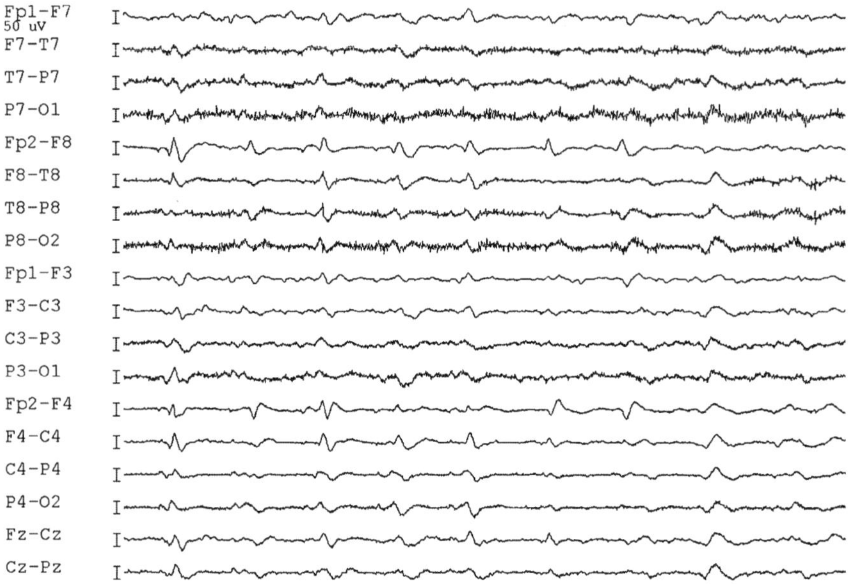


**Fig. 1.1** Focal right PLEDS in a patient with HSV encephalitis (EEG courtesy of Deepak Lachhwani, M.D.)

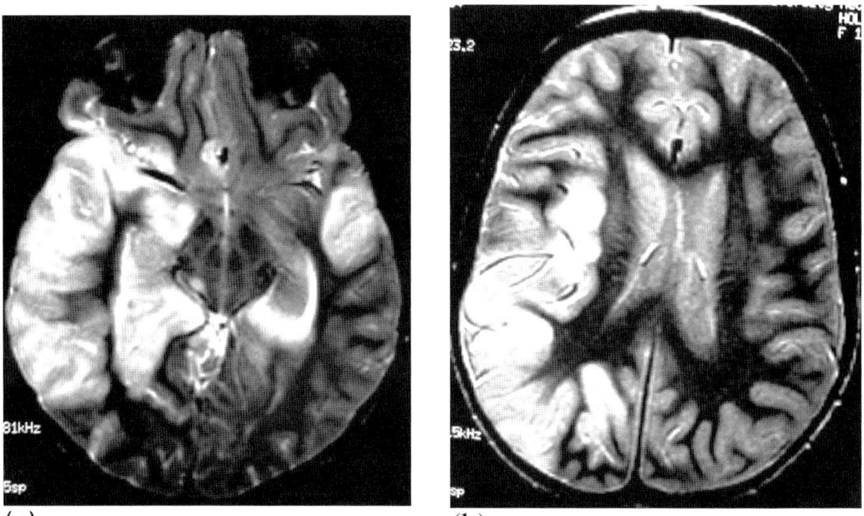


**Fig. 1.2** Head MRI scan, T2-weighted axial images, of a 9-year-old girl with sporadic HSV encephalitis demonstrates temporal lobe inflammation (**a**) and parietooccipital lobe inflammation (**b**), both with mass effect.

## Meningitis

HSV-induced aseptic meningitis syndrome is typically caused by HSV-2, usually as a complication of primary genital infection. Signs of meningitis appear shortly after genital lesions are noted, and include headache, photophobia, and nuchal rigidity. Seizures and focal CNS findings are generally absent. CSF findings demonstrate pleocytosis (300–2600 white blood cells/$mm^3$) with lymphoid predominance and occasionally hypoglycorrhachia [22]. Recovery is spontaneous and complete, requiring no specific antiviral therapy. However, this syndrome may recur with genital recurrences.

HSV is now thought to be the major agent responsible for benign recurrent lymphocytic meningitis (Mollaret's meningitis) [24]. This syndrome involves recurrent attacks of fever and meningismus with CSF demonstrating lymphocytic pleocytosis (48–1600 cells/$mm^3$), normal glucose, and elevated protein (41–240 mg/dL). HSV-2 DNA has been detected in CSF of patients with Mollaret's meningitis while the patients are symptomatic but not in asymptomatic patients or in healthy controls [10,24].

## Other Neurological Disease

HSV is also associated with diseases of the peripheral nervous system, generally as a result of recurrence within the dermatome of primary infection. However, recurrent disease does not necessarily occur at precisely the same anatomic location [25]. Common sites of infection and the associated diseases are listed in Table 1.3. HSV-1 seems to be the most likely cause of peripheral facial nerve palsy (Bell's palsy), although multiple infectious agents and clinical syndromes are also possible. Patients with HSV encephalitis may also develop acute retinal necrosis syndrome [26–28], parainfectious encephalomyeloradiculitis, recurrent encephalitis, ascending myelitis, and postinfectious encephalopathy [29,30]. Although usually associated with encephalitis, acute HSV cerebellitis has been demonstrated in the absence of previous CNS infection [31].

**Table 1.3** HSV infections of the peripheral nervous system [25]

| Nerve | Disease manifestation |
|---|---|
| Vth cranial nerve | Gingivostomatitis |
| | Recurrent cold sores |
| | Corneal infections |
| | HSV gladiatorum[a] |
| VIIth cranial nerve | Facial paralysis |
| Cervical and thoracic sensory nerves | Herpetic whitlow |
| | Nipple infection |
| Lumbosacral sensory nerves | Genital herpes |

[a] Can also affect cervical and thoracic sensory nerves.

## *Diagnosis*

Culture remains the most sensitive method for diagnosing active infection of non-CNS sites, such as skin, eyes, and mucous membranes. Samples should be obtained by swabbing the base of denuded lesions with premoistened cotton swabs followed by direct inoculation into either viral transport or culture media. HSV cytopathic effect may be observed from between 24 hours and 5 days, depending on the viral load of the sample. More rapid diagnosis is available through direct detection methods, most commonly direct immunofluorescent staining. This method is more sensitive (80–90%) and specific than the Tzanck test [32]. Serologic evaluation is possible via enzyme-linked immunosorbent assays (ELISA) or latex agglutination procedures. However, these results are difficult to interpret because detectable IgM may occur in both reactivated disease and new disease, and infected infants may demonstrate diminished or absent production of IgM. Mothers of infected infants may be seronegative or seropositive. However, many assays do not distinguish between HSV-1 and HSV-2. Thus, new infection by one type may be obscured by serologic evidence of previous infection with the other type.

The gold standard for diagnosis of HSV-associated CNS disease has been isolation of HSV obtained at brain biopsy. However, polymerase chain reaction (PCR) testing now has replaced brain biopsy as the diagnostic test of choice for HSV encephalitis. HSV PCR of CSF carries a sensitivity and specificity of 98% and 96%, respectively [33], and now is widely available in commercial laboratories. False negative results may occur early in the course of CNS disease. However, detection of HSV in CSF by PCR remains possible for up to 10 days in the setting of concurrent antiviral therapy [34]. HSV PCR has, thus, become an extremely useful tool in the diagnosis of a variety of neurological disorders, including encephalitis, meningitis, Mollaret's meningitis, myelitis, and Bell's palsy [35].

## *Treatment*

Acyclovir remains the drug of choice for most HSV infections. It is available for parenteral, oral, and topical delivery. Oral preparations of its prodrug improve the bioavailability of active drug. Use of acyclovir for non-CNS HSV disease or recurrence is of unclear benefit in most cases. Treatment decisions in such cases must, therefore, be individualized. Preliminary research has shown a clinical benefit from use of both corticosteroids and acyclovir together in patients with Bell's palsy, although this finding remains to be confirmed [10]. Data regarding dose and duration is lacking, although initiation early in the course of disease seems more beneficial than when a treatment delay occurs. Use of acyclovir has significant positive impact on HSV encephalitis mortality. The currently accepted treatment of non-neonatal HSV encephalitis is parenteral acyclovir 30 mg/kg/d, divided every 8 hours, for 21 days. Neonates with HSV disease localized to skin, eye, and mouth require parenteral acyclovir 60 mg/kg/d, divided every 8 hours, for 14 days. However, neonates with evidence of disseminated disease or encephalitis may require 21 days of treatment. Higher doses (90 mg/kg/d) currently are being studied to assess the possibility of added benefit. Acyclovir is well tolerated. It rarely has been associated with renal dysfunction and neutropenia [36]. The possibility of a HSV vaccine remains enticing and is the subject of considerable research interest [37].

## Cytomegalovirus

### *Introduction*

Cytomegalovirus (CMV) is the most common cause of congenital infection in the United States, a leading infectious cause of brain damage and sensorineural hearing loss in children in developed countries [38], and an important opportunistic pathogen in patients with abnormal immune function. It has been called "a ubiquitous agent with protean clinical manifestations [39],"a testimony to the difficulty of recognizing and predicting its potential for neurological disease.

### *Epidemiology*

CMV transmission occurs primarily through exposure to urine, respiratory secretions, and sexual contact, and, rarely, via blood and blood products. Vertical transmission from mother to fetus occurs transplacentally and via exposure to cervical secretions. Breast milk has been identified as a significant source of postnatal acquisition of symptomatic CMV disease in very low birth weight infants [40]. CMV causes congenital infection in 0.2 to 2.5% of all live births in the world [41]. In the United States, approximately 1% of newborns shed CMV in the urine at birth, leading to approximately 40,000 new cases of congenital CMV per year [42]. Most of these infections are asymptomatic; however 10% of congenitally infected infants will demonstrate clinically apparent disease [42].

### *Pathogenesis*

CMV is the largest and slowest growing member of the *Herpesviridae* family of DNA viruses. Inoculation of CMV usually takes place via a mucosal surface in the upper respiratory or genital tract and is likely followed by viremia, accounting for dissemination to many different organs and viral shedding from saliva, urine, and genital secretions. Disease may be caused by a primary cytopathic effect, immunopathologic process, or both. The extent of brain injury induced by primary infection is very variable and most often affects the periventricular subependymal matrix, especially in the lateral ventricles. Necrosis and accompanying calcification can be associated with these lesions [42].

## *Clinical Manifestations*

### Congenital CMV Infection

The spectrum of symptomatic congenital CMV infection is wide, and can include mild disease as well as intrauterine growth retardation, hepatitis, hepatosplenomegaly, pneumonitis, hyperbilirubinemia, thrombocytopenia, hemolytic anemia, petechiae, and purpura. Associated CNS and ocular abnormalities are noted in Table 1.4. Five to 17% of infants with asymptomatic congenital CMV at birth are also at risk for development of neurological sequelae, including microcephaly, developmental and intellectual impairment, mental retardation, and sensorineural deafness. This risk drops significantly if the child demonstrates normal development at 12 months of age [43]. However, congenitally acquired CMV remains a leading cause of sensorineural deafness and mental retardation in the United States [38,44,45]. In patients with both symptomatic and asymptomatic congenital CMV infection, evidence of viremia during infancy is associated with development of hearing loss [190,191].

### Perinatal CMV Infection

CMV acquired in the perinatal period typically causes infection in infants from 1 to 4 months of age. Although most of these infections are asymptomatic, approximately one third of infants may demonstrate some signs and symptoms. These include

**Table 1.4** CNS and ocular abnormalities associated with congenital CMV disease [41]

| |
|---|
| Anomaly of optic disc, optic atrophy [a] |
| Anterior chamber malformation |
| Cerebellar aplasia |
| Cerebral cyst formation |
| Chorioretinitis [a] |
| Encephalomalacia |
| Microcephaly [a] |
| Microgyria |
| Microphthalmia |
| Periventricular leukomalacia, calcifications [a] |
| Psychomotor retardation |
| Sensorineural hearing loss [a] |
| Spongiosis of brain |
| Strabismus |
| Ventriculomegaly with hydrocephalus |

[a] Most commonly observed.

self-limited lymphadenopathy, hepatosplenomegaly, hepatitis, and pneumonitis. Perinatal CMV infection has not been shown to cause sensorineural hearing loss or neurodevelopmental disease [46].

### Acquired CMV Infection

CMV acquired by both immunocompetent and immunosuppressed children and adolescents most often manifests as mononucleosis syndrome. Typical CMV-induced mononucleosis is characterized by fever, severe fatigue, and malaise, for approximately 3 to 4 weeks duration. Associated laboratory manifestations include mild elevation of liver enzymes and peripheral lymphocytosis with atypical lymphocytes seen on smear. In contrast to the more commonly recognized Epstein-Barr virus (EBV)-induced mononucleosis, CMV-induced mononucleosis rarely causes pharyngitis or splenomegaly. Neurological complications of CMV-induced mononucleosis are rare and include Guillain-Barré syndrome and meningoencephalitis [47].

### Neurological Manifestations

CNS disease is a well recognized and described component of symptomatic congenital CMV disease. A review of 106 neonates with symptomatic congenital CMV infection identified 54 (53%) infants with microcephaly, 28 (27%) with lethargy/hypotonia, 20 (19%) with poor suck, and 7 (7%) with seizures. Seventy-two (68%) had one or more of these findings [48]. Direct viral infection of neural tissue probably plays a significant role in CNS disease from congenital CMV infection, although infectious vasculitis and thrombocytopenia-related intracranial hemorrhage may also contribute (Fig. 1.3) [49]. Findings on neuroimaging include intracranial calcifications, dilated lateral ventricles, enlarged subarachnoid space, oligo/pachygyria, abnormal myelination, and periventricular cysts (Fig. 1.4). Intracranial calcifications may be visualized in up to 40% of symptomatic infants [42]. The magnitude of the prenatal insult is suggested by the presence of microcephaly, cerebral calcification, and intrauterine growth retardation [50,51]. It may take years to realize the full neurological impact of congenital CMV infection. Ultimately, 50 to 90% of patients with symptomatic congenital CMV infection will develop CNS impairment, including cognitive defects or mental retardation, as will 7 to 25% of asymptomatic CMV infected patients [38]. Early findings demonstrated to be predictive of later CNS impairment include microcephaly, chorioretinitis, lethargy, poor feeding, or abnormalities on cranial CT scan [44,52,53]. Of these, microcephaly at birth seems to be the most specific predictor of poor cognitive outcome, with a highly significant positive correlation between head size at birth and the intelligence–developmental quotient. Conversely, symptomatic children with normal findings on cranial CT scan and a head circumference proportional to their weight seem to exhibit good cognitive outcome [53].

Congenitally CMV-infected infants with no initial signs of disease may develop signs or symptoms of neurological disease within the first 1 to 2 years of life, manifesting as mental retardation, motor disabilities (e.g., spastic diplegia or quadriplegia),

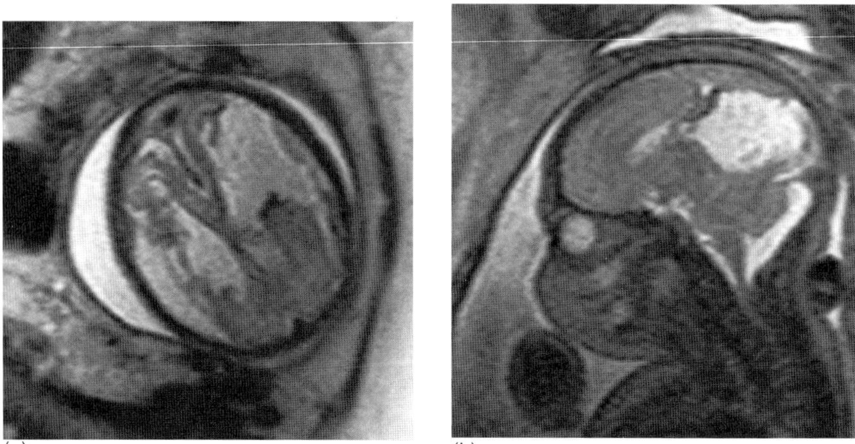

(a) (b)

**Fig. 1.3** Axial (**a**) and parasagittal (**b**) single-shot fast spin echo T2-weighted half-Fourier-acquisition single-shot turbo-spin-echo MRI scan of the brain of a third trimester fetus infected with CMV in the early second trimester shows brain destruction, colpocephaly, and periventricular magnetic susceptibility consistent with calcification (images courtesy of Janet Reid, M.D.; reproduced with permission from: Faerber E. TORCH infections. In: Reid JR, ed. Pediatric radiology curriculum [Internet]. Cleveland, OH: Cleveland Clinic Center for Online Medical Education and Training; 2005. Available from: https://www.cchs.net/pediatricradiology).

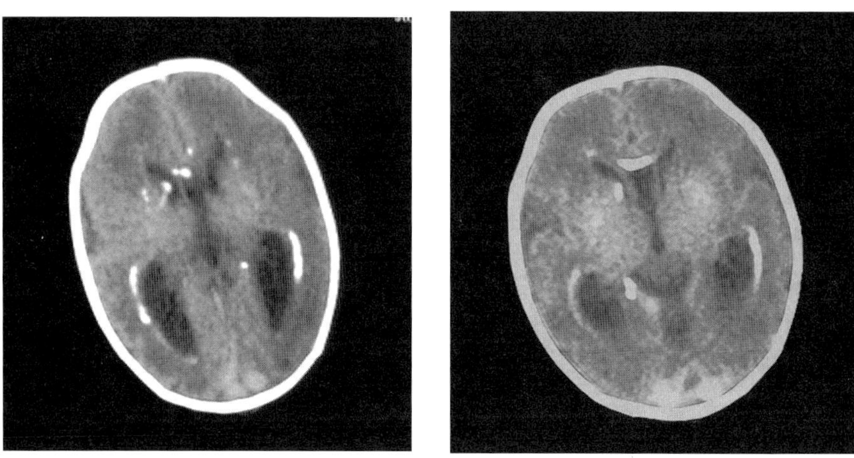

**Fig. 1.4** Head CT scan, axial images, of two patients with congenital CMV demonstrates periventricular calcifications and dilated lateral ventricles.

sensorineural hearing impairment, or microcephaly. It is currently estimated that 2 to 7% of infants with initial asymptomatic congenital CMV infection will develop microcephaly with various degrees of mental retardation and neuromuscular defects by 2 years of age [50]. Long-term, prospective evaluation of the intellectual and neurological development of children with asymptomatic congenital CMV infections has shown conflicting results. Although some studies suggest that asymptomatic CMV disease may be associated with a broad range of subtle neurodevelopmental sequelae [45], others find no significant differences in comparison with patient controls [46]. Thus, a need exists for identification and longitudinal follow-up of infants with asymptomatic congenital CMV, with careful assessments of psychomotor development and sensorineural hearing abilities, to identify those children deserving of corrective and supportive measures.

Primary meningoencephalitis may occur in patients with acquired CMV infection [49] or as a primary or recurrent infection in immunocompromised hosts. Symptoms include headache, photophobia, nuchal rigidity, memory deficits, and inability to concentrate; fever is not prominent [47]. CSF may demonstrate mild mononuclear pleocytosis and slightly elevated protein, but normal or slightly low glucose. Neuroimaging studies may demonstrate periventricular enhancement and ventricular enlargement but may also be normal [34]. The differential diagnosis of CMV meningoencephalitis in an immunocompetent host includes other viruses with neurotropism: HSV, EBV, varicella-zoster virus (VZV), enteroviruses, and arboviruses.

CMV encephalitis is increasingly recognized in patients with acquired immunodeficiency syndrome (AIDS) and may be seen in transplant recipients. Pathologic studies of patients with end-stage AIDS suggest that 20 to 30% patients have evidence of CMV infection of the brain, although not all will demonstrate clinical signs of this [34]. CMV disease will occur in 50 to 100% of solid organ transplant recipients if either donor or recipient is CMV seropositive [54]. However, primary CMV encephalitis in this population remains rare. Clinical manifestations of CMV encephalitis in an immunocompromised host include rapid deterioration of cognition, occasionally accompanied by cranial nerve palsies. CSF findings are similar to those found in immunocompetent patients with CMV encephalitis. CMV has also been associated with peripheral neuropathy in patients with AIDS [55], as well as an ascending paralysis similar to Guillain-Barré syndrome and polyradiculopathy [47]. However, direct causality is difficult to establish, because HIV may also produce similar neurological disease.

As with other neurotropic viruses, CMV is suspected to be associated with many other diseases of the CNS, either via a primary infection of neural tissue or via a postinfectious inflammatory cascade. An association of CMV with Rasmussen's syndrome, lissencephaly-pachygyria, infantile spasms, Guillain-Barré syndrome, and such neuropsychiatric disorders as schizophrenia has been reported [47,49,51,56]. However, difficulties in demonstrating CMV presence in affected tissues have precluded confirmation of a causal relationship for these diseases.

### Chorioretinitis

Ocular involvement by CMV is primarily retinal and can involve all layers of the retina. Strabismus, optic atrophy, microphthalmos, cataracts, retinal necrosis and calcification, blindness, anterior chamber and optic disk malformations, and papillary membrane vestige have also been described [50]. Fifteen percent (range 5–30%) of newborns with symptomatic congenital CMV will have CMV chorioretinitis [57,58], although this entity is rarely seen in asymptomatic congenitally infected newborns. Most retinal lesions in congenitally infected infants appear inactive at birth. Recent observations suggest the possibility of progression as well as late-onset new retinal lesions [47,58]. CMV retinitis is a far greater problem in severely immunocompromised patients. Fifteen percent to 30% of patients with AIDS will develop retinal lesions from CMV, usually in the more advanced stages, in which CD4 counts drop below 50 cells/μl in adults and 100 cells/μl in children [57,59]. Similarly, CMV retinitis may occur in solid organ and bone marrow transplant patients, especially those who experience primary infection with viremia or who receive T-lymphocyte suppressive therapy [54]. Because younger children may not complain of vision changes, ophthalmologic screening is essential in immunocompromised pediatric patients.

CMV produces characteristic white, perivascular lesions and hemorrhage (Fig. 1.5), descriptively called cottage cheese and ketchup, or brushfire retinitis [60]. Progressive retinitis can cause blurred vision, decreased visual acuity, visual field defects, strabismus, and blindness. Although the ophthalmologic appearance of CMV chorioretinitis is characteristic, laboratory diagnosis by PCR of vitreous fluid may be performed in unusual cases. Of note, detection of CMV DNA in an ocular sample does not exclude presence of another infectious agent, and dual infections have been reported [57].

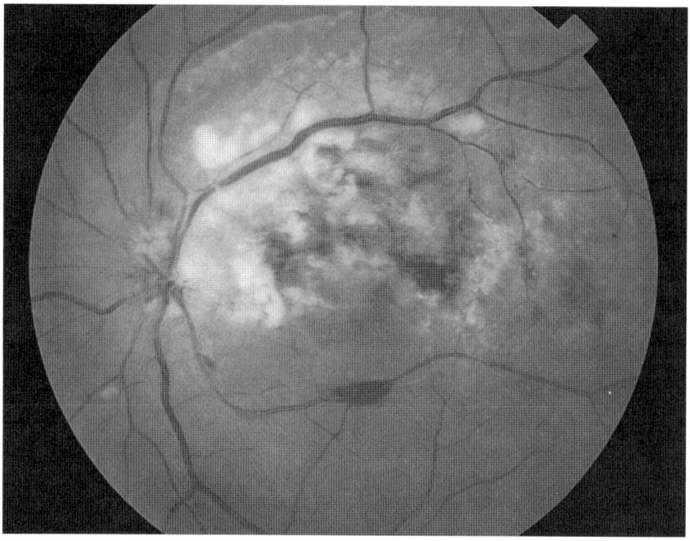

**Fig. 1.5** CMV retinitis with characteristic white, perivascular lesions and hemorrhage.

### Sensorineural Hearing Loss

Sensorineural hearing loss is present at birth in 25 to 50% of infants with symptomatic congenital CMV infection and in 15% of infants with otherwise asymptomatic CMV infection [47,61]. One follow-up study of children with asymptomatic congenital CMV infection demonstrated subsequent development of hearing loss in 18% of children [62]. With the large number of infants born with congenital CMV infection each year in the United States, congenitally acquired CMV thus represents the most common cause of nonhereditary sensorineural deafness and is estimated to account for at least one third of sensorineural hearing loss in young children [50].

Approximately two thirds of all congenitally CMV-infected infants experience postnatal deterioration of their hearing deficit [61–63]. Although presence of intrauterine growth retardation and petechiae are independently associated with presence of hearing loss at birth, neither seems predictive of hearing loss progression. Of interest, one study demonstrated a significant association between hearing loss at any time and depressed cognitive and motor function in children with confirmed congenitally acquired CMV infection [53]. Thus, children with congenital CMV infection, whether symptomatic or not, deserve careful, serial audiometric examinations and those children in whom deficits are discovered should undergo cognitive and neuromotor evaluation.

## *Diagnosis*

CMV presence is best confirmed by viral cultures from urine or mucosal tissues, especially the oropharynx or nasopharynx. However, a positive culture from these sites does not necessarily confirm active disease or recent infection, because viral shedding may occur intermittently over a prolonged period after initial infection. Regardless, CMV isolated from the urine of an infant younger than 2 weeks of age strongly indicates congenital infection, with only a slight chance of postnatal acquisition. Detection of CMV IgM or CMV IgG in a previously seronegative patient may also suggest recent infection. However, false-positive and false-negative CMV IgM antibody results are common, making interpretation of these results problematic. PCR assays are commercially available to detect CMV in both blood and CSF samples; some laboratories will also perform this test on vitreous fluid to identify CMV chorioretinitis. Because CMV may not grow in culture from these sites, PCR is a useful, rapid, diagnostic tool in patients with suspected neurological or systemic disease. Rapid diagnosis is also available using DNA hybridization. The gold standard for diagnosis of CMV infection or reactivation in solid organs is histopathology. CMV may be identified by presence of typical inclusion bodies or by immunohistochemical analysis.

### *Treatment*

Prevention remains the most important factor in controlling CMV infection, because antiviral agents have limited proven impact once disease is established. Vaccine discovery is in progress and includes such products as the Towne vaccine, and DNA, glycoprotein B, and subunit vaccines [194–197]. However, none are licensed currently for clinical use. Limited evidence demonstrates some benefit to CMV-specific hyperimmune globulin in prevention and treatment of congenital CMV infection when administered to pregnant women with primary CMV infection [192]. Antiviral agents currently licensed for treatment of CMV in pediatric patients include ganciclovir and foscarnet. Ganciclovir therapy for infants with symptomatic congenital CMV infection remains controversial, with few studies demonstrating significant benefit in outcome or resolution of disease. A Phase II trial comparing ganciclovir at two different doses was remarkable for significant adverse effects and no long-lasting impact on CMV viruria [64]. However, hearing improvement or stabilization occurred in 16% of babies at 6 months, a finding suggested previously by others [65]. Preferred treatment of serious CMV infection in immunocompromised hosts involves use of parenteral ganciclovir or foscarnet, although demonstration of direct antiviral benefit frequently is obscured by simultaneous recovery of immune function in recovering patients. The best evidence for treatment efficacy is demonstrated in CMV retinitis, in which ganciclovir, foscarnet, and cidofovir all seem to be efficacious. After induction therapy for at least 2 weeks, most patients require lifelong therapy to avoid the risk of relapse. Oral valganciclovir seems to be as effective as parenteral ganciclovir in induction therapy for adults with CMV retinitis [66]. Therapy of CMV disease with ganciclovir is limited by adverse effects, such as severe neutropenia and transaminitis, whereas foscarnet may be associated with renal failure and metabolic disturbances with secondary cardiac arrhythmias. Given the lack of proven benefit in most cases, careful consideration of CMV treatment should be undertaken before initiation.

## Varicella-Zoster Virus

### *Introduction*

Varicella-zoster virus (VZV) causes primary disease (chickenpox) and resultant latent disease, which can reactivate, causing zoster (shingles). Although both diseases are usually well tolerated by immunocompetent children and adolescents, significant neurological complications can occur, with associated hospitalization and neurological morbidity. VZV, thus, occupies a prominent place in lists of infectious pathogens with potential for severe neurological disease.

## *Epidemiology*

Primary VZV infection nearly always results in chickenpox and is highly communicable during acute disease, with a secondary attack rate of more than 90% among household contacts [67]. Transmission occurs by exposure to varicella lesions or respiratory secretions. Vertical transmission from mother to fetus occurs transplacentally. Before varicella vaccine was available, nearly every person in the United States was infected with varicella, resulting in approximately 4 million cases annually and causing 10,000 hospitalizations and 100 deaths [68]. Ninety percent of infections occur in children. These numbers have dropped considerably in the post vaccine licensure era, but vaccine coverage is not yet universal and evaluation of breakthrough cases and adult disease is ongoing.

## *Pathogenesis*

VZV is a member of the *Herpesviridae* family of DNA viruses and is most closely related to HSV. Unlike other herpesviruses, however, VZV can release infectious virus into respiratory droplets during primary disease, accounting for its high degree of infectiousness. Inoculation of VZV occurs via mucosal surfaces, resulting in replication in regional lymph nodes and a primary viremia inoculating the liver and other cells of the reticuloendothelial system. A secondary viremia occurs during the last several days of the 10 to 23 day incubation period, permitting viral spread to cutaneous cells where vesicles then form. After this primary chickenpox, latent infection occurs in dorsal root ganglia. VZV reactivation causes a localized vesicular rash involving the dermatomal distribution of a single sensory nerve with infectious VZV present in herpes zoster lesions but not respiratory secretions [69,70].

## *Clinical Manifestations*

### Congenital VZV Syndrome

Varicella acquired during pregnancy can have severe consequences for both the mother and fetus. The highest risk for congenital VZV syndrome accompanies maternal varicella in the first 20 weeks of gestation and is reported to occur in 2 to 5% of maternal cases [69,71]. Clinical manifestations are severe (Table 1.5). Neurological abnormalities include microcephaly and cortical atrophy, likely secondary to intrauterine VZV encephalitis. Seizures and mental retardation commonly accompany these findings. Ocular abnormalities and dysfunction of the autonomic nervous system also occur.

**Table 1.5** Clinical manifestations of congenital varicella syndrome [69]

| | |
|---|---|
| Skin | Cutaneous defects |
| | Cicatricial scars[a] |
| | Hypopigmentation |
| | Bullous lesions |
| Extremities | Hypoplastic limbs |
| | Muscular atrophy and denervation |
| | Joint abnormalities |
| | Absent or malformed digits |
| Eye | Chorioretinitis |
| | Microphthalmia |
| | Anisocoria |
| CNS | Intrauterine encephalitis |
| | Microcephaly |
| | Cortical atrophy |
| | Seizures |
| | Mental retardation |
| Urinary tract | Hydronephrosis/hydroureter |
| | Neurogenic bladder |
| Gastrointestinal | Esophageal dilation |
| | Gastroesophageal reflux/aspiration |

[a]Most prominent stigmata.

Neonatal varicella can occur in infants born within 2 days before to 5 days after onset of maternal varicella. Exposure to secondary viremia without sufficient transfer of maternal VZV antibodies places these infants at risk for progressive varicella, with an attack rate of 20% and an untreated mortality rate of 30% [71,72].

## Complications of Varicella

The most frequent complication of primary varicella in a normal host is secondary bacterial infection of the skin with *Staphylococcus aureus* or group A β-hemolytic streptococci, causing cellulitis, fasciitis, lymphadenitis, and subcutaneous abscesses. Such infections can progress to multisystem disease via hematogenous spread. Neurological diseases are the second most common complication of varicella, comprising 18 to 20% of all complications, with an estimated incidence of 1 to 3 per 10,000 cases.67,69,70,73–76 Encephalitis and cerebellar ataxia are most frequently described and often lead to hospitalization.

## *Neurological Manifestations*

### Encephalitis

Varicella accounted for 13% of reported encephalitis cases with known etiology between 1972 and 1977 [77], but more recent studies suggest this percentage has increased to 17 to 28% [10,78–81]. Varicella encephalitis is the most serious CNS complication of varicella and has an incidence of 1 to 2 episodes per 10,000 varicella cases [76]. The pathogenesis remains unclear, with some histopathologic studies suggesting a postinfectious demyelinating process and others demonstrating direct viral cytopathology [82–85]. Patients develop symptoms 5 to 7 days after onset of varicella rash, although numerous reports describe pre-eruptive varicella encephalitis, with neurological disease occurring up to 2 to 3 weeks before onset of the typical varicella rash [86–89].

Varicella encephalitis typically presents with headache, fever, vomiting, and altered sensorium. Seizures occur in 29 to 52% of cases and are most frequently generalized [83,90]. Most patients will have cerebellar ataxia and may also demonstrate hypertonia or hypotonia, hyperreflexia or hyporeflexia, positive plantar reflexes, hemiparesis, and sensory changes [76,80]. CSF findings typically include increased opening pressure, mild-to-moderate lymphocytic pleocytosis (<100 cells/mm$^3$), mildly elevated protein (50–100 mg/dL) and normal glucose levels. EEG shows slow wave activity reflective of a diffuse encephalopathy. MRI scan is the most sensitive of available neuroimaging modalities and may show edema and/or areas of demyelination [82,91,92].

The mortality for varicella encephalitis is 5 to 10%, without clear benefit from antiviral therapy [77]. Historic rates of mortality are higher, likely reflecting confusion with Reye's syndrome. Most cases have complete or near complete recovery, but long-term sequelae occur in 10 to 20% of survivors and include epilepsy, persistent ataxia, and mild motor, cognitive, and behavioral deficits [80,93].

### Cerebellar Ataxia

Cerebellar ataxia has an incidence of approximately 1 episode per 10,000 cases [94]. Because this syndrome is rarely fatal, few pathologic studies exist to clarify its pathogenesis. However, cerebellar ataxia is likely similar to varicella encephalitis, resulting either from a direct viral infection or a para-infectious, immunologically mediated demyelinating process [87,95–97]. Ataxia may develop up to 2 weeks after onset of primary varicella, but pre-eruptive cases are also described [76,87,88]. This syndrome has also been described after varicella vaccination [98].

Cerebellar ataxia is frequently accompanied by headache, vomiting, dysphasia, and lethargy. Nystagmus and nuchal rigidity occur in 25% of patients [76,88]. CSF is typically normal but may show moderate lymphocytic pleocytosis (<100 cells/mm$^3$) with mildly elevated protein in 20 to 30% of cases [76,95]. MRI scan may demonstrate multiple areas of high signal intensity in the white matter of the cerebellum [98]. Varicella-associated cerebellar ataxia is self-limited, with recovery typically occurring within 1 to 3 weeks. Severe sequelae are not reported.

### Other Neurological Disease

Additional neurological diseases that accompany or follow primary varicella infection include aseptic meningitis, transverse myelitis, facial nerve palsy (Ramsay Hunt syndrome), and Guillain-Barré syndrome [67,69,70,76,99]. Cases of hemiplegia resulting from varicella-induced cerebral vasculopathy are also described [100,101]. Varicella infection seems to be a risk factor for childhood arterial ischemic stroke, with data demonstrating a threefold increase in cases with preceding varicella infection [198]. Varicella reactivation from sensory ganglia causes zoster (shingles) in the related dermatomal distribution and may be accompanied by CSF pleocytosis and MRI scan findings suggestive of inflammation in the brainstem. Adult patients may experience postherpetic neuralgia but this entity is rare in pediatric patients.

Patients with immunodeficiency are at risk for progressive varicella encephalitis and dissemination. Initial CSF and MRI scan evaluation may not demonstrate typical findings suggestive of encephalitis, thus delaying diagnosis [102]. Presence of intense abdominal pain seems to suggest dissemination to multiple sites, including brain, liver, and lungs [103]. Varicella also causes retinal disease in patients with AIDS. This syndrome is known as progressive outer retinal necrosis and has a rapid, progressive, clinically distinct course leading to blindness in most cases [104]. Rapid recognition and initiation of antiviral therapy with appropriate surgical intervention may improve visual outcome [105].

## *Diagnosis*

Laboratory diagnosis is not usually necessary for primary varicella in healthy hosts because the varicella exanthem has a classic appearance. However, specific diagnosis is often important to guide treatment decisions in patients with immunodeficiency or pre-eruptive neurological disease. Rapid diagnosis of cutaneous VZV disease is available by fluorescent antibody staining of epithelial cells obtained from the base of a newly formed vesicle with a cotton- or Dacron-tipped swab. A cytologic method to detect multinucleated giant cells in lesion specimens (Tzanck smear) is nearly as sensitive as fluorescent antibody staining but does not differentiate between VZV and HSV. VZV is difficult to grow in cell culture and typically requires 5 to 7 days before viral presence can be recognized. Sensitivity of viral culture is 36%, compared with 86 to 100% for fluorescent antibody staining [106]. Serologic assays are rarely used for diagnosis, because VZV IgG rarely is detectable for the first 3 to 4 days of illness and VZV IgM assays have high rates of false-positive and false-negative results. However, VZV IgG results are useful in determining immune status of an immunocompromised,

VZV-exposed patient. VZV can be detected by PCR in ocular and CSF samples, but well-standardized assays are only available in research laboratories [34,97,107].

### *Treatment*

Acyclovir is the most common drug used to treat VZV disease. Because oral absorption is limited, prodrug forms (valacyclovir and famciclovir) are more often considered for outpatient management. However, antiviral therapy is not routinely recommended for treatment of uncomplicated varicella in healthy children because of its marginal therapeutic benefit, cost, and potential for emergence of resistance [108]. Intravenously administered acyclovir is recommended for treatment of primary or recurrent varicella in immunocompromised patients to reduce risk of dissemination and death. Intravenous acyclovir should be dosed in these patients at 1500 mg/m$^2$/d divided into doses every 8 hours for at least 7 days, or until no new lesions have appeared for 48 hours, and should be initiated within 24 hours of initial lesions appearance for maximal efficacy. Use of acyclovir in immunocompetent patients with neurological complications of varicella is of unclear benefit, especially if symptoms of primary VZV disease have resolved by the time of neurological disease onset. However, intravenously administered acyclovir is reasonable in these situations because direct viral infection may contribute to the pathogenesis of neurological disease. Concurrent use of systemic acyclovir and corticosteroids is common in patients with Ramsay Hunt syndrome, although dosing, duration, and efficacy are variable.

### *Prevention*

VZV vaccination is the best way to reduce disease burden and has been shown to be very effective [68]. The currently licensed varicella vaccine contains live, attenuated Oka strain varicella virus, which, although infectious, causes far milder disease than wild-type varicella. Although universally recommended for all susceptible children and adolescents without a contraindication, barriers to varicella vaccine administration remain, limiting theoretic benefits from a universal vaccination plan.

## Epstein-Barr Virus

### *Introduction*

EBV, the etiologic agent of classic infectious mononucleosis, contributes significantly to a diversity of diseases in both immunocompetent and immunocompromised children and adults. EBV-associated neurological disease generally occurs as a complication of infectious mononucleosis but may also be associated with potentially fatal EBV-related lymphoproliferative diseases and CNS lymphomas. The neurological manifestations may, in fact, be the only recognizable clinical features of EBV infection, thus, necessitating a high index of suspicion to make an accurate diagnosis.

## *Epidemiology*

EBV transmission occurs via exposure to oropharyngeal secretions during acute infectious mononucleosis and, rarely, via blood, blood products, and transplanted tissues. EBV is ubiquitous, causing seroconversion in up to 90% of children in developing countries. In higher socioeconomic groups, 40 to 50% of adolescents have antibodies to EBV, and 10 to 20% of susceptible individuals contract EBV every year thereafter [109,110].

## *Pathogenesis*

EBV is a gammaherpesvirus with the unique ability to immortalize B lymphocytes (i.e., confer the ability to grow continuously in cell culture). Inoculation of EBV occurs in the epithelial cells of the buccal mucosa or salivary glands and is followed by infection of B lymphocytes in the lymphoid tissues of the pharynx, with subsequent dissemination to the entire lymphoid system. A general depression of cellular immunity can occur during acute primary EBV infection. The atypical lymphocytes commonly seen in the blood of mononucleosis patients are thought to be mostly T lymphocytes responding to the B lymphocyte infection [111]. The various components of the immune response likely contribute significantly to the clinical manifestations of EBV infection. EBV-associated neurological disease, thus, may be caused by primary infection or by an immunopathologic process that may precipitate demyelinating disease.

## *Clinical Manifestations*

EBV acquired by immunocompetent hosts most often causes infectious mononucleosis syndrome. Typical disease is characterized by a 5-day prodromal illness, consisting of malaise and fatigue, followed by onset of fever, sore throat, worsening malaise, and fatigue, with accompanying tonsillopharyngitis and lymphadenopathy. Many patients will demonstrate mononuclear leukocytosis with atypical lymphocytes, and up to 50% will develop splenic enlargement. EBV-induced mononucleosis is usually less severe in younger patients, who may remain asymptomatic. However,

20% of patients may develop significant complications involving mainly the pulmonary, neurological, and hematologic systems [112].

## Neurological Manifestations

Neurological complications may develop during or shortly after the peak of clinical illness and often comprise the only clinical symptoms in younger children with primary EBV infection. Neurological complications have been reported in 1 to 2% of mononucleosis patients overall, in 5.5% of hospitalized patients, and in 4 to 7.1% of pediatric patients with mononucleosis [109,112–114]. These complications are diverse and include meningoencephalitis, cerebellitis, aseptic meningitis, transverse myelitis, Guillain-Barré syndrome and cranial neuritis (especially Bell's palsy) [113,115].

### Meningoencephalitis

Meningoencephalitis was the first described neurological complication of infectious mononucleosis, but occurs in less than 1% of cases [116]. EBV-associated encephalitis causes up to 5% of all encephalitis cases of known etiology 117 Although the pathogenesis of EBV meningoencephalitis has been ascribed to postinfectious inflammation, reports of isolation of EBV and its specific antibodies from CSF argue for a more direct infection of the CNS [118–120]. Patients present with rapid onset of neurological symptoms, but classic signs and symptoms of infectious mononucleosis are frequently absent. Acute neurological manifestations are diverse and include combative or bizarre behavior, headache, meningismus, lethargy, transient global amnesia, generalized seizures, choreoathetosis, and, rarely, coma [113,115,116,121–124]. Patients with pure brainstem encephalitis caused by EBV may present with diplopia, ptosis, nystagmus, and ataxia [116,125]. CSF may demonstrate mild protein elevation and mononuclear pleocytosis, with cell counts frequently measuring less than 22 cells/$mm^3$. EEG findings are variable, with focal or generalized high-voltage slow wave activity reported [122]. MRI scan is the most sensitive neuroimaging modality and most commonly demonstrates lesions consistent with demyelination [126,127]. EBV meningoencephalitis is usually associated with complete recovery within several weeks, but reported neurological sequelae include hydrocephalus resulting from aqueductal stenosis, cerebral edema with herniation, chorea, global cognitive impairment, and hyperactivity [113,115,122,193].

The "Alice in Wonderland" syndrome is an encephalopathy that presents with perceptual defects concerning size, shape, color and spatial relationships (metamorphopsia) that has been described in patients with infectious mononucleosis [113,128,129]. Metamorphopsia is related to lesions of the occipital, occipitotemporal, and parietooccipital regions. Patients may demonstrate EEG abnormalities in the parietooccipital region but no other specific findings. The "Alice in Wonderland" syndrome associated with EBV infection seems to be benign, with complete, spontaneous recovery.

## Cerebellitis

Acute cerebellar ataxia can present as the sole manifestation of infectious mononucleosis, although many patients experience a prodromal illness or other accompanying systemic signs typical of acute EBV. The incidence of EBV-associated cerebellar ataxia is difficult to assess, because most clinical cases do not undergo laboratory confirmation of etiology. Neurological symptoms typically peak within 1 week of onset and include disequilibrium, gait and truncal ataxia, and, frequently, behavioral changes. Cerebellar dysarthria occurs in approximately 50% of cases. Nystagmus rarely is present in children, but may be more common in young adults [130]. CSF findings are nonspecific and may demonstrate mild mononuclear pleocytosis [131]. Results of neuroimaging by CT or MRI scan are usually normal. The prognosis is excellent, with complete recovery demonstrated within 4 months [113].

## Other Neurological Diseases

Guillain-Barré syndrome is perhaps the best-known neurological complication of EBV disease. It is an ascending paralysis of the extremities with albuminocytologic dissociation of the CSF (high CSF protein and lack of CSF pleocytosis). Unusual variants occur, including the Miller Fisher syndrome (ophthalmoplegia, ataxia, and areflexia). Pediatric patients are more likely to demonstrate evidence of infection with EBV than adults, who are more likely to have had CMV disease [132], but the list of infections associated with Guillain-Barré syndrome is extensive.

Additional neurological complications of EBV-associated infectious mononucleosis include cranial nerve palsy (most often affecting the VIIth cranial nerve—Bell's Palsy), optic nerve disease (blurred vision, papilledema, optic neuritis, papilloretinal edema, and retrobulbar neuritis), peripheral neuropathy, and transverse myelitis [111,113,133]. The ability of EBV infection to cause both acute and chronic demyelinating disease has raised suspicion that EBV may precipitate such diseases as multiple sclerosis and subacute sclerosing panencephalitis, likely in combination with other infections, but this link has not been confirmed [113,124,134]. Studies have demonstrated a positive correlation between specific EBV serologic patterns and eventual onset of multiple sclerosis [135,136], but confirmation of causality is difficult because of technical limitations of brain tissue evaluation for EBV.

EBV has been associated with oncologic disease since 1970, when EBV DNA was detected in tissue from patients with nasopharyngeal carcinoma. EBV was found subsequently to be associated with non-Hodgkin's lymphoma and oral hairy leukoplakia in patients with AIDS and is present in nearly all primary CNS lymphomas arising in immunocompromised patients [137]. EBV has now been found in additional cancers, including T-cell lymphomas and Hodgkin's disease, and is also associated with lymphoproliferative diseases in patients with severe combined immunodeficiency, AIDS, and recipients of organ or bone marrow transplants [138].

### *Diagnosis*

EBV does not grow in routine cell cultures and, although its presence can be inferred by the ability of patient's cells to immortalize cultured EBV-negative lymphocytes, this technique is time consuming and not generally available [139]. Instead, detection of heterophil antibody response by commercially available, rapid heterophil slide tests is the mainstay of diagnosis. EBV infection can also be diagnosed by EBV-specific serologic tests, which detect antibodies to three different groups of EBV antigens: viral capsid antigen, early antigen, and nuclear antigen. Antibodies to these antigens appear at different times and for different durations and, thus, can be used to estimate timing of infection. EBV DNA can be detected by PCR in peripheral blood or CSF leukocytes [140,141], and some laboratories have developed PCR-based assays to estimate quantities of EBV DNA [119]. EBV can be demonstrated in pathologic samples by Southern hybridization, in situ hybridization, and PCR [110]. However, most of these techniques are generally not necessary for routine cases of EBV-associated infectious mononucleosis or for its neurological complications.

### *Treatment*

Treatment is largely supportive because EBV-associated infectious mononucleosis and its neurological complications are usually self-limited, with no major sequelae. Short-term corticosteroids are considered for patients with severe manifestations and respiratory embarrassment from tonsillar hypertrophy. Antiviral agents (acyclovir and ganciclovir) inhibit EBV replication transiently but have no demonstrated clinical benefit in immunocompetent patients [110,111,115,142]. Ganciclovir may have some benefit in treatment of EBV encephalitis in immunocompromised patients [143,144]. On-going evaluation of anti-B-cell monoclonal antibodies and EBV-specific cytotoxic T cells has demonstrated some benefit in treatment of EBV lymphoproliferative disease [111,138].

## Human Herpesviruses 6 and 7

### *Introduction*

Human Herpesviruses (HHV) 6 and 7 (HHV-6/7) are recently described ß-herpesviruses that infect almost all individuals in early childhood, causing both undifferentiated febrile illness and roseola infantum. Although the complete scope and nature of disease caused by these viruses remains to be fully described, both seem to cause disease in neonatal, transplant, and AIDS patients. Ongoing investigation additionally suggests a significant role in febrile seizures, meningoencephalitis, and possibly multiple sclerosis.

## *Epidemiology*

HHV-6/7 transmission likely occurs via exposure to oral secretions. Vertical transmission and transmission via blood, blood products and transplanted organs have been documented serologically, but specific disease syndromes are difficult to describe because of the persistence of virus in almost all adults [145–147]. Both viruses seem to be ubiquitous, causing seroconversion in most children and 80 to 100% of adults in many parts of the world [146,148–150].

## *Pathogenesis*

HHV-6/7 are ß-herpesviruses and are, thus, related to CMV. HHV-6 exists in two subtypes (A and B), but no pathogenic differences between the two are known. HHV-6/7 are T-cell lymphotropic viruses that replicate in peripheral blood mononuclear cells. After primary infection, viral DNA can be detected in these cells as well as in saliva, CSF, and brain tissue, implicating these areas as additional sites of viral latency or persistence [151]. Latent virus has the potential to be shed asymptomatically in the saliva and to reactivate in immunosuppressed patients [152].

## *Clinical Manifestations*

Primary HHV-6 infection is a major cause of acute febrile illness and emergency unit visits in young children [153]. Roseola infantum (exanthem subitum) is the classic illness caused by HHV-6 and affects most children by age 3 years (peak onset 6–15 months). Patients develop fever for 2 to 4 days, followed by defervescence and onset of papular, macular, or maculopapular rash. Roseola may be accompanied by diarrhea (68%), Nagayama spots (erythematous papules on the soft palate; 65%), cough (50%), cervical adenopathy (31%), edematous eyelids (30%), bulging fontanelle (26%), and seizures (8%) [154]. However, not every patient with primary HHV-6 infection develops an exanthem, complicating clinical diagnosis. Primary HHV-7 infection occurs in slightly older children (ages 2 to 5 yr) and seems to cause both an unspecified febrile illness and roseola [148,155].

## *Neurological Manifestations*

### Febrile Seizures

Roseola has been associated with classic febrile seizures in infants and young children. Seizures typically occur in the pre-eruptive phase of illness. In one large, prospective study, HHV-6 accounted for 31% of first-time febrile seizures in children up to 2 years old, whereas 13% of children with HHV-6 primary infection developed seizures [153]. Multiple smaller studies also suggest that acute HHV-6 is a frequent cause of febrile seizures [156–158]. However, some research suggests that the fever associated with HHV-6 infection and not the virus itself is the true cause of this association [159,160]. Because HHV-7 primary infection seems similar to HHV-6, it is suspected to play a significant role in febrile seizures as well, although few rigorous studies exist to confirm this [148,150,155].

Patients with an initial febrile seizure caused by primary HHV-6 infection do not seem to demonstrate an increased risk for recurrent seizures when compared with patients with febrile seizures from other causes [161]. However, primary HHV-6 infection seems to be associated more frequently with severe convulsions and postictal paralysis than other causes of febrile seizures [158,162]. No differences exist in long-term sequelae of patients with febrile seizures caused by HHV-6/7 compared with other causes [161].

### Meningoencephalitis

Similar to other herpesviruses, HHV-6 is neurotropic and is thought to have clinical manifestations associated with both primary and reactivation disease. The first case of HHV-6 infection with encephalitis was reported in 1990 [163], prompting recognition that some patients with primary HHV-6 infection and more complex seizures may have active viral disease in the CNS. One subsequent series examined 21 infants with virologically confirmed HHV-6 infection (pre-eruptive phase) and complex seizures (15 generalized and 6 focal) and demonstrated 4 infants with encephalitis. These infants showed more severe clinical features, CSF pleocytosis (14 to 28 cells/mm$^3$, lymphocyte predominance), mild CSF protein elevation (58 to 66 mg/dL), EEG abnormalities in paroxysmal and background reading, and CT scan findings of low-density lesions in the frontotemporal region [164]. Additional studies demonstrate evidence of HHV-6 DNA in CSF of patients with meningoencephalitis and no other proven cause of disease [81,146,165–171] and in brain tissue of patients with primary HHV-6 infection [149,172]. However, a study of 31 normal brain tissues demonstrated HHV-6 DNA in approximately one third of specimens [173], and other studies have demonstrated persistence of HHV-6 DNA and antibodies in the CSF after primary infection [147,150,151], thus, calling into question the significance of these findings. Until active viral replication in the brain can be demonstrated, proof of causality will remain elusive. Despite this, patients with evidence of primary HHV-6 infection and meningoencephalitis continue to be described, with clinical, radiologic and laboratory findings similar to patients with meningoencephalitis caused by other herpesviruses and with similar rates of death and severe neurological sequelae [167,174,175].

### Other Neurological Diseases

An etiologic role of HHV-6/7 has been evaluated for many neurological diseases. As with meningoencephalitis, proof of causality is difficult because HHV-6 is ubiquitous and likely remains present in the CNS long after primary infection. HHV-6 DNA has been demonstrated in the CSF of patients with acute disseminated/demyelinating encephalomyelitis [176], encephalitis-associated hypersensitivity syndrome [177,178], and influenza-associated encephalopathy [179], although this latter association remains controversial [180]. Investigation of brains from patients with multiple sclerosis demonstrates expression of HHV-6 virion proteins in the nuclei of oligodendrocytes but not in control patients [181], and HHV-6 has been proposed as a possible cofactor for such demyelinating diseases as multiple sclerosis [181–184], Guillain-Barré syndrome [185], and acute disseminated encephalomyelitis [176]. However, these associations remain far from clear and will remain the focus of ongoing research. Reports of HHV-7 and CNS disease are rare, but several cases of acute hemiplegia have been described in patients with serologic evidence of HHV-7 infection [189].

## *Diagnosis*

Primary HHV-6/7 infection is generally a clinical diagnosis, and laboratory diagnosis is usually reserved for atypical or severe cases. HHV-6/7 can be isolated in cell culture, but this method is slow, technically challenging, and not performed routinely [186]. Commercially available serologic diagnostic techniques include immunofluorescent assays and enzyme immunoassays and are used primarily for epidemiologic and pathologic studies. Demonstration of seroconversion from negative to positive IgG response or detection of IgM antibody during primary infection can establish HHV-6/7 infection, but should be interpreted cautiously because infection with other herpesviruses may cause increases in HHV-6/7-specific IgG. In addition, HHV-6/7-specific IgM can appear during both primary and reactivated infections and persist for extended periods. PCR assays and in situ immunofluorescence assays allow direct detection of HHV-6 DNA and antigens in numerous sites, but cannot differentiate between active and latent infection. New methods to measure active viral replication are anticipated to resolve this problem, but require further study [186].

## *Treatment*

Treatment of primary HHV-6/7 infection is supportive, because recovery is complete in several days, with few sequelae. However, because the scope of HHV-6/7 infections continues to broaden, interest in effective treatment options may increase. HHV-6 in vitro sensitivity has been assessed to four antiviral drugs (acyclovir, ganciclovir, phosphonoformic acid, and zidovudine). HHV-6 multiplication is inhibited by ganciclovir at concentrations easily attained in humans and by the other three only in nearly toxic concentrations [187,188]. However, no antiviral drug has been approved specifically for treatment of HHV-6/7 infection.

## References

1. Smith JS, Robinson NJ. Age-Specific Prevalence of Infection with Herpes Simplex Virus Types 2 and 1: A Global Review. *J Infect Dis* 2002; 186:S3–S28.
2. Fleming DT, McQuillan GM, Johnson RE. Herpes Simplex Virus Type 2 in the United States, 1976–1994. *N Engl J Med* 1997; 337:1105–1111.
3. Adam E, Kaufman RH, Mirkovic RH. Persistence of Virus Shedding in Asymptomatic Women after Recovery from Herpes Genitalis. *Obstet Gynecol* 1979; 54:171–173.
4. Sullivan-Bolyai J, Hull HF, Wilson C, Corey L. Neonatal Herpes Simplex Virus Infection in King County, Washington: Increasing Incidence and Epidemiologic Correlates. *JAMA* 1983; 250:3059–3062.
5. Gutierrez KM, Falkovitz Halpern MS, Maldonado Y, Arvin AM. The Epidemiology of Neonatal Herpes Simplex Virus Infections in California from 1985 to 1995. *J Infect Dis* 1999; 180:199–202.
6. Brown ZA, Wald A, Morrow RA, Selke S, Zeh J, Corey L. Effect of Serologic Status and Cesarean Delivery on Transmission Rates of Herpes Simplex Virus from Mother to Infant. *JAMA* 2003; 289:203–209.
7. Diamond C, Mohan K, Hobson A, Frenkel L, Corey L. Viremia in Neonatal Herpes Simplex Virus Infections. *Pediatr Infect Dis J* 1999; 18: 487–489.
8. Whitley RJ, Kimberlin DW. Viral Encephalitis. *Pediatr Rev* 1999; 20:192–198.
9. Johnson RT. Acute Encephalitis. *Clin Infect Dis* 1996; 23:219–226.
10. Schmutzhard E. Viral Infections of the CNS with Special Emphasis on Herpes Simplex Infections. *J Neurol* 2001; 248:469–477.
11. Annunziato PW, Gershon A. Herpes Simplex Virus Infection. *Pediatr Rev* 1996; 17: 415–423.
12. Brown ZA, Benedetti J, Ashley R, Selke S, Berry S, Vontver LA. Neonatal Herpes Simplex Virus Infection in Relation to Asymptomatic Maternal Infection at the Time of Labour. *N Engl J Med* 1991; 324:1247–1252.
13. Whitley RJ. Neonatal Herpes Simplex Virus Infections. *J Med Virol* 1993; Supplement 1: 13–21.
14. Kimberlin DW, Lin C-Y, Jacobs RF, Powell D, Frenkel L, Gruber W, Rathore M, Bradley JS, Diaz PS. Natural History of Neonatal Herpes Simplex Virus Infections in the Acyclovir Era. *Pediatrics* 2001; 108:223–229.
15. Arvin AM, Whitley RJ, Gutierrez, KM. Herpes Simplex Virus Infections. In: Remington JS, Klein JO, Wilson CB & Baker CJ, eds., *Infectious Diseases of the Fetus and Newborn Infant*, 6th ed., Philadelphia: Elsevier Saunders, 2006; 845–865.

16. Hutto C, Arvin AM, Jacobs RF, Steele R, Stagno S, Lyrene R, Willett L, Powell D, Andersen RD, Werthammer J, Ratcliff G, Nahmias A, Christy C, Whitley RJ. Intrauterine Herpes Simplex Virus Infections. *J Pediatr* 1987; 110:97–101.
17. Nahmias A, Josey WE, Naib JM, Freeman ME, Fernandez RJ, Wheeler JH. Perinatal Risk Associated with Maternal Genital Herpes Simplex Virus Infection. *Am J Obstet Gynecol* 1971; 110:825.
18. Overall JC. Herpes Simplex Virus Infection of the Fetus and Newborn. *Pediatr Ann* 1994; 23: 131–136.
19. Kimberlin DW, Powell D, Gruber W, Diaz PS, Arvin AM, Kumar ML, Jacobs RF, Van Dyke R. Administration of Oral Acyclovir Suppressive Therapy after Neonatal Herpes Simplex Virus Disease Limited to the Skin, Eyes and Mouth: Results of a Phase I/Ii Trial. *Pediatr Infect Dis J* 1996; 15:247–254.
20. Bale JF, Andersen RD, Grose C. Magnetic Resonance Imaging of the Brain in Childhood Herpesvirus Infections. *Pediatr Infect Dis J* 1987; 6:644–647.
21. Nahmias A, Whitley RJ, Visintine AN. Herpes Simplex Virus Encephalitis: Laboratory Evaluations, and Their Diagnostic Significance. *J Infect Dis* 1982; 145:829–836.
22. Arvin AM. Herpes Simplex Virus 1 and 2. In: Feigin, RD, Cherry, JD, Demmler, GJ & Kaplan, SL, eds., *Textbook of Pediatric Infectious Diseases*, 5th ed., Philadelphia: Elsevier Saunders, 2004; 1884–1912.
23. Demaeral PH, Wilms G, Robberecht W. MRI of Herpes Simplex Encephalitis. *Neuroradiology* 1992; 34:490–493.
24. Tedder DG, Ashley R, Tyler KL. Herpes Simplex Virus Infection as a Cause of Benign Recurrent Lymphocytic Meningitis. *Ann Intern Med* 1994; 121:334–338.
25. Simmons A. Clinical Manifestations and Treatment Considerations of Herpes Simplex Virus Infection. *J Infect Dis* 2002; 186:S71–S77.
26. Ganatra JB, Chandler D, Santos C, Kuppermann B, Margolis TP. Viral Causes of the Acute Retinal Necrosis Syndrome. *Am J Ophthalmol* 2000; 129:166–172.
27. Gain P, Chiquet C, Thuret G, Drouet E, Antoine J-C. Herpes Simplex Virus Type 1 Encephalitis Associated with Acute Retinal Necrosis Syndrome in an Immunocompetent Patient. *Acta Ophthalmol Scand* 2002; 80:546–549.
28. Maertazdorf J, Van der Lelij A, Baarsma GS, Osterhaus ADME, Verjans GMGM. Herpes Simplex Virus Type 1 (Hsv-1)-Induced Retinitis Following Herpes Simplex Encephalitis: Indications for Brain-to-Eye Transmission of Hsv-1. *Ann Neurol* 2000; 48:936–939.
29. Ito Y, Kimura H, Yabuta Y, Ando Y, Murakami T, Shiomi M, Morishima T. Exacerbation of Herpes Simplex Encephalitis after Successful Treatment with Acyclovir. *Clin Infect Dis* 2000; 30:185–187.
30. Kusuhara T, Nakajima M, Inoue H, Takahashi M, Yamada T. Parainfectious Encephalomyelo radiculitis Associated with Herpes Simplex Virus 1 DNA in Cerebrospinal Fluid. *Clin Infect Dis* 2002; 34:1199–1205.
31. Ciardi M, Giacchetti G, Fedele CG, Tenorio A, Brandi A, Libertone R, Ajassa C, Borgese L, Delia S. Acute Cerebellitis Caused by Herpes Simplex Virus Type 1. *Clin Infect Dis* 2003; 36: e50–e54.
32. Corey L, Spear PG. Infections with Herpes Simplex Viruses. *N Engl J Med* 1986; 314: 686–692.
33. Lakeman FD, Whitley RJ, Diagnosis of Herpes Simplex Encephalitis: Application of Polymerase Chain Reaction to Cerebrospinal Fluid from Brain-Biopsied Patients and Correlation with Disease. *J Infect Dis* 1995; 171:857–863.
34. Storch GA. Central Nervous System Infections. In: Storch, GA, ed. *Essentials of Diagnostic Virology*. Philadelphia: Churchill Livingstone, 2000; 37–58.
35. Atkins JT. HSV PCR for CNS Infections: Pearls and Pitfalls. *Pediatr Infect Dis J* 1999; 18: 823–824.
36. Feder HM, Goyal RK, Krause PJ. Acyclovir-Induced Neutropenia in an Infant with Herpes Simplex Encephalitis: Case Report. *Clin Infect Dis* 1995; 20.

37. Stanberry LR, Cunningham AL, Mindel A, Scott LL, Spruance SL, Aoki FY, Lacey CJ. Prospects for Control of Herpes Simplex Virus Disease Through Immunization. *Clin Infect Dis* 2000; 30:549–566.
38. Arav-Boger R, Pass RF. Diagnosis and Management of Cytomegalovirus Infection in the Newborn. *Pediatr Ann* 2002; 31:719–724.
39. Weller TH. The Cytomegaloviruses: Ubiquitous Agents with Protean Clinical Manifestations. *N Engl J Med* 1971; 285:203–214.
40. Maschmann J, Hamprecht K, Dietz K, Jahn G, Speer CP. Cytomegalovirus Infection of Extremely Low-Birth Weight Infants Via Breast Milk. *Clin Infect Dis* 2001; 33: 1998–2003.
41. Hanshaw JB. Cytomegalovirus Infections. *Pediatr Rev* 1995; 16: 43–48.
42. Griffith B, Booss J. Neurologic Infections of the Fetus and Newborn. *Neurol Clin* 1994; 12: 541–564.
43. Ivarsson S-A, Lernmark B, Svanberg L. Ten-Year Clinical, Developmental, and Intellectual Follow-up of Children with Congenital Cytomegalovirus Infection without Neurologic Symptoms at One Year of Age. *Pediatrics* 1997; 99:800–803.
44. Conboy TJ, Pass RF, Stagno S, Alford CA, Myers GJ, Britt WJ, McCollister FP, Summers MN, McFarland CE, Boll TJ. Early Clinical Manifestations and Intellectual Outcome in Children with Symptomatic Congenital Cytomegalovirus Infection. *J Pediatr* 1987; 111: 343–348.
45. Williamson WD, Percy AK, Yow MD, Gerson P, Catlin FI, Koppelman ML, Thurbery S. Asymptomatic Congenital Cytomegalovirus Infection; Audiologic, Neuroradiologic, and Neurodevelopmental Abnormalities During the First Year. *Am J Dis Child* 1990; 144: 1365–1368.
46. Kumar ML, Nankervis GA, Jacobs IB, Ernhart CB, Glasson CE, McMillan PM, Gold E. Congenital and Postnatally Acquired Cytomegalovirus Infections: Long-Term Follow-Up. *J Pediatr* 1984; 104:674–679.
47. Demmler GJ. Cytomegalovirus. In: Feigin, RD, Cherry, JD, Demmler, GJ & Kaplan, SL, eds., *Textbook of Pediatric Infectious Diseases*, 5th ed., Philadelphia: Elsevier Saunders, 2004; 1912–1932.
48. Boppana SB, Pass RF, Britt WJ, Stagno S, Alford CA. Symptomatic Congenital Cytomegalovirus Infection: Neonatal Morbidity and Mortality. *Pediatr Infect Dis J* 1992; 11:93–99.
49. Bale JF. Human Cytomegalovirus Infection and Disorders of the Nervous System. *Arch Neurol* 1984; 41:310–320.
50. Stagno S, Britt W. Cytomegalovirus Infections. In: Remington JS, Klein JO, Wilson CB & Baker CJ, eds., *Infectious Diseases of the Fetus and Newborn Infant*, 6th ed., Philadelphia: Elsevier Saunders, 2006; 739–772.
51. Hayward JC, Titelbaum DS, Clancy RR, Zimmerman RA. Lissencephaly-Pachygyria Associated with Congenital Cytomegalovirus Infection. *J Child Neurol* 1991; 6:109–114.
52. Boppana SB, Fowler KB, Vaid Y, Hedlund G, Stagno S, Britt WJ, Pass RF. Neuroradiologic Findings in the Newborn Period and Long-Term Outcome in Children with Symptomatic Congenital Cytomegalovirus Infection. *Pediatrics* 1997; 99:409–414.
53. Noyola DE, Demmler GJ, Nelson CT, Griesser C, Williamson WD, Atkins JT, Rozelle J, Turcich M, Llorente AM, Sellers-Vinson S, Reynolds A, Bale JF, Gerson P, Yow MD. Early Predictors of Neurodevelopmental Outcome in Symptomatic Congenital Cytomegalovirus Infection. *J Pediatr* 2001; 138:325–331.
54. Pass RF. Cytomegalovirus. In: Long, SS, Pickering, LK & Prober, CG, eds. *Principles and Practice of Pediatric Infectious Diseases*, 2nd ed., Philadelphia: Churchill Livingstone, 2003: 1050–1059.
55. Fuller GN, Jacobs JM, Guiloff RJ. Association of Painful Peripheral Neuropathy in AIDS with Cytomegalovirus Infection. *Lancet* 1989; 2:937–940.
56. McLachan RS, Levin S & Blume WT. Treatment of Rasmussen's Syndrome with Ganciclovir. *Neurology* 1996; 47:925–928.

57. Lim-Bon-Siong R, Pepose JS. Ocular Infections. In: Storch, GA, ed. *Essentials of Diagnostic Virology*. Philadelphia: Churchill Livingstone, 2000; 139–153.
58. Boppana SB, Amos C, Britt WJ, Stagno S, Alford CA, Pass RF. Late Onset and Reactivation of Chorioretinitis in Children with Congenital Cytomegalovirus Infection. *Pediatr Infect Dis J* 1994; 13:1139–1142.
59. Kempen JH, Jabs DA, Wilson LA, Dunn JP, West SK, Tonascia J. Mortality Risk for Patients with Cytomegalovirus Retinitis and Acquired Immune Deficiency Syndrome. *Clin Infect Dis* 2003; 37:1365–1373.
60. Bloom JN, Palestine AG. The Diagnosis of Cytomegalovirus Retinitis. *Ann Intern Med* 1988; 109:963–969.
61. Rivera LB, Boppana SB, Fowler KB, Britt WJ, Stagno S, Pass RF. Predictors of Hearing Loss in Children with Symptomatic Congenital Cytomegalovirus Infection. *Pediatrics* 2002; 110: 762–767.
62. Fowler KB, McCollister FP, Dahle AJ, Boppana SB, Britt WJ, Pass RF. Progressive and Fluctuating Sensorineural Hearing Loss in Children with Asymptomatic Congenital Cytomegalovirus Infection. *J Pediatr 1997*; 130:624–630.
63. Williamson WD, Demmler GJ, Percy AK, Catlin FI. Progressive Hearing Loss in Infants with Asymptomatic Congenital Cytomegalovirus Infection. *Pediatrics* 1992; 90:862–866.
64. Whitley RJ, Cloud G, Gruber W, Storch GA, Demmler GJ, Jacobs RF, Dankner W. Ganciclovir Treatment of Symptomatic Congenital Cytomegalovirus Infection: Results of a Phase II Study. *J Infect Dis* 1997; 175:1080–1086.
65. Nigro G, Scholz H, U. B. Ganciclovir Therapy for Symptomatic Congenital Cytomegalovirus Infection in Infants: A Two-Regimen Experience. *J Pediatr* 1994; 124:318–322.
66. Martin DF, Sierra-Madero J, Walmsley S, Wolitz RA, Macey K, Georgiou P, Rovinson CA. A Controlled Trial of Valganciclovir as Induction Therapy for Cytomegalovirus Retinitis. *N Engl J Med* 2002; 346:1119–1126.
67. Straus SE, Ostrove JM, Inchauspe G, Felser JM, Freifeld A, Croen KD, Sawyer MH. Varicella-Zoster Infections. *Ann Intern Med* 1988; 108:221–237.
68. AAP Committee of Infectious Diseases. Varicella Vaccine Update. *Pediatrics* 2000; 105: 136–140.
69. Arvin AM. Varicella-Zoster Virus. In: Long, SS, Pickering, LK & Prober, CG, eds., *Principles and Practice of Pediatric Infectious Diseases,* 2nd ed., Philadelphia: Churchill Livingstone, 2003; 1041–1050.
70. Gershon A. Varicella-Zoster Virus. In: Feigin, RD, Cherry, JD, Demmler, GJ & Kaplan, SL, eds., *Textbook of Pediatric Infectious Diseases*, 5th ed., Philadelphia: Elsevier Saunders, 2004; 1962–1971.
71. Brunell PA. Varicella in Pregnancy, the Fetus and the Newborn: Problems in Management. *J Infect Dis* 1992; 166:S42–47.
72. Prober CG, Gershon A, Grose C, McCracken GH, Nelson JD. Consensus: Varicella-Zoster Infections in Pregnancy and the Perinatal Period. *Pediatr Infect Dis J* 1990; 9: 865–869.
73. Fleisher G, Henry W, McSorley M, Arbeter A, Plotkin S. Life-Threatening Complications of Varicella. *Am J Dis Child* 1981; 135:896–899.
74. Ziebold C, von Kries R, Lang R, Weigl J, Schmitt HJ. Severe Complications of Varicella in Previously Healthy Children in Germany: A 1-Year Survey. *Pediatrics* 2001; 108:e79.
75. Peterson CL, Mascola L, Chao SM, Lieberman JM, Arcinue EL, Blumberg DA, Kim KS, Kovacs A, Wong VK, Brunell PA. Children Hospitalized for Varicella: A Prevaccine Review. *J Pediatr* 1996; 129:529–536.
76. Gnann JW. Varicella-Zoster Virus: Atypical Presentations and Unusual Complications. *J Infect Dis* 2002; 186:S91–98.
77. Preblud S, Orenstein W, Bart K. Varicella: Clinical Manifestations, Epidemiology, and Health Impact in Children. *Pediatr Infect Dis J* 1984; 3:505–509.
78. Cizman M, Jazbec J. Etiology of Acute Encephalitis in Childhood in Slovenia. *Pediatr Infect Dis J* 1993; 12:903–908.

79. Rantala H, Uhari M. Occurrence of Childhood Encephalitis: A Population-Based Study. *Pediatr Infect Dis J* 1989; 8:426–430.
80. Rantala H, Uhari M, Uhari M, Saukkonen A-L, Sorri M. Outcome after Childhood Encephalitis. *Dev Med Child Neurol* 1991; 33:858–867.
81. Koskiniemi M, Korppi M, Mustonen K, Rantala H, Muttilainen M, Herrgard E, Ukkonen P, Vaheri A. Epidemiology of Encephalitis in Children. A Prospective Multicenter Study. *Eur J Pediatr* 1997; 156:541–545.
82. Bauman ML, Bergman I. Postvaricella Encephalitis. *Arch Neurol* 1984; 41: 556–558.
83. Kleinschmidt-DeMasters BK, Amlie-Lefond C, Gilden DH. The Patterns of Varicella Zoster Virus Encephalitis. *Hum Pathol* 1996; 27:927–937.
84. McCormick WF, Rodnitzky RL, Schochet SS, McKee AP. Varicella-Zoster Encephalomyelitis. *Arch Neurol* 1969; 21:559–569.
85. Kennedy PGE, Barrass JD, Graham DI, Clements GB. Studies on the Pathogenesis of Neurological Diseases Associated with Varicella-Zoster Virus. *Neuropathol Appl Neurobiol* 1990; 16:305–316.
86. Wagner HJ, Seidel A, Grande-Nagel I, Kruse K, Sperner J. Pre-Eruptive Varicella Encephalitis: Case Report and Review of the Literature. *Eur J Pediatr* 1998; 157:814–815.
87. Dangond F, Engle E, Yessayan L, Sawyer MH. Pre-Eruptive Varicella Cerebellitis Confirmed by PCR. *Pediatr Neurol* 1993; 9:491–493.
88. Liu GT, Urion DK. Pre-Eruptive Varicella Encephalitis and Cerebellar Ataxia. *Pediatr Neurol* 1992; 8:69–70.
89. Maguire JF, Meissner HC. Onset of Encephalitis Early in the Course of Varicella Infection. *Pediatr Infect Dis J* 1985; 4:699–701.
90. Gibbs F, Gibbs E, Spies H, Carpenter P. Common Types of Childhood Encephalitis. *Arch Neurol* 1964; 10:15–25.
91. Darling CF, Larsen MB, Byrd SE, Radkowski MA, Palka PS, Allen ED. MR and CT Imaging Patterns in Post-Varicella Encephalitis. *Pediatr Radiol* 1995; 25:241–244.
92. Tenorio G, Whitaker JN. Steroid-Dependent Postvaricella Encephalomyelitis. *J Child Neurol* 1991; 6.
93. Wetzel K, Asholt I, Herrmann E, Kratzer C, Masuhr F, Schielke E. Good Cognitive Outcome of Patients with Herpes Zoster Encephalitis: A Follow-up Study. *J Neurol* 2002; 249: 1612–1614.
94. Guess H. Population-Based Studies of Varicella Complications. *Pediatrics* 1986; 78: 723–727.
95. Gieron-Korthals MA, Westberry KR, Emmanuel PJ. Acute Childhood Ataxia: 10-Year Experience. *J Child Neurol* 1994; 9:381–384.
96. Snodgrass SR. Syndromic Diagnosis in Para-Infectious Neurologic Disease: Varicella Ataxic Syndrome. *J Child Neurol* 1998; 13:83–85.
97. Puchhammer-Stockl E, Popow-Kraupp T, Heinz FX, Mandl CW, Kunz C. Detection of Varicella-Zoster Virus DNA by Polymerase Chain Reaction in the Cerebrospinal Fluid of Patients Suffering from Neurological Complications Associated with Chicken Pox or Herpes Zoster. *J Clin Microbiol* 1991; 29:1513–1516.
98. Sunaga Y, Hikima A, Ostuka T, Morikawa A. Acute Cerebellar Ataxia with Abnormal MRI Lesions after Varicella Vaccination. *Pediatr Neurol* 1995; 13:340–342.
99. White HH. Varicella Myelopathy. *N Engl J Med* 1962; 266:772–773.
100. Yilmaz K, Caliskan M, Akdeniz C, Aydinli N, Karabocuoglu M, Uzel N. Acute Childhood Hemiplegia Associated with Chickenpox. *Pediatr Neurol* 1998; 18:256–261.
101. Gilden DH, Lipton HL, Wolf JS, Akenbrandt W, Smith JE, Mahalingam R, Forghani B. Two Patients with Unusual Forms of Varicella-Zoster Virus Vasculopathy. *N Engl J Med* 2002; 347:1500–1503.
102. Silliman CC, Tedder DG, Ogle JW, Simon J, Kleinschmidt-DeMasters BK, Manco-Johnson M, Levin MJ. Unsuspected Varicella-Zoster Virus Encephalitis in a Child with Acquired Immunodeficiency Syndrome. *J Pediatr* 1993; 123:418–422.
103. Morgan ER, Smalley LA. Varicella in Immunocompromised Children. *Am J Dis Child* 1983; 137:883–885.

104. Moorthy R, Weinberg D, Teich S, Berger B, Minturn J, Kumar S, Rao N, Fowell S, Loose I, Jampol L. Management of Varicella Zoster Virus Retinitis in AIDS. *Br J Ophthalmol* 1997; 81:189–194.
105. Purdy KW, Heckenlively JR, Church JA, Keller MA. Progressive Outer Retinal Necrosis Caused by Varicella-Zoster Virus in Children with Acquired Immunodeficiency Syndrome. *Pediatr Infect Dis J* 2003; 22:384–385.
106. Storch GA. Skin and Mucous Membrane Infections. In: Storch, GA, ed., *Essentials of Diagnostic Virology*. Philadelphia: Churchill Livingstone, 2000; 93–103.
107. Read SJ, Kurtz JB. Laboratory Diagnosis of Common Viral Infections of the Central Nervous System by Using a Single Multiplex PCR Screening Assay. *J Clin Microbiol* 1999; 37: 1352–1355.
108. AAP Committee on Infectious Diseases. The Use of Oral Acyclovir in Otherwise Healthy Children with Varicella. *Pediatrics* 1993; 91:674–676.
109. Chetham MM, Roberts KB. Infectious Mononucleosis in Adolescents. *Pediatr Ann* 1991; 20: 206–212.
110. Katz BZ. Epstein-Barr Virus (Mononucleosis and Lymphoproliferative Disorders). In: Long, SS, Pickering, LK & Prober, CG, eds., *Principles and Practice of Pediatric Infectious Diseases*, 2nd ed., Philadelphia: Churchill Livingstone, 2003; 1059–1068.
111. Leach CT, Sumaya CV. Epstein-Barr Virus. In: Feigin, RD, Cherry, JD, Demmler, GJ & Kaplan, SL, eds., *Textbook of Pediatric Infectious Diseases*, 5th ed., Philadelphia: Elsevier Saunders, 2004; 1932–1956.
112. Sumaya CV, Ench Y. Epstein-Barr Virus Infectious Mononucleosis in Children. I. Clinical and General Laboratory Findings. *Pediatrics* 1985; 75:1003–1010.
113. Connelly KP, DeWitt LD. Neurologic Complications of Infectious Mononucleosis. *Pediatr Neurol* 1994; 10:181–184.
114. Alpert G, Fleisher GR. Complications of Infection with Epstein-Barr Virus During Childhood: A Study of Children Admitted to the Hospital. *Pediatr Infect Dis J* 1984; 3:304–307.
115. Domachowske JB, Cunningham CK, Cummings DL, Crosley CJ, Hannan WP, Weiner LB. Acute Manifestations and Neurologic Sequelae of Epstein-Barr Virus Encephalitis in Children. *Pediatr Infect Dis J* 1996; 15:871–875.
116. North K, de Silva L, Procopis P. Brain-Stem Encephalitis Caused by Epstein-Barr Virus. *J Child Neurol* 1993; 8:40–42.
117. Kennard C, Swash M. Acute Viral Encephalitis. Its Diagnosis and Outcome. *Brain* 1981; 104:129–148.
118. Halsted CC, Chang RS. Infectious Mononucleosis and Encephalitis: Recovery of EB Virus from Spinal Fluid. *Pediatrics* 1979; 64:257–258.
119. Weinberg A, Li S, Palmer M, Tyler KL. Quantitative CSF PCR in Epstein-Barr Virus Infections of the Central Nervous System. *Ann Neurol* 2002; 52:543–548.
120. Cotton MF, Reiley T, Robinson C, Pedneault L, Alfieri C, Simoes EAF. Acute Aqueductal Stenosis in a Patient with Epstein-Barr Virus Infectious Mononucleosis. *Pediatr Infect Dis J* 1994; 13:224–227.
121. Pommer B, Pilz P, Harrer G. Transient Global Amnesia as a Manifestation of Epstein-Barr Virus Encephalitis. *J Neurol* 1983; 229:125–127.
122. Friedland R, Yahr MD. Meningoencephalopathy Secondary to Infectious Mononucleosis. *Arch Neurol* 1977; 34:186–188.
123. Demey HE, Martin J-J, Leus RM, Moeremans CJ, Bossaert LL. Coma as a Presenting Sign of Epstein-Barr Encephalitis. *Arch Intern Med* 1988; 148:1459–1461.
124. Bray PF, Culp KW, McFarlin DE, Panitch HS, Torkelson RD, Schlight JP. Demyelinating Disease after Neurologically Complicated Primary Epstein-Barr Virus Infection. *Neurology* 1992; 42:278–282.
125. Angelini L, Bugiani M, Zibordi F, Cinque P, Bizzi A. Brainstem Encephalitis Resulting from Epstein-Barr Virus Mimicking an Infiltrating Tumor in a Child. *Pediatr Neurol* 2000; 22: 130–132.

126. Donovan WD, Zimmerman RD. MRI Findings of Severe Epstein-Barr Virus Encephalomyelitis. *J Comput Assist Tomogr* 1996; 20:1027–1029.
127. Shian WJ, Chi CS. Epstein-Barr Virus Encephalitis and Encephalomyelitis: MR Findings. *Pediatr Radiol* 1996; 26:690–693.
128. Cinbis M, Aysun S. "Alice in Wonderland" Syndrome as an Initial Manifestation of Epstein-Barr Virus Infection. *Br J Ophthalmol* 1992; 76:316.
129. Liaw S-B, Shen E-Y. Alice in Wonderland Syndrome as a Presenting Symptom of EBV Infection. *Pediatr Neurol* 1991; 7:464–466.
130. Pitts J, Norris ADC. Cerebellar Encephalitis Following Epstein-Barr Virus Infection. *Int J Clin Pract* 1998; 52:276–277.
131. Erzurum S, Kalausky SM, Watanakunakorn C. Acute Cerebellar Ataxia and Hearing Loss as Initial Symptoms of Infectious Mononucleosis. *Arch Neurol* 1983; 40:760–762.
132. Grose C, Henle W, Henle G, Feorino PM. Primary Epstein-Barr Virus Infections in Acute Neurologic Diseases. *N Engl J Med* 1975; 292:392–395.
133. Hyden D, Roberg M, Forsberg P, Fridell E, Gryden A, Linde A, Odkvist L. Acute "Idiopathic" Peripheral Facial Palsy: Clinical, Serological, and Cerebrospinal Fluid Findings and Effects of Corticosteroids. *Am J Otolaryngol* 1993; 14:179–186.
134. Shoji H, Kusuhara T, Honda Y, Hino H, Kojima K, Abe T, Watanabe M. Relapsing Acute Disseminated Encephalomyelitis Associated with Chronic Epstein-Barr Virus Infection: MRI Findings. *Neuroradiology* 192; 34:340–342.
135. Larsen PD, Bloomer LC, Bray PF. Epstein-Barr Nuclear Antigen and Viral Capsid Antigen Antibody Titers in Multiple Sclerosis. *Neurology* 1985; 35:435–438.
136. Levin LI, Munger KL, Rubertone MV, Peck CA, Lennette ET, Spiegelman D, Ascherio A. Multiple Sclerosis and Epstein-Barr Virus. *JAMA* 2003; 289:1533–1536.
137. Makhleh RE, Manivel MC, Copenhaver CM. In Situ Hybridization for the Detection of Epstein-Barr Virus in Central Nervous System Lymphomas. *Cancer* 1991; 67:444–448.
138. Cohen JI. Epstein-Barr Virus Infection. *N Engl J Med* 2000; 343:481–492.
139. Storch GA. Infectious Mononucleosis. In: Storch, GA, ed. *Essentials of Diagnostic Virology*. Philadelphia: Churchill Livingstone, 2000; 159–166.
140. Tang Y-W, Espy MJ, Persing DH, Smith TF. Molecular Evidence and Clinical Significance of Herpesvirus Coinfection in the Central Nervous System. *J Clin Microbiol* 1997; 35: 2869–2872.
141. Studahl M, Hagberg L, Rekabdar E, Bergstrom T. Herpesvirus DNA Detection in Cerebral Spinal Fluid: Differences in Clinical Presentation between Alpha-, Beta-, and Gamma-Herpesviruses. *Scand J Infect Dis* 2000; 32:237–248.
142. Tynell E, Aurelius E, Brandell A. Acyclovir and Prednisolone Treatment of Acute Infectious Mononucleosis: A Multicenter, Double-Blind, Placebo-Controlled Study. *J Infect Dis* 1996; 174:324–331.
143. Dellemijn PLI, Branderburg A, Niesters HGM. Successful Treatment with Ganciclovir of Presumed Epstein-Barr Meningo-Encephalitis Following Bone Marrow Transplant. *Bone Marrow Transplant* 1995; 16:311–312.
144. Garamendi I, Montejo M, Cancelo L, Lopez L, Aguirrebengoa K, Martin A, Zarraga S. Encephalitis Caused by Epstein-Barr Virus in a Renal Transplant Recipient. *Clin Infect Dis* 2002; 34:287–288.
145. Boutolleau D, Cointe D, Gautheret-Dejean A, Mace M, Agut H, Grangeot-Keros L, Ingrand D. No Evidence for a Major Risk of Roseolovirus Vertical Transmission During Pregnancy. *Clin Infect Dis* 2003; 36:1634–1635.
146. Jones CA, Isaacs D. Human Herpesvirus-6 Infections. *Arch Dis Child* 1996; 74:98–100.
147. Caserta MT, Mock DJ, Dewhurst S. Human Herpesvirus 6. *Clin Infect Dis* 2001; 33:829–833.
148. Pohl-Koppe A, Blay M, Jager G, Weiss M. Human Herpes Virus Type 7 DNA in the Cerebrospinal Fluid of Children with Central Nervous System Diseases. *Eur J Pediatr* 2001; 160:351–358.

149. Yoshikawa T, Asano Y. Central Nervous System Complications in Human Herpesvirus-6 Infection. *Brain & Development* 2000; 22:307–314.
150. Lyall EGH. Human Herpesvirus 6: Primary Infection and the Central Nervous System. *Pediatr Infect Dis J* 1996; 15:693–696.
151. Caserta MT, Breese Hall C, Schnabel K, McIntyre K, Long C, Costanzo M, Dewhurst S, Insel R, Epstein LG. Neuroinvasion and Persistence of Human Herpesvirus 6 in Children. *J Infect Dis* 1994; 170:1586–1589.
152. Campadelli-Fiume G, Mirandola P, Menotti L. Human Herpesvirus 6: An Emerging Pathogen. *Emerg Infect Dis* 1999; 5:353–366.
153. Breese Hall C, Long CE, Schnabel KC, Caserta MT, McIntyre KM, Costanzo MA, Knott A, Dewhurst S, Insel R, Epstein LG. Human Herpesvirus-6 Infection in Children: A Prospective Study of Complications and Reactivation. *N Engl J Med* 1994; 331: 432–438.
154. Asano Y, Yoshidawa T, Suga S. Clinical Features of Infants with Primary Human Herpes Virus 6 Infection (Exanthem Subitum, Roseola Infantum). *Pediatrics* 1994; 93: 104–108.
155. Torigoe S, Kumamoto T, Koide W, Taya K, Yamanishi K. Clinical Manifestations Associated with Human Herpesvirus 7 Infection. *Arch Dis Child* 1995; 72:518–519.
156. Bonthius DJ, Karacay B. Meningitis and Encephalitis in Children. An Update. *Neurol Clin* 2002; 20:1013–1038.
157. Barone SR, Kaplan MH, Krilov LR. Human Herpesvirus-6 Infection in Children with First Febrile Seizures. *J Pediatr* 1995; 127:95–97.
158. Kondo K, Nagafuji H, Hata A, Tomomori C, Yamanishi K. Association of Human Herpesvirus 6 Infection of the Central Nervous System with Recurrence of Febrile Convulsions. *J Infect Dis* 1993; 167:1197–1200.
159. Teach SJ, Wallace HL, Evans MJ, Duffner PK, Hay J, Faden HS. Human Herpesviruses Types 6 and 7 and Febrile Seizures. *Pediatr Neurol* 1999; 21:699–703.
160. Hukin J, Farrell K, MacWilliam LM, Colbourne M, Waida E, Tan R, Mroz L, Thomas E. Case-Control Study of Primary Human Herpesvirus 6 Infection in Children with Febrile Seizures. *Pediatrics* 1998; 101:e3.
161. Jee SH, Long CE, Schnabel KC, Sehgal N, Epstein LG, Breese Hall C. Risk of Recurrent Seizures after a Primary Human Herpesvirus 6-Induced Febrile Seizure. *Pediatr Infect Dis J* 1998; 17:43–48.
162. Suga S, Suzuki K, Ihira M, Yoshikawa T, Kajita Y, Ozaki T, Iida K, Saito Y, Asano Y. Clinical Characteristics of Febrile Convulsions During Primary HHV-6 Infection. *Arch Dis Child* 2000; 82:62–66.
163. Ishiguro N, Yamada S, Takahashi T, Takahashi Y, Togashi T, Okuno T, Yamanishi K. Meningo-Encephalitis Associated with HHV-6 Related Exanthem Subitum. *Acta Paediatr Scand* 1990; 79:987–989.
164. Suga S, Yoshikawa T, Asano Y, T. K, Nakashima T, Kobayashi I, Yazaki T. Clinical and Virological Analyses of 21 Infants with Exanthem Subitum (Roseola Infantum) and Central Nervous System Complications. *Ann Neurol* 1993; 33:597–603.
165. McCullers JA, Lakeman FD, Whitley RJ. Human Herpesvirus 6 Is Associated with Focal Encephalitis. *Clin Infect Dis* 1995; 21:571–576.
166. Moschettini D, Balestri P, Fois A, Valensin PE. Acute Encephalitis Due to Human Herpesvirus 6. *Clin Infect Dis* 1996; 23:397–398.
167. Rantala H, Mannonen L, Ahtiluoto S, Linnavuori K, Herva R, Vaheri A, Koskiniemi M. Human Herpesvirus-6 Associated Encephalitis with Subsequent Infantile Spasms and Cerebellar Astrocytoma. *Dev Med Child Neurol* 2000; 42:418–421.
168. Jones CMV, Dunn HG, Thomas EE, Cone RW, Weber JM. Acute Encephalopathy and Status Epilepticus Associated with Human Herpes Virus 6 Infection. *Dev Med Child Neurol* 1994; 36:646–650.
169. Patnaik M, Peter JB. Intrathecal Synthesis of Antibodies to Human Herpesvirus 6 Early Antigen in Patients with Meningitis/Encephalitis. *Clin Infect Dis* 1995; 21:715–716.

170. Yoshikawa T, Nakashima T, Suga S, Asano Y, Yazaki T, Kimura H, Morishima T, Kondo K, Yamanishi K. Human Herpesvirus-6 DNA in Cerebrospinal Fluid of a Child with Exanthem Subitum and Meningoencephalitis. *Pediatrics* 1992; 89:888–890.
171. Glaser CA, Gilliam S, Schnurr D, Forghani B, Honarmand S, Khetsuriani N, Fischer M, Cossen CK, Anderson LJ. In Search of Encephalitis Etiologies: Diagnostic Challenges in the California Encephalitis Project, 1998-2000. *Clin Infect Dis* 2003; 36:731–742.
172. Ahtiluoto S, Mannonen L, Paetau A, Vaheri A, Koskiniemi M. In Situ Hybridization Detection of Human Herpesvirus 6 in Brain Tissue from Fatal Encephalitis. *Pediatrics* 2000; 105: 431–433.
173. Cuomo L, Trivedi P, Cardillo MR. Human Herpesvirus 6 Infection in Neoplastic and Normal Brain Tissue. *J Med Virol* 2001; 63:45–51.
174. Asano Y, Yoshikawa T, Kajita Y, Ogura R, Suga S, Yazaki T, Nakashima T, Yamada A, Kurata T. Fatal Encephalitis/Encephalopathy in Primary Human Herpesvirus-6 Infection. *Arch Dis Child* 1992; 67:1484–1485.
175. Yanagihara K, Tanaka-Taya K, Itagaki Y, Toribe Y, Arita K, Yamanishi K, Okada S. Human Herpesvirus 6 Meningoencephalitis with Sequelae. *Pediatr Infect Dis J* 1995; 14: 240–241.
176. Kamei A, Ichinohe S, Onuma R, Hiraga S, Fujiwara T. Acute Disseminated Demyelination Due to Primary Human Herpesvirus-6 Infection. *Eur J Pediatr* 1997; 156:709–712.
177. Fujino Y, Nakajima M, Inoue J, Kusuhara T, Yamada T. Human Herpesvirus 6 Encephalitis Associated with Hypersensitivity Syndrome. *Ann Neurol* 2002; 51:771–774.
178. Descamps V, Collot S, Houhou N, Ranger-Rogez S. Human Herpesvirus-6 Encephalitis Associated with Hypersensitivity Syndrome. *Ann Neurol* 2003; 53:280.
179. Sugaya N, Yoshikawa T, Miura M, Ishizuka T, Kawakami C, Asano Y. Influenza Encephalopathy Associated with Infection with Human Herpesvirus 6 and/or Human Herpesvirus 7. *Clin Infect Dis* 2002; 34:461–466.
180. Kawada J-I, Kimura H, Hara S, Ito Y, Kawashima H, Okuno T, Morishima T. Absence of Associations between Influenza-Associated Encephalopathy and Human Herpesvirus 6 or Human Herpesvirus 7. *Pediatr Infect Dis J* 2003; 22:115–119.
181. Challoner M, Smith KT, Parker JD, Macleod DL. Plaque-Associated Expression of Human Herpesvirus 6 in Multiple Sclerosis. *PNAS* 1995; 92:7440–7444.
182. Wilborn F, Schmidt CA, Brinkmann V, Jendroska K, Oettle H, Siegert W. A Potential Role for Human Herpesvirus Type 6 in Nervous System Disease. *J Neuroimmunol* 1994; 49: 213–214.
183. Goodman AD, Mock DJ, Powers JM, Baker JV, Blumberg BM. Human Herpesvirus 6 Genome and Antigen in Acute Multiple Sclerosis Lesions. *J Infect Dis* 2003; 187: 1365–1376.
184. Tyler KL. Human Herpesvirus 6 and Multiple Sclerosis: The Continuing Conundrum. *J Infect Dis* 2003; 187:1360–1364.
185. Merelli E, Sola P, Faglioni P, Poggi M, Montorsi M, Torelli G. Newest Human Herpesvirus (HHV-6) in the Guillain-Barré Syndrome. *Acta Neurol Scand* 1992; 85:334–336.
186. Hodinka RL, Moshal KL. Childhood Infections. In: Storch, GA, ed. *Essentials of Diagnostic Virology*. Philadelphia: Churchill Livingstone, 2000; 167–186.
187. Grose C. Human Herpesviruses 6, 7, and 8. In: Feigin, RD, Cherry, JD, Demmler, GJ & Kaplan, SL, eds., *Textbook of Pediatric Infectious Diseases*, 5th ed., Philadelphia: Elsevier Saunders, 2004; 1957–1962.
188. Agut H, Collandre H, Aubin JT. In Vitro Sensitivity of Human Herpesvirus-6 to Antiviral Drugs. *Res Virol* 1989; 140:219–228.
189. Torigoe S, Koide W, Yamada M, Miyashiro E, Tanaka-Taya K, Yamanishi K. Human Herpesvirus-7 Infection Associated with Central Nervous System Manifestations. *J Pediatr* 1996; 129:301–305.
190. Bradford RD, Cloud G, Lakeman AD, Boppana S, Kimberlin DW, Jacobs R, et al. Detection of Cytomegalovirus (CMV) DNA by Polymerase Chain Reaction Is Associated with Hearing Loss in Newborns with Symptomatic Congenital CMV Infection Involving the Central Nervous System. *J Infect Dis* 2005; 191:227–233.

191. Boppana SB, Fowler KB, Pass RF, Rivera LB, Bradford RD, Lakeman FD, Britt WJ. Congenital Cytomegalovirus Infection: Association Between Virus Burden in Infancy and Hearing Loss. *J Pediatr* 2005; 146:817–823.
192. Nigro G, Adler SP, La Torre R, Best AM. Passive Immunization during Pregnancy for Congenital Cytomegalovirus Infection. *N Engl J Med* 2005; 353:1350–1362.
193. Cotton MF, Reiley T, Robinson CC, Pedneault L, Alfieri C, Simoes EAF. Acute Aqueductal Stenosis in a Patient with Epstein-Barr Virus Infectious Mononucleosis. *Pediatr Infect Dis J* 1994; 13:224–227.
194. Jacobson MA, Sinclair E, Bredt B, Agrillo L, Black D, Epling CL et al. Safety and Immunogenicity of Towne Cytomegalovirus Vaccine with or without Adjuvant Recombinant Interleukin-12. *Vaccine* 2006; 24:5311–5319.
195. Wang Z, La Rosa C, Lacey SF, Maas R, Mekhoubad S, Britt WJ, Diamond DJ. Attenuated Poxvirus Expressing Three Immunodominant CMV Antigens as a Vaccine Strategy for CMV Infection. *J Clin Virol* 2006; 35:324–331.
196. Zhang C, Buchanan H, Andrews W, Evans A, Pass RF. Detection of Cytomegalovirus Infection During a Vaccine Clinical Trial in Healthy Young Women: Seroconversion and Viral Shedding. *J Clin Virol* 2006; 35:338–342.
197. Schleiss M. Progress in Cytomegalovirus Vaccine Development. *Herpes* 2005; 12:66–75.
198. Askalan R, Laughlin S, Mayank S, Chan A, MacGregor D, Andrew M, Curtis R, Meaney B, deVeber G. Chickenpox and Stroke in Childhood: A Study of Frequency and Causation. *Stroke* 2001; 32:1257–1262.

# Chapter 2
# Myxoviruses

**Jason G. Newland, M.D., F.A.A.P. and José R. Romero, M.D., F.A.A.P.**

## Paramyxoviruses

The *Paramyxoviridae* are enveloped, nonsegmented, negative-sense RNA viruses. The family is divided into two subfamilies, the *Paramyxovirinae* and *Pneumovirinae*. Of the five genera that comprise the *Paramyxovirinae*, three are known to cause disease in humans: *Respirovirus*, *Rubulavirus*, and *Morbillivirus*. The *Pneumovirinae*, in turn, consist of two genera pathogenic for humans, *Pneumovirus*, and the recently identified *Metapneumovirus* [1].

## Parainfluenza

### *Epidemiology*

The parainfluenza viruses (PIV) are members of the *Respirovirus* genus. Although four serotypes of PIV have been identified, PIV4 is infrequently isolated from clinical samples. Transmission of PIV occurs through large droplets that inoculate the eyes and nose via respiratory aerosols or autoinoculation [2]. By 2 years of age, more than 90% of children have been infected with PIV3. PIV1 and PIV2 infection is normally not encountered until after 2 years of age. PIV4 is also found in this age group, with more than 50% of children younger than 5 years of age possessing antibodies to PIV4 [3].

PIV are ubiquitous worldwide. They cause disease throughout the year, but peak activity is observed during the spring and fall months.

### *Clinical Manifestations*

PIV can cause both upper and lower respiratory tract disease, with the former predominating. Up to 50% of PIV-related upper respiratory tract infections are complicated by otitis media. PIV, in particular PIV1, typically cause croup that may

L.L. Barton and N.R. Friedman (eds.), *The Neurological Manifestations of Pediatric Infectious Diseases and Immunodeficiency Syndromes.*

be severe enough to warrant treatment with corticosteroids and hospitalization. PIV3 infection can cause pneumonia and bronchiolitis, predominantly in infants younger than 1 year of age. PIV can also cause laryngitis, tracheitis, and a nonfocal febrile illness [3].

## *Neurological Manifestations*

PIV have been causally linked to multiple neurological syndromes, including meningitis, meningoencephalitis, Guillain-Barré, Reye, and demyelinating syndromes. The reported ages of patients have ranged from newborn to elderly adults. However, more than half of the reported patients have been younger than 2 years of age. Reported underlying conditions or concurrent illnesses have included severe combined immunodeficiency, *Haemophilus influenzae b* meningitis, human immunodeficiency virus infection, and malignancy [4–16].

The principle neurological diagnosis among patients with PIV central nervous system (CNS) infections has been aseptic meningitis. The most common reported clinical presentation consisted of fever, rhinorrhea, and emesis. Other symptoms observed include headache, lethargy, irritability, and vertigo [4,10–13]. Nuchal rigidity has been infrequently reported [11,13]. PIV have also been linked to febrile seizures. In one study, 11% of patients with febrile seizure were associated with PIV infection. Most patients seem to recover without neurological sequelae. However, in patients in whom profound underlying immunodeficiency exists, death may occur [5].

## *Neuropathology*

Because of the generally favorable outcome of neurological illnesses resulting from PIV infection, little is known regarding the pathophysiology and neuropathology of PIV-associated neurological syndromes. Even in a patient who died of disseminated PIV3, autopsy revealed no abnormalities within the brain despite isolation of the virus from the cerebrospinal fluid (CSF) [5].

## *Diagnosis*

Cytochemical analysis of the CSF reveals a predominantly mononuclear pleocytosis that ranges from 10 to 913 cells/$mm^3$. In almost all cases, the CSF protein and glucose levels are normal [4,6,7,9,11–13]. In all cases of neurological disease reported, PIV was isolated from the CSF using cell culture. Although all PIV serotypes, with the exception of PIV1, have been isolated from the CSF, PIV3 has been the overwhelmingly dominant serotype identified.

All four types of PIV were isolated from children with PIV-associated febrile seizures in one study, but none were from the CSF [17]. In a separate report, two patients with simple febrile seizures yielded PIV3 and PIV2 from the CSF [18].

### *Treatment*

Neurological disease, similar to respiratory disease that results from PIV, is self-limiting. As such, only supportive care is required as treatment.

## Mumps

### *Introduction*

The earliest descriptions of mumps dates to Hippocrates in the fifth century BC. Hamilton et al. published the initial report of CNS involvement with mumps in 1790, describing mumps-associated neurological findings in a patient who succumbed to the disease. In the early 19th century, Hintz observed an association between epidemic parotitis and deafness [19,20].

### *Epidemiology*

Mumps is a member of the genus Rubulavirus within the subfamily *Paramyxovirinae*. Before the introduction of an effective mumps vaccine in 1967, cases were seen annually, with epidemics approximately every 3 to 4 years in the United States. In epidemic years, the rate of infection reached as high as 250 cases per 100,000 population [19,20]. In temperate climates, mumps infections are observed during the winter and spring months. This seasonality does not hold true for the tropical regions. Currently, because of widespread use of mumps vaccine, no seasonality is observed among mumps cases in the United States. Other countries around the world that have implemented vaccination programs have observed a reduction in mumps cases exceeding 85% [21].

In 2003, the total number of mumps cases in the United States was only 270, the lowest number ever reported [22,23]. Although significant strides have been made in reducing the annual number of mumps cases, outbreaks continue to occur [24,25]. Two large outbreaks of mumps in Great Britain (2004–2005) and the United States (2005–2006) attest to the latter.

In Great Britain, the outbreak was attributed to decreased immunization rates secondary to vaccine shortages in combination with the lack of use of a booster dose of mumps vaccine. The outbreak in the United States was thought to be the result of multiple factors that included a large susceptible population because of lack of 100% effectiveness of the two-dose measles, mumps, rubella (MMR) vaccine regimen, delayed diagnosis by physicians, and close living quarters (i.e., college dormitories) among the people most affected [24,25].

Mumps is considered one of the classic diseases of childhood. Typically, children between the ages of 5 and 9 years were most commonly affected, with children younger than the age of 5 years comprising the next largest group. However, since institution of mumps vaccination, many more cases now occur in individuals older than the age of 10 years.

## Clinical Manifestations

Mumps is a highly contagious disease that is transmitted via respiratory droplets. Infectivity rates approach 60 to 100% among susceptible individuals. An important source of virus spread is persons experiencing asymptomatic infections. The incubation period for mumps is 16 to 18 days, but ranges from 14 to 24 days. Individuals experiencing mumps are infectious 3 days before and 4 days after parotid enlargement. Shedding of virus in the urine may occur for 10 to 14 days after the onset of parotid enlargement [26].

The classic patient with mumps presents with a prodrome consisting of headache, anorexia, vomiting, malaise, and fever 1 to 2 days before the onset of parotitis, the hallmark of the disease. The fever can be as high as 103°F but, in some cases, is low grade or completely absent. After the prodrome, swelling of the parotid gland(s) begins. In 70 to 80% of cases, the parotid enlargement is bilateral. The parotid swelling reaches its maximum on the third day and persists for 2 days before receding.

Up to 30% of infections are asymptomatic or so mild as to go unrecognized. Other associated clinical manifestations of mumps are diverse. Up to 38% of postpubertal males develop epididymoorchitis. In postpubertal females, oophoritis occurs in 7%. Other reported manifestations include pancreatitis, myocarditis, nephritis, arthropathy, and rash [20].

## Neurological Manifestations

Mumps virus should be recognized as an important etiologic agent of neurological disease. CNS involvement in mumps infection has been reported to occur in 0.5 to 10% of all mumps infections. The reported rates of meningitis and encephalitis per mumps case are 1 and 2.6 per 1000, respectively. During epidemics, as many as 30% of mumps-infected patients experience neurological illnesses [21,26–28].

During the pre-vaccine era, mumps was the leading cause of both meningitis and encephalitis. Meyers et al. reported that mumps was the second most common cause of aseptic meningitis as well as the most common cause of encephalitis between 1953 and 1958 [29]. Mumps virus was responsible for up to 25% of known causes of viral meningitis [28,30]. Among reportable cases of encephalitis to the Centers for Disease Control and Prevention (CDC) in 1967, mumps was the most common etiology, comprising approximately 36% of the cases. Nine years after the inception of the mumps vaccine, only 3.5% of encephalitis cases reported to the CDC were caused by mumps virus, a testament to the effectiveness of the vaccine [28]. Although clinical data regarding the 2006 mumps outbreak in the United States remains incomplete, at least 21 of the 3860 cases had reported neurological complications. These included meningitis in 10, encephalitis in 5 and deafness in 6 patients.

CNS involvement during mumps infection occurs most commonly in children. Children younger than 10 years of age account for more than 70% of the cases [31–33]. Interestingly, CNS involvement occurs three times more often in male than in female patients.

Mumps meningitis and/or encephalitis may occur with or without associated parotitis. Approximately 50% of patients do not have parotitis. Typically, in patients with parotitis, the meningitis presents during the first week after its onset. However, the onset of the meningitis may occur as late as 3 weeks after parotitis or may even precede it [32–34]. In contrast, mumps-associated encephalitis typically appears weeks later.

Although it is common to describe the CNS involvement in mumps as either meningitis or encephalitis, many patients have combinations of both, or rather, meningoencephalitis. In patients with mumps aseptic meningitis alone, the commonly reported signs and symptoms include fever, headache, vomiting, and neck stiffness. Azimi et al. observed the fever to last, on average, 3.1 days, but could persist for as long as 7 days. Other associated signs and symptoms may include abdominal pain, diarrhea, and sore throat [31].

In their report, Koskiniemi et al. described patients with mumps-associated encephalitis alone. These patients were primarily boys (4:1) and had a mean age of 7.3 years (range 1.2–13.7 yr). As with meningitis, patients presented with fever and commonly had parotitis before the onset of encephalitis. Neurological signs and symptoms consisted of impaired locomotion and balance (36%), seizures (24%), psychic disorder (22%), and sensory disturbance (12%). Progression to coma was reported in 7%. The average length of hospitalization was 10.9 days (3–41 d) [35].

Mumps-associated deafness has been estimated to occur in 0.5 to 5 per 100,000 cases of mumps. It is typically unilateral and results in permanent hearing loss [20,36]. The presence of meningitis or encephalitis is not a prerequisite for its development and it has been reported to occur even in patients with asymptomatic mumps infection. Other neurological diseases attributed to mumps infection include Guillain-Barré syndrome, transverse myelitis, cerebellitis, facial palsy, and an illness similar to subacute sclerosing panencephalitis (SSPE) [20,37–39].

Neurological sequelae after mumps meningitis are rare. Azimi et al. [31] and Johnstone et al. [40] reviewed the outcomes of 181 patients with mumps meningitis and found that all recovered without sequelae. Additionally, among patients followed for up to 40 months after recovery from their illness, none developed deafness.

In contrast, the outcome is less favorable in patients with encephalitis, in whom sequelae are observed in 25%. These sequelae include behavioral disturbances, impaired ability to concentrate, ataxia, and dysarthria. Overall, mortality is rare and has been associated with infections in immunocompromised hosts or individuals with severe underlying conditions [35,41].

Hydrocephalus has been reported in 16 cases after mumps meningitis and/or encephalitis. This complication has been diagnosed from 1 day to 19 years after the initial mumps infection [42].

## *Neuropathology*

Because death from mumps-associated CNS disease is rare, limited reports exist that discuss its pathology. A serofibrinous leptomeningitis with hyperemia and edema primarily localized at the base of the brain has been described. Donohue et al. found pathology similar to that of CNS-associated measles infection, consisting of perivascular edema and inflammation. Areas of demyelination have been identified in the cerebrum, cerebellum, basal ganglia, thalamus, midbrain, pons, and medulla [43,44].

In 1968, Johnson and colleagues provided a potential explanation for the development of hydrocephalus by demonstrating that suckling mice developed aqueductal stenosis after intracerebral injection of mumps virus. Additionally, nucleocapsids of the mumps virions have been visualized within ependymal cells of the CNS in both animal models and patients with mumps meningitis and/or encephalitis [45–48].

## *Diagnosis*

Cytochemical analysis of the CSF in mumps meningitis reveals a predominant lymphocytic pleocytosis. The CSF leukocyte count is commonly less than 500 cells/mm$^3$ but has been reported to be as high as 5000 cells/mm$^3$ [31,34]. In some, a polymorphonuclear majority may be observed [40]. Pleocytosis has also been reported in patients with clinically apparent mumps infection in the absence of neurological signs or symptoms [43]. Abnormalities in the CSF protein concentration are reported in up to one third of cases and can be as high as 200 mg/dl [31,34]. In the majority of patients, the CSF glucose concentration is normal. However, hypoglycorrhachia has been reported to occur in 6 to 28% of cases [31,34,40]. In one report, persistent hypoglycorrhachia was observed for as long as 4 days [32].

In patients with encephalitis, CSF pleocytosis of less than 500 cells/mm$^3$ (range 0–1853 cells/mm$^3$) in association with a normal protein concentration and a slightly depressed glucose concentration is generally seen [35].

Electroencephalograms (EEGs) are abnormal in patients with mumps-associated encephalitis. Koskiniemi et al. noted that EEG abnormalities were present in all patients evaluated during the first week of illness [35]. The characteristic EEG findings in the majority of cases have been classified as moderate to severe slowing. However, lateralization and even focal temporal lobe slow wave changes have been reported. An abnormal EEG persisted for as long as 2 weeks in almost one third of the cases [35,49].

Magnetic resonance imaging (MRI) scanning has greater sensitivity than computed tomographic (CT) scanning in identifying brain abnormalities in patients with mumps-associated CNS disease. Findings on neuroimaging of patients with mumps meningitis and/or encephalitis are varied and include cerebral edema, transverse myelitis, and demyelinated areas, including the thalamus, caudate, and cerebellum [50]. Hydrocephalus has been identified in association with aqueductal stenosis.

The diagnosis of mumps occurs through isolation of the virus by cell culture, amplification of its genome by polymerase chain reaction (PCR), or evidence of a fourfold rise in serologic titers. Mumps is easily cultured from CSF, saliva, or throat swabs [20]. Recent data have shown that PCR is an effective and more rapid diagnostic methodology. Poggio and colleagues demonstrated that reverse transcriptase (RT)-PCR was equivalent to culture in detecting mumps from the CSF [51]. In situations in which cell culture or PCR are unsuccessful in establishing the diagnosis, a fourfold rise in serologic titers using either hemagglutination, complement fixation, or enzyme-linked immunosorbent assay (ELISA) assays can be used. Caution must be taken in interpreting these results because antibodies to mumps may cross-react with those to PIV [52].

## *Treatment and Prevention*

No specific therapy is available for the treatment of mumps infection. Immunoglobulin has been shown to be beneficial in the prevention of orchitis, but a similar effect has not been observed for other mumps-related complications [53,54]. The lack of an effective treatment for mumps and its complications emphasizes the importance of the mumps vaccine in preventing this illness. Mumps vaccine is a live attenuated virus that is commonly administered concomitantly with measles and rubella virus vaccines (i.e., MMR vaccine). In controlled studies, the efficacy of mumps vaccine after a single dose approached 95%. In the United States, administration of the vaccine occurs in children after their first birthday and again between 4 and 6 years of age.

A recognized complication of the use of mumps vaccine is the development of aseptic meningitis. In the United States, where the Jeryl Lynn strain of mumps virus is used, the reported rate of aseptic meningitis is 1 in 800,000 doses. In contrast, the Urabe strain used in Japan has reported rates of aseptic meningitis as high as 1 in 2000 doses. The onset of mumps vaccine strain-associated meningitis occurs 2 to 3 weeks after immunization and seems to be clinically similar to that observed with natural infection [19,55,56]. Wakefield et al. have also suggested that the MMR vaccine is associated with the subsequent onset of autism. Numerous published studies have refuted this hypothesis [57,58].

## Measles

### *Introduction*

Measles, a disease caused by a paramyxovirus in the genus *Morbillivirus*, was first described in the 7th century [59]. Cell culture isolation of measles virus, however, was not possible until 1954. Shortly thereafter, the measles virus was adapted to grow in chick embryo tissue culture, paving the way for vaccine development [60,61].

### *Epidemiology*

Before the licensure of inactivated measles vaccine in 1963, measles was a common illness in the United States, resulting in up to 500,000 cases and 500 deaths a year [62,63]. Epidemics occurred every 2 to 5 years during the winter–spring months, and were more frequent in urban populations. Children were most commonly affected, with more than 50% of the measles cases reported occurring in those 5 to 9 years of age [64,65].

Pneumonia caused up to 60% of deaths, whereas encephalitis contributed another 20%. Children younger than 5 years of age and adults older than 20 years had the greatest risk of mortality [63].

After introduction of the live attenuated measles vaccine in United States in 1965, a dramatic decrease in the incidence of measles was observed. Most significantly, since 1992, only one measles-associated death has been reported in the United States [66]. Measles, however, remains a frequent cause of illness and death in developing countries. More than 30 million people worldwide are infected with measles virus every year, resulting in more than 700,000 deaths. Measles is the fifth leading cause of death among children younger than 5 years of age and the leading cause of death caused by a vaccine-preventable disease.

### *Clinical Disease*

Measles has an incubation period of 8 to 12 days. Two to 4 days before the onset of rash, a prodrome consisting of fever, cough, coryza, conjunctivitis, and generalized malaise begins. During the prodromal period, a pathognomonic enanthem, Koplik spots, appears in the oropharynx. These blue and/or white papules on an erythematous base are initially located on the buccal mucosa opposite the first lower molar. They generally spread to involve most of the buccal and labial mucosa [64,67].

The classic exanthem of measles becomes apparent approximately 14 days after exposure. The rash initially erupts on the ears and forehead as erythematous macules and papules that spread in a centrifugal pattern to cover the face, neck, trunk, upper extremities, buttocks, and lower extremities sequentially. Three to 4 days after the onset of the rash, the rash begins to fade in the same progression as it appeared, such that by day 6 or 7 it has completely resolved. In some cases, the rash may be present for up to 10 days [67,68]. As the rash resolves, a fine desquamation may be noted. During the evolution of the rash, the fever reaches its peak by the second or third day and normally resolves, as does the conjunctivitis and rhinorrhea, 24 hours thereafter. The cough may persist for as long as 10 days.

Atypical measles was observed in individuals immunized with the killed measles vaccine and subsequently infected with natural measles. Use of the killed vaccine was abandoned in 1968 in the United States. Atypical measles is characterized by the lack of a typical prodrome and by an erythematous, maculopapular rash, which begins on the wrists and ankles and progresses cephalad. Prominent symptoms in atypical measles are headache, abdominal pain, and myalgias. Almost all cases have pulmonary involvement. The illness typically lasts 1 to 2 weeks [69,70].

Modified measles occurs in patients who are partially immunized. Clinically it is a milder form of classic measles. The incubation period is similar to that of classic measles. However, the prodromal period is of shorter duration and milder. Koplik spots are rarely present [69]. The exanthem is similar to typical measles in distribution and progression; however, it does not coalesce.

Complications associated with measles involve numerous organ systems. Otitis media is the most frequent complication and occurs in up to 15% of cases. Pulmonary involvement has been observed in more than 50% of children with measles [68,71]. Myocarditis and pericarditis have also been reported [69]. Measles infects the intestines in most patients and has been associated with diarrhea. In developing nations, malnourished children with measles frequently die because of persistent diarrhea [68].

## *Neurological Manifestations*

Neurological complications are a common and potentially fatal consequence of measles infection. Acute postinfectious encephalitis (APE) occurs in 0.5 to 1 of every 1000 cases of measles. Although previously it was thought that the incidence of SSPE was 1 in 100,000 natural infections [72–74], a more recent report, based on data from the 1989 to 1999 measles resurgence in the United States, indicates that the true incidence is approximately 7 to 11 cases per 100,000 case of measles [75]. In a review of measles deaths from 1964 to 1971, a neurological cause was found in 21% of cases [63]. Of the 165 measles deaths reported in the United States from 1987 to 1992, 11% were attributed to APE [66]. Measles inclusion body encephalitis (MIBE) is an even rarer complication that has been described almost exclusively in immunosuppressed individuals [76].

## Acute Postinfectious Encephalitis

APE occurs most often in children younger than 10 years of age, with a majority of cases occurring in children between 2 and 8 years of age. Male and female patients are equally affected [72,77,78].

In the majority of cases, the onset of APE occurs after the fourth day of the exanthem and generally no later than the eighth day. Less commonly, APE has been observed as early as the prodromal phase or as late as after the resolution of the rash [72,79]. In immunosuppressed patients, the presentation may be delayed to as long as 6 months after the acute illness [80]. The pathophysiology of APE is unknown, although it is hypothesized to be an immune-mediated complication.

The clinical presentation of APE is variable. Typically, a child with a resolving rash and normal temperature will have recrudescence of high fever and onset of drowsiness and listlessness. Frequently, patients recover and never require hospital admission [78,81]. However, some may develop sudden onset of seizures and rapidly progress to coma. The most common symptoms are convulsions, lethargy, coma, and irritability (Table 2.1). Convulsions have been noted in approximately 50% of patients with APE. Progression to coma occurs in up to 30% of patients. Additional signs and symptoms include cranial nerve defects, abnormal reflexes, and paralysis [72,77,79]. The outcome of APE is generally poor. Mortality has been reported to range from 10 to 38% [66,77–79,81,82]. In immunocompromised children, APE almost universally results in death. As many as 69% of children may experience neurological sequelae after APE [77,82]. These have included a decrease in cognitive function, recurrent seizures, paresis, choreoathetoid movements, and behavioral disorders [77,82].

**Table 2.1** Signs and symptoms associated with acute postinfectious encephalitis secondary to measles [72,77,79]

| Symptoms | Percent |
|---|---|
| Convulsions | 43% |
| Lethargy/drowsiness | 35% |
| Coma | 30% |
| Irritability | 21% |
| Stupor | 20% |
| Headache | 10% |
| Delirium | 8% |
| Nuchal rigidity | 35% |
| Babinski sign | 24% |
| Nystagmus | 9% |
| Clonus | 7% |
| Ataxia | 6% |

## *Neuropathology*

Attempts to isolate measles virus or detect its genome or viral proteins from the brain tissue of patients with APE have been unsuccessful. Additionally, no intrathecal production of measles virus specific antibodies has been documented. This has led to the speculation that APE may be an immune-mediated complication of measles [83–85]. The finding of antibodies to myelin basic protein in the CSF of these patients supports this hypothesis [85]. Potential mechanisms for the induction of autoimmunity include altered presentation of myelin antigens, molecular mimicry by measles viral proteins with those of myelin antigens, and dysregulation of host immune responses to measles virus [83]. Histologic examination of the brains of cases of APE reveals perivascular lymphocytic infiltration and perivenular demyelination [84,85].

### Subacute Sclerosing Panencephalitis

In the early 1930s, Dawson noted viral-like inclusion bodies in the neurons of two patients who died of an insidious neurodegenerative disease. To differentiate this from epidemic encephalitis, it was named "inclusion encephalitis [86]." In 1945, van Bogaert described a similar entity as "subacute sclerosing leukencephalitis" (SSPE) [87]. In 1950, the name subacute sclerosing panencephalitis was suggested [88]. A tentative link between SSPE and measles was made when Bouteille et al. noted viral structures in the brains of patients with SSPE similar to measles virus on electron microscopy (EM) [87]. A definitive link between measles and SSPE was established in 1967 when Connelly and colleagues reported the presence of measles antigens in brain specimens of patients with SSPE [89]. Cocultivation techniques eventually led to the recovery of the measles virus from the brains of patients with SSPE [90]. PCR techniques and in situ RNA hybridization have further substantiated the role of measles virus in SSPE [65].

SSPE primarily affects children and adolescents. The average age at onset is 9 years, and boys are more frequently affected than girls, in a ratio of 2–4:1 [74,91,92]. Children who acquire natural measles infection at an early age are at increased risk of developing SSPE. Those who develop measles at younger than 1 year of age have, in fact, a 16 times greater risk of suffering from SSPE than those who acquire measles at 5 years of age or older [87].

The mean interval to onset of SSPE after measles infection is 7 years. However, onset may occur as soon as 2 years or as late as 10 years after infection. Although the initial reports describe SSPE as a disease that occurs in three stages [93,94], clear demarcation of each stage is not possible. Initial subtle personality changes and progressive intellectual decline are followed by motor involvement. Myoclonic jerks are initially observed in the head and subsequently involve the trunk, arms, and legs. Generalized tonic-clonic and partial seizures may develop.

Ocular involvement has been observed in 10 to 50% of the cases. Ophthalmologic findings may include papilledema, papillitis, optic atrophy, chorioretinitis, or cortical blindness [87,95].

As the disease inexorably progresses, the patient becomes increasingly stuporous and eventually enters into a comatose state. Motor involvement progresses to quadriplegia, spasticity, and myoclonus may disappear. Decerebrate and decorticate posturing may be observed. Autonomic dysregulation occurs at the advanced stages of SSPE, and death often is a result of hyperpyrexia, cardiovascular collapse, or hypothalamic dysfunction. On average, the length of time from onset of symptoms to death is 1 to 3 years [87,96]. A spontaneous remission rate has been documented in up to 10% of the cases and can occur at any stage of the disease. Factors that favor remission are age at onset younger than 12 years, disappearance of periodic complexes and normalization of background on EEG, and an increase in measles titers in the CSF [97].

## *Neuropathology*

As stated previously, defective measles virus can only be recovered, and with great difficulty, from the brain tissue of patients with SSPE [83,90]. Brain tissue from these patients has been found to contain interfering particles, which may play a role in viral persistence. Moreover, mutations in specific viral genes result in mutant viruses that are unable to replicate and bud from the cell membrane [98]. Multiple abnormalities in the M protein of measles virus are considered to be a hallmark of the disease. However, abnormalities of the fusion (F), or hemagglutinin (H), proteins have also been associated with persistent viral infection.

Both the grey and white matter are involved in the disease. During the early phases of SSPE, there is mild inflammation of the meninges and parenchyma of the brain. Neuronal degeneration, perivascular cuffing, infiltration by plasma cells and lymphocytes, astrocyte proliferation, gliosis, and demyelination can be seen. Intranuclear and intracytoplasmic inclusion bodies, which are composed of measles virus nucleocapsids, may be observed within neurons and glial cells [87].

As the disease progresses, there is evidence of atrophy of the cerebral cortex. Widespread neuronal degeneration is evident. The meninges and parenchyma have focal or diffuse perivascular infiltrates composed of lymphocytes, plasma cells, and phagocytes [87].

### Measles Inclusion Body Encephalitis

MIBE, first described in the 1970s, occurs almost exclusively in immunosuppressed individuals [76]. MIBE has been associated with wild-type measles virus as well as vaccine strains of measles virus [99].

The overwhelming majority of cases have occurred in children and adolescents. The onset of MIBE occurs within 1 year (typically, 1 to 7 mo) after acute measles infection or immunization with live, attenuated measles vaccine [76]. It may also occur after a clinically inapparent measles infection. In one review, nearly 20% of cases had no exposure to individuals with measles or history of clinical measles [76].

An altered level of consciousness is seen in all cases. Fever is typically absent. Difficult to control seizures are an almost universal finding. Seizures may be focal, or may take the form of epilepsia partialis continua in up to one third of the cases. Death occurs in approximately 85% of individuals with MIBE within 1 year of diagnosis. The majority of survivors are left with significant neurological sequelae [76].

## *Neuropathology*

The pathogenesis of MIBE is unknown, but suspected to be similar to that of SSPE. On light microscopy, lymphocytic perivascular infiltration, neuronal loss, and astrocyte and microglial proliferation are seen in the presence of minimal inflammation. Glial cells and neurons are found to contain eosinophilic intranuclear and intracytoplasmic inclusions. EM reveals paramyxovirus nucleocapsids [76].

## *Diagnosis*

### Acute Postinfectious Encephalitis

In patients with APE, cytochemical analysis of the CSF demonstrates a mild mononuclear cell pleocytosis. In the majority of cases, the CSF white blood cell count is between 10 and 99 cells/mm$^3$, but can be as high as 700 cells/mm$^3$ [72,77]. The CSF protein concentration may also be elevated, whereas the glucose level is typically normal [72 Measles virus or its genome has been isolated from the CSF and brain by cell culture and PCR techniques in patients with APE [100–102].

All patients with APE have abnormal EEG findings. Even in patients without overt clinical evidence of encephalitis, abnormal EEGs were observed in 51% of cases [103]. EEG findings include diffuse slowing with asynchronous bursts of delta waves, and diffuse, irregular slow waves and spikes. Repeat EEGs years after APE may continue to show abnormalities [72,104].

MRI scan findings have consisted of high signal intensity lesions throughout the brain on T2-weighted imaging. Cortical lesions have been observed in all regions of the cerebral cortex. Multiple lesions may be seen in the basal ganglia and thalami. Additional areas involved have included the deep white matter, corpus callosum, external capsule, striata, and centrum semiovale [105,106]. Using single-photon emission computed tomography, Kim et. al. demonstrated that patients with measles encephalitis have multiple areas of hypoperfusion, even in the face of a normal MRI scan result [106].

### Subacute Sclerosing Panencephalitis

The diagnosis of SSPE can be established based on clinical history, serologic testing, molecular diagnostics, and EEG. Hemagglutination inhibition or complement fixation assays document extremely elevated (>1:1280) antibody titers [107]. Measles antibody can also be detected in the CSF. Cytochemical analysis of the CSF is normal in most cases. However, on closer analysis of the CSF protein, an increase in gammaglobulin may be observed. This may be evaluated by the presence of an oligoclonal band in the CSF [87,108]. With the advent of molecular techniques, RT-PCR has recently been used to identify measles virus in brain tissue of patients in whom the diagnosis of SSPE is suspected.

EEG is an important diagnostic modality in SSPE. During the early stages of the disease, the EEG results may be normal. However, in the presence of myoclonus, the EEG finding of periodic complexes is diagnostic. Three types of periodic complexes have been observed. Type 1 complexes consist of high voltage (200–500 mV) discharges of polyphasic, stereotyped delta waves with or without background suppression. The interval between complexes is 4 to 10 seconds and as the disease progresses the interval shortens. Type 2 has similar delta waves as type 1, but is intermixed with rapid spikes. Type 3 complexes are characterized by prolonged spike waves that are interrupted by giant delta waves [87,109].

The role of neuroimaging in diagnosis is not clearly defined. Several studies have shown no clinical correlation between disease severity and MRI and CT scan abnormalities [110–112]. Findings present on MRI scans in patients with SSPE have consisted of periventricular white matter lesions, cortical gray matter changes, cerebral atrophy, and basal ganglia involvement.

### Inclusion Body Encephalitis [76]

In MIBE, the CSF analysis generally fails to reveal any abnormalities. If abnormal, the CSF changes are generally limited to mild pleocytosis and increased CSF protein concentration. Unlike SSPE, high measles antibody titers in the CSF are unusual. Findings on EEG examination consist of diffuse slowing and spike wave activity. At the time of presentation, results of neuroimaging studies are generally normal. Subsequent neuroimaging abnormalities have included cerebral edema, atrophy, and ventricular dilation.

Similar to SSPE, measles viruses associated with MIBE are replication-deficient variants. As would be expected, their detection by cell culture would be the exception rather than the rule. The definitive diagnosis of MIBE requires brain biopsy to search for the presence of measles virus particles, antigens, or nucleic acid in tissue. Measles genome has been detected in the brain tissue of MIBE patients using RT-PCR.

## *Treatment*

### Acute Postinfectious Encephalitis

Supportive care is the cornerstone of therapy for APE. Anticonvulsants for seizures, intravenous fluids for management of electrolytes, and antipyretic medications and cooling techniques for fever are important in the care of these patients. Additionally, patients with increased intracranial pressure should be monitored closely. The use of mannitol may be indicated in the setting of cerebral edema [69,113].

#### Subacute Sclerosing Panencephalitis

Attempts to treat SSPE have relied on the use of antivirals or immunomodulating agents. Amantadine was one of the first antiviral agents to show a beneficial effect in preventing the progression of disease. Inosiplex has provided the greatest benefit in terms of long-term survival and remission [114–116]. Inosiplex acts by inhibiting viral replication and augmenting the immune response of host cells [96]. Gascon et al. have demonstrated that inosiplex alone was as effective as the combination of inosiplex and intrathecal interferon-$\alpha$ in improving outcome or stabilizing neurological status of patients with SSPE. Additionally, it was demonstrated that both treatments led to improvement or stabilization of neurological symptoms in approximately 30% of patients, a substantial improvement over a spontaneous remission rate of 5 to 10% [117].

#### Inclusion Body Encephalitis

Therapy is supportive and focused on controlling the associated seizures. If the patient is receiving immunosuppressive therapy, an attempt to withhold immunomodulating medications should be made. Ribavirin has been used in the therapy of MIBE with very limited success [76,118].

### *Prevention*

The greatest impact on APE and SSPE has been the prevention of measles infection. Measles vaccine should be administered to children older than 1 year of age. Although there may be a risk of SSPE after vaccination, it is extraordinarily rare, occurring in 1 per 1 million vaccines versus 7 to 11 per 100,000 unvaccinated children [75]. Use of measles vaccine should be avoided in severely immunosuppressed children.

## Nipah and Hendra Viruses

### *Introduction*

Nipah and Hendra viruses are closely related viruses in a newly created genus *Henipavirus* within the *Paramyxoviridae* family. Unlike other paramyxoviruses, these are zoonotic viruses that have been recently identified as a cause of severe and often times fatal disease in humans [119].

## Epidemiology

The natural reservoirs of Nipah and Hendra viruses are the fruit bats of the pteropid bat species, commonly referred to as "flying-foxes." Animals infected by these viruses include dogs, cats, horses, and pigs.

Outbreaks of Hendra virus have occurred among horses in Australia. The equine disease is characterized by a severe respiratory disease in association with ataxia that is often fatal [119]. Disease in humans caused by Hendra virus has only been observed in persons who have handled or worked closely with infected animals. No human-to-human transmission has been documented [119]. To date, only three human cases have been reported, and all have been in workers closely involved in the care of horses with Hendra virus infections. Two fatalities have been reported, one as a result of severe respiratory disease and the other from encephalitis [120,121].

In contrast, Nipah virus has been associated with a larger number of cases of human disease. Similar to Hendra virus, almost all cases have occurred in persons working with infected animals. The first reported human outbreak of Nipah virus occurred among pig farmers in Malaysia. Disease occurred predominantly in male patients who had an average age of 37 years (range 13–68 yr). A striking feature of this disease was its severity; it had a mortality rate of 32% [122].

## Clinical Disease

The clinical manifestations of Hendra virus infection are not well characterized because of the paucity of cases that have been reported. Two patients suffered fever, myalgias, and lethargy 1 week after contact with the infected horses. One patient was ill for 6 weeks but had a complete recovery. The other suffered severe respiratory disease and died 6 days after the onset of illness [120,123].

In Nipah virus infection, clinical disease is apparent within 2 weeks of the initial contact with the infected animal, but may occur as late as 2 months after exposure. The initial presenting signs and symptoms consist of fever, headache, dizziness, and emesis. In individuals with severe disease, signs of multisystem organ failure are present [122].

## Neurological Manifestations

Neurological involvement in human Hendra virus infection has been reported in only one case. This patient initially suffered from fever, headache, sore throat, and neck stiffness and was diagnosed with aseptic meningitis. Although full recovery was achieved, 13 months later he developed fever, recurrent seizures, coma, respiratory failure, and, ultimately, death [121].

Unlike Hendra virus infections, cases of Nipah virus infection are commonly associated with neurological complications. A decreased level of consciousness and brainstem dysfunction have been observed in up to 55% of patients. Seizures, primarily generalized, were present in 23% of cases. Clinical signs of cerebellar dysfunction are common [122]. Other reported neurological signs and symptoms include areflexia, segmental myoclonus, hypertension, hypotension, tachycardia, dysarthria, and dysphagia [122].

Patients who survive Nipah virus encephalitis may develop a repeat episode of encephalitis as long as 1 year after the initial infection. The clinical presentation in these patients is one of acute onset characterized by fever, headache, seizures, dizziness, focal neurological signs, myoclonus, and an altered level of consciousness. Fatalities have been reported in 18% of these patients [124,125]. Lastly, some individuals who initially had asymptomatic or nonencephalitic Nipah virus infection may develop encephalitis up to 1 year after their initial infection.

## *Neuropathology*

Little data exist on the pathogenesis and pathology of Hendra and Nipah virus infections because of their recent identification as human pathogens. In the sole patient with Hendra virus encephalitis, autopsy of the brain revealed a leptomeningitis characterized by lymphocytic and plasma cell infiltrates. Additionally, foci of necrosis were noted in the neocortex, basal ganglia, brainstem, and cerebellum. Nucleocapsids of the Hendra virions were observed in cell remnants by EM, and immunohistochemical staining of brain tissue detected the presence of Hendra virus [121].

Autopsies of patients with Nipah virus encephalitis reveal a diffuse vasculitis with the most severely affected organ being the brain. The vascular endothelium has evidence of vessel-wall necrosis, thrombosis, as well as neutrophil and mononuclear cell infiltration. Syncytial giant cell formation is also observed in affected vessels. Viral and eosinophilic cytoplasmic inclusions can be observed in neurons by EM and light microscopy, respectively. Additionally, immunohistochemical staining can identify Nipah viral antigens within infected endothelial and brain cells [126].

## *Diagnosis*

In Hendra virus encephalitis, initial CSF cytochemical analysis may reveal a polymorphonuclear pleocytosis with an elevated protein concentration [121]. Subsequent CSF analyses demonstrate a lymphocytic predominant pleocytosis with elevated protein concentration. In cell culture, Hendra virus produces syncytial formation when grown in Vero cells. The Hendra virus genome may be detected from clinical specimens using PCR. Viral inclusions are identified using EM within infected tissue. ELISAs are available to detect the presence of IgG and IgM antibodies against Hendra virus [119,120].

In Nipah virus encephalitis, CSF cytochemical analysis reveals a predominantly lymphocytic pleocytosis (0–842 cells/$mm^3$). Nipah virus-specific antibodies may be found in the CSF in one third of patients. The virus can be isolated from the CSF, but typically only in the most severe cases. Additionally, virus has been cultured from respiratory secretions and urinary specimens of acutely infected patients [122,125,127].

In the Hendra virus-infected individual, MRI scan findings consisted of increased signal within the grey matter that progressed to be more diffuse and pronounced within 1 week of onset of illness [121].

MRI scan findings can be suggestive of Nipah virus infection. Typically, findings consist of multiple, small (2–7 mm) lesions throughout the subcortical and deep white matter of the cerebral hemispheres on T2-weighted images. Additional areas where lesions may be located include the cortex, brainstem, thalamus, and corpus callosum [122]. In patients with relapsed encephalitis, MRI scan findings demonstrated patchy confluent cortical gray matter lesions [124].

EEGs in patients with Nipah virus infection are often abnormal. Goh et al. reported that the most common finding was diffuse slow wave activity with focal sharp waves. Focal abnormalities are primarily located in the temporal region. In comatose patients, EEG demonstrated bilateral temporal periodic complexes consisting of sharp and slow waves every 1 to 2 seconds [122].

### *Treatment*

Supportive care is the principle treatment for both Hendra and Nipah virus infections. Close monitoring of the neurological status as well as the potential for respiratory failure is imperative. Additionally, cardiovascular support may be indicated in the most severe cases.

No antiviral agent has been approved for use in the treatment of Hendra or Nipah virus infections. Chong et al. administered ribavirin in an open label study of patients with acute Nipah virus encephalitis. They observed a 36% reduction in mortality among treated patients. However, because of the small number of cases in this series, it is still not clear whether this treatment should be routinely used [128].

## Orthomyxovirus

### *Introduction*

Influenza A and B viruses are common respiratory pathogens associated with significant morbidity and mortality. Although their target organ is the respiratory tract, involvement of the CNS is known to occur. As in the case of respiratory disease, neurological complications may result in death or permanent neurological sequelae.

### *Epidemiology*

Influenza viruses are single-stranded RNA viruses in the *Orthomyxoviridae* family. They are divided into three distinct antigenic types: A, B, and C. Influenza A and

B are the major human pathogens. In the United States, annual winter epidemics occur that last approximately 6 weeks. Children have the highest attack rates and transmit the disease to adults, resulting in a secondary peak of disease. Children under the age of 2 years and the elderly are at greatest risk for severe influenza disease. Additionally, individuals with preexisting medical conditions (e.g., asthma, heart disease, and diabetes) are at increased risk for fatality as a result of influenza infection [129,130].

Transmission of influenza virus occurs through respiratory droplets. Sneezing and coughing are the most common mechanisms of viral spread. Transmission may also occur through direct and indirect contact with respiratory secretions. The incubation period is 2 to 3 days but can be as long as 7 days. The peak of viral shedding occurs simultaneously with the most severe symptoms. Viral shedding persists for 1 week in influenza A and up to 2 weeks in influenza B infections [130].

## *Clinical Manifestations*

Constitutional and respiratory signs and symptoms comprise the most common clinical manifestations of influenza disease. Typically, children present with acute onset of fever, headache, cough, and rhinorrhea. In comparison with adults, children are more likely to experience anorexia, abdominal pain, vomiting, and nausea. Influenza B virus-associated illness presents similarly, except that adults typically have a milder respiratory disease than children. Complications associated with influenza infection include laryngotracheobronchitis (croup), myositis, secondary bacterial infections, and myocarditis [129,130].

## *Neurological Manifestations*

Neurological complications have been observed after both influenza A and B infections. The most commonly reported neurological complication is febrile seizures. [131]. Additionally, influenza virus infections have been associated with encephalopathy/encephalitis. Because of the uncertain pathogenesis of this entity, the remainder of this section will use the term encephalopathy. Other less commonly associated neurological diseases include the Guillain-Barré syndrome and transverse myelitis, both of which have been observed after influenza immunization [132–134]. From the mid-1960s to mid-1980s, encephalopathy was primarily reported in patients with Reye syndrome. Today this syndrome is rarely observed [135].

Febrile seizures have been observed in 19.5% of hospitalized patients with influenza A infection, with equal prevalence in male and female patients. In comparison with adenovirus or PIV, patients hospitalized with influenza A seem to be both at greater risk for febrile seizures (odds ratio [OR] 1.97), as well as for recurrent seizures during the same admission (OR 4.3) [131].

Encephalopathy is a rare complication of both influenza A and B virus infection. Initial reports of influenza A encephalopathy appeared in the 19th century [136]. However, it was not until the H2N2 influenza A pandemic of 1958 that cell culture and serologic confirmation of influenza A virus-associated encephalopathy was reported [137]. Nearly 10 years later, a link between influenza B virus and encephalopathy was established [138]. Recently, avian influenza virus (influenza A H5N1) was shown to cause a fatal encephalopathy in two children [139]. The pathogenesis remains unknown. Children, especially those 5 years of age or younger, seem to be at greatest risk for influenza-associated encephalopathy [140–142].

Influenza-associated encephalopathy may occur from within the first days to weeks after the onset of respiratory symptoms. Reports from Japan indicate that the onset of the encephalopathy is commonly very early, typically occurring within 1 week of the onset of respiratory disease. Morishima and colleagues observed that in approximately 80% of patients, CNS disease developed within 1 day of the onset of influenza symptoms [143]. A report from the United States indicates that approximately 60% of patients with influenza A virus-associated encephalopathy developed neurological symptoms within 4 days of the onset of respiratory symptoms [144]. However, neurological symptoms may present as late as 3 weeks after the onset of illness [144,145]. Similar to influenza A virus, almost all patients with influenza B virus-associated encephalopathy present during the first week after the onset of their illness [142,146].

Individuals with influenza-associated encephalopathy initially present with the signs and symptoms of typical influenza: fever, headache, cough, and vomiting. The onset of neurological disease is heralded by altered mental status and/or seizures. During the 1998 to 1999 influenza season in Japan, 100% of patients with encephalopathy had altered level of consciousness, and 80% experienced seizures [143]. In contrast, among eight children with influenza A-associated encephalopathy during the 2003–2004 season in the United States, one half presented with seizures and one quarter presented with altered mental status [144]. Interestingly, 27% of patients with influenza B virus-associated encephalitis had speech abnormalities [142]. Other reported neurological signs and symptoms include abnormal deep tendon reflexes, meningismus, abnormal movements, facial nerve palsy, and paresthesias [142–145].

The hospital course of patients with influenza virus-associated encephalitis also seems to be very variable. In Japan, many patients rapidly deteriorate to a state of coma that may be associated with multisystem organ failure. Fatality rates in that country have been reported to be as high as 25 to 37%. Influenza A virus-associated encephalopathy accounts for a majority of the fatal cases [141,143,147]. Although severe disease with onset of coma and multisystem organ failure has been observed in other parts of the world, its incidence and mortality rate have been dissimilar. In a report from Austria, a 10% mortality was associated with influenza A virus-associated encephalopathy [145]. In the largest case series of patients with influenza A-associated encephalopathy from the United States, no deaths occurred and only one patient had neurological sequelae, consisting of severe static encephalopathy [144].

The risk of fatality seems to be significantly less in patients with influenza B virus-associated encephalopathy. To date, only two deaths have been reported. One death was in a patient with concomitant respiratory syncytial virus infection and a second patient died of acute necrotizing encephalopathy [138,146]. Significant neurological sequelae, including cognitive difficulty and speech delay, have been reported in survivors of influenza B virus-associated encephalitis [142].

## Neuropathology

The neuropathology of influenza-associated encephalopathy is variable. Autopsy findings in acute necrotizing encephalopathy demonstrates petechial hemorrhages and congestion of thalamic vessels surrounded by tissue necrosis [148]. In a case of influenza A-associated encephalopathy, influenza virus was detected within brain tissue by both RT-PCR and immunohistochemistry. In this case, although edema was noted, no inflammatory cells were present in the involved areas [149]. In contrast, other investigators have been unable to detect the influenza genome in the brain tissue of cases despite the presence of massive cerebral edema [143]. Because of the lack of fatalities in cases of influenza B virus, little is known regarding its neuropathology.

## Diagnosis

Evaluation of the CSF may reveal a mild lymphocytic pleocytosis, but as many as 90% of cases have normal CSF cell counts [143]. However, in one report, CSF pleocytosis was observed in 67% of patients [145]. The mean white blood cell count was 268 cells/$mm^3$. Abnormal CSF glucose and protein concentrations are rare.

Although an infrequent finding, the influenza genome has been amplified from the CSF using RT-PCR in patients with influenza A- and B-associated encephalopathy [143,145,150–152]. In Japan, hyperammonemia and hypoglycemia have been observed in 11% and 4% of patients, respectively. Additionally, increased liver transaminases, elevated lactate dehydrogenase levels, and thrombocytopenia have been associated with a poor prognosis [143].

EEG examination commonly demonstrates diffuse slowing. Focal slowing, periodic lateralized epileptiform discharges, and generalized and focal spikes have also been reported [144,145,153].

Abnormalities in neuroimaging are frequently observed in patents with influenza A virus-associated encephalopathy. The most notable findings on CT or MRI scan are edema, hemorrhage, and symmetric lesions. Although the latter are commonly seen in the thalamus, they may also occur in the cerebral white matter, cerebellum, and brainstem [154]. Morishima and colleagues observed findings of acute necrotizing encephalopathy in approximately 10% of cases they studied [143]. Additional findings observed in cases of influenza A virus-associated encephalopathy include cerebral edema in association with low-density cerebral lesions, single or multifocal cerebral lesions, and reversible splenium lesions in the corpus callosum [145,155]. Influenza B virus-associated encephalopathy seems to have fewer abnormalities present on MRI or CT scan. In addition to acute necrotizing encephalopathy, the only additional abnormality reported has been cerebral edema [142,146].

## *Treatment*

Supportive care is the primary treatment for influenza-associated encephalopathy. Amantadine may be used in cases of influenza A virus-associated encephalopathy, although no studies have evaluated its effectiveness, and resistance has been increasingly noted. Oseltamivir, a neuraminidase inhibitor, active against both influenza A and B viruses, has also been used. However, unlike amantadine, drug could not be detected in the CSF after oral administration in one reported case [156].

## References

1. Lamb RA, Collins PL, Kolakofsky D, Melero JA, Nagai Y, Oldstone MBA, Pringle CR, Rima BK. Family Paramyxoviridae. Virus Taxonomy. *Seventh Report of the International Committe on Taxonomy of Viruses*. 2000. Van Regenmortel MHV, Fauquet CM, Bishop DHL, Carstens EB, Estes MK, Lemon SM, Maniloff J, Mayo MA, McGeoch DJ, Pringle CR, Wickner RB (eds). Academic Press, San Diego, CA.
2. Hall CB. Respiratory syncytial virus and parainfluenza virus. *N Engl J Med* 2001; 344:1917–1928.
3. Hall CB. Parainfluenza Viruses. *Textbook of Pediatric Infectious Diseases*. 2004. Feigin RD, Cherry JD, Demmler GJ, Kaplan SL (eds). Saunders, Philadelphia, pp 2270–2283.
4. Craver RD, Gohd RS, Sundin DR, Hierholzer JC. Isolation of parainfluenza virus type 3 from cerebrospinal fluid associated with aseptic meningitis. *Am J Clin Pathol* 1993; 99: 705–707.
5. Frank JA, Jr., Warren RW, Tucker JA, Zeller J, Wilfert CM. Disseminated parainfluenza infection in a child with severe combined immunodeficiency. *Am J Dis Child* 1983; 137:1172–1174.
6. Isaia G, Teodosiu O, Popescu G, Dinca A, Niculescu R, Toma E, Paun L, Popescu E. Isolation of parainfluenza virus type 3 from an infant with meningoencephalitis. *Virologie* 1980; 31:191–195.
7. Jantausch BA, Wiedermann BL, Jeffries B. Parainfluenza virus type 2 meningitis and parotitis in an 11-year-old child. *South Med J* 1995; 88:230–231.
8. Lindquist SW, Darnule A, Istas A, Demmler GJ. Parainfluenza virus type 4 infections in pediatric patients. *Pediatr Infect Dis J* 1997; 16:34–38.
9. Roman G, Phillips CA, Poser CM. Parainfluenza virus type 3: isolation from CSF of a patient with Guillain-Barré syndrome. *JAMA* 1978; 240:1613–1615.
10. Vreede RW, Schellekens H, Zuijderwijk M. Isolation of parainfluenza virus type 3 from cerebrospinal fluid. *J Infect Dis* 1992; 165:1166.
11. Wong VK, Steinberg E, Warford A. Parainfluenza virus type 3 meningitis in an 11-month-old infant. *Pediatr Infect Dis J* 1988; 7:300–301.
12. Arisoy ES, Demmler GJ, Thakar S, Doerr C. Meningitis due to parainfluenza virus type 3: report of two cases and review. *Clin Infect Dis* 1993; 17:995–997.
13. Arguedas A, Stutman HR, Blanding JG. Parainfluenza type 3 meningitis. Report of two cases and review of the literature. *Clin Pediatr* (Phila) 1990; 29:175–178.
14. Rubin EE, Quennec P, McDonald JC. Infections due to parainfluenza virus type 4 in children. *Clin Infect Dis* 1993; 17:998–1002.
15. Powell HC, Rosenberg RN, McKellar B. Reye's syndrome: isolation of parainfluenza virus. Report of three cases. *Arch Neurol* 1973; 29:135–139.
16. McCarthy VP, Zimmerman AW, Miller CA. Central nervous system manifestations of parainfluenza virus type 3 infections in childhood. *Pediatr Neurol* 1990; 6:197–201.

17. Downham MA, McQuillin J, Gardner PS. Diagnosis and clinical significance of parainfluenza virus infections in children. *Arch Dis Child* 1974; 49:8–15.
18. Rantala H, Uhari M, Tuokko H. Viral infections and recurrences of febrile convulsions. *J Pediatr* 1990; 116:195–199.
19. Plotkin S. Mumps Vaccine. *Vaccines*. 2004. Plotkin S, Orenstein W (eds). 4th ed. Saunders, Philadelphia, pp 441–469.
20. Cherry JD. Mumps Virus. *Textbook of Pediatric Infectious Diseases*. 2004. Feigin R, Cherry J, Demmler G, Kaplan S (eds). 5th ed. Saunders, Philadelphia, pp 2305–2314.
21. Galazka AM, Robertson SE, Kraigher A. Mumps and mumps vaccine: a global review. *Bull World Health Organ* 1999; 77:3–14.
22. Summary of Notifiable Diseases, United States, 1998. *MMWR* 1999; 47:ii-92.
23. Summary of Notifiable Diseases, United States, 2002. *MMWR* 2004; 51:1–84.
24. Update: multistate outbreak of mumps, United States, January 1-May 2, 2006. *MMWR* 2006; 55:559–563.
25. Mumps epidemic—United kingdom, 2004–2005. *MMWR* 2006; 55:173–175.
26. Jubelt B. Enterovirus and mumps virus infections of the nervous system. *Neurol Clin* 1984; 2:187–213.
27. Russell RR, Donald JC. The neurological complications of mumps. *Br Med J* 1958; 30:27–30.
28. Control CfD. Mumps-United States. *MMWR* 1978; 27:379–381.
29. Meyer HM, Jr., Johnson RT, Crawford IP, Dascomb HE, Rogers NG. Central nervous system syndromes of "vital" etiology. A study of 713 cases. *Am J Med* 1960; 29:334–347.
30. Lennette EH, Magoffin RL, Knouf EG. Viral central nervous system disease. An etiologic study conducted at the Los Angeles County General Hospital. *JAMA* 1962; 179: 687–695.
31. Azimi PH, Cramblett HG, Haynes RE. Mumps meningoencephalitis in children. *JAMA* 1969; 207:509–512.
32. Wilfert CM. Mumps meningoencephalitis with low cerebrospinal-fluid glucose, prolonged pleocytosis and elevation of protein. *N Engl J Med* 1969; 280:855–859.
33. Levitt LP, Rich TA, Kinde SW, Lewis AL, Gates EH, Bond JO. Central nervous system mumps. A review of 64 cases. *Neurology* 1970; 20:829–834.
34. Strussberg S, Winter S, Friedman A, Benderly A, Kahana D, Freundlich E. Notes on mumps meningoencephalitis. Some features of 199 cases in children. *Clin Pediatr (Phila)* 1969; 8:373–374.
35. Koskiniemi M, Donner M, Pettay O. Clinical appearance and outcome in mumps encephalitis in children. *Acta Paediatr Scand* 1983; 72:603–609.
36. Kanra G, Kara A, Cengiz AB, Isik P, Ceyhan M, Atas A. Mumps meningoencephalitis effect on hearing. *Pediatr Infect Dis J* 2002; 21:1167–1169.
37. Pollack S, Bar-On E, Enat R. Guillain-Barré syndrome; association with mumps. *N Y State J Med* 1981; 81:795–797.
38. Majda-Stanislawska E. Mumps cerebellitis. *Eur Neurol* 2000; 43:117.
39. Ghosh S. Guillain-Barré syndrome complicating mumps. *Lancet* 1967; 1:895.
40. Johnstone JA, Ross CA, Dunn M. Meningitis and encephalitis associated with mumps infection. A 10-year survey. *Arch Dis Child* 1972; 47:647–651.
41. Bakshi N, Lawson J, Hanson R, Ames C, Vinters HV. Fatal mumps meningoencephalitis in a child with severe combined immunodeficiency after bone marrow transplantation. *J Child Neurol* 1996; 11:159–162.
42. Cinalli G, Spennato P, Ruggiero C, Aliberti F, Maggi G. Aqueductal stenosis 9 years after mumps meningoencephalitis: treatment by endoscopic third ventriculostomy. *Childs Nerv Syst* 2004; 20:61–64.
43. Bang HO, Bang J. Involvement of the central nervous system in mumps. *Acta Meica Scandinavica* 1943; 113:487–505.
44. Donohue WL, Playfair FD, Whitaker L. Mumps encephalitis; pathology and pathogenesis. *J Pediatr* 1955; 47:395–412.

45. Johnson RT, Johnson KP. Hydrocephalus as a sequela of experimental myxovirus infections. *Exp Mol Pathol* 1969; 10:68–80.
46. Johnson RT, Johnson KP, Edmonds CJ. Virus-induced hydrocephalus: development of aqueductal stenosis in hamsters after mumps infection. *Science* 1967; 157:1066–1067.
47. Wolinsky JS. Mumps virus-induced hydrocephalus in hamsters. Ultrastructure of the chronic infection. *Lab Invest* 1977; 37:229–236.
48. Herndon RM, Johnson RT, Davis LE, Descalzi LR. Ependymitis in mumps virus meningitis. Electron microscopical studies of cerebrospinal fluid. *Arch Neurol* 1974; 30:475–479.
49. Zysno E, Reichnmiller HE, Dold U. EEG changes in mumps meningoencephalitis of the adult. *Electroencephalogr Clin Neurophysiol* 1967; 23:184.
50. Tarr RW, Edwards KM, Kessler RM, Kulkarni MV. MRI of mumps encephalitis: comparison with CT evaluation. *Pediatr Radiol* 1987; 17:59–62.
51. Poggio GP, Rodriguez C, Cisterna D, Freire MC, Cello J. Nested PCR for rapid detection of mumps virus in cerebrospinal fluid from patients with neurological diseases. *J Clin Microbiol* 2000; 38:274–278.
52. Afzal MA, Marsden SA, Hull RM, Pipkin PA, Bentley ML, Minor PD. Evaluation of the neurovirulence test for mumps vaccines. *Biologicals* 1999; 27:43–49.
53. Gellis S, McGuiness A, M P. A study of the prevention of mumps orchitis by gammaglobulin. *Am J Med Sci* 1945; 210:661–664.
54. Rotbart HA. Viral meningitis. *Semin Neurol* 2000; 20:277–292.
55. Nalin DR. Mumps vaccine complications: which strain? *Lancet* 1989; 2:1396.
56. Sugiura A, Yamada A. Aseptic meningitis as a complication of mumps vaccination. *Pediatr Infect Dis J* 1991; 10:209–213.
57. DeStefano F, Thompson WW. MMR vaccine and autism: an update of the scientific evidence. *Expert Rev Vaccines* 2004; 3:19–22.
58. Smeeth L, Cook C, Fombonne E, Heavey L, Rodrigues LC, Smith PG, Hall AJ. MMR vaccination and pervasive developmental disorders: a case-control study. *Lancet* 2004; 364:963–969.
59. Black FL. Measles. *Viral Infections of Humans: Epidemiology and Control*. 1989. Evans AS (ed). 3rd ed. Plenum Medical, New York, pp 451–469.
60. Enders JF, Peebles TC. Propagation in tissue cultures of cytopathogenic agents from patients with measles. *Proc Soc Exp Biol Med* 1954; 86:277–286.
61. Milovanovic MV, Enders JF, Mitus A. Cultivation of measles virus in human amnion cells and in developing chick embryo. *Proc Soc Exp Biol Med* 1957; 95:120–127.
62. Langmuir AD. Medical importance of measles. *Am J Dis Child* 1962; 103:224–226.
63. Barkin RM. Measles mortality. Analysis of the primary cause of death. *Am J Dis Child* 1975; 129:307–309.
64. Babbott FL, Jr., Gordon JE. Modern measles. *Am J Med Sci* 1954; 228:334–361.
65. Strebel PM, Papania MJ, Halsey NA. Measles Vaccine. *Vaccines*. 2004. Plotkin SA, Orenstein WA (eds). 4th ed. Saunders, Philadelphia, pp 389–440.
66. Gindler J, Tinker S, Markowitz L, Atkinson W, Dales L, Papania MJ. Acute measles mortality in the United States, 1987–2002. *J Infect Dis* 2004; 189 Suppl 1:S69–77.
67. Robbins FC. Measles: clinical features. Pathogenesis, pathology and complications. *Am J Dis Child* 1962; 103:266–273.
68. Perry RT, Halsey NA. The clinical significance of measles: a review. *J Infect Dis* 2004; 189 Suppl 1:S4–16.
69. Cherry JD. Measles Virus. *Textbook of Pediatric Infectious Diseases*. 2004. Feigin RD, Cherry JD, Demmler GJ, Kaplan SL (eds). 5th ed. Saunders, Philadelphia, pp 2283–2304.
70. Cherry JD, Feigin RD, Lobes LA, Jr., Shackelford PG. Atypical measles in children previously immunized with attenuated measles virus vaccines. *Pediatrics* 1972; 50:712–717.
71. Kohn J, Koiransky H. Successive roentgenograms of the chest of children during measles. *Am J Dis Child* 1929; 38:258–270.
72. La Boccetta AC, Tornay AS. Measles Encephalitis. Report of 61 Cases. *Am J Dis Child* 1964; 107:247–255.

73. Miller DL. Frequency of Complications of Measles, 1963. Report on a National Inquiry by the Public Health Laboratory Service in Collaboration with the Society of Medical Officers of Health. *Br Med J* 1964; 5401:75–78.
74. Modlin JF, Jabbour JT, Witte JJ, Halsey NA. Epidemiologic studies of measles, measles vaccine, and subacute sclerosing panencephalitis. *Pediatrics* 1977; 59:505–512.
75. Bellini WJ, Rota JS, Lowe LE, Katz RS, Dyken PR, Zaki SR, Shieh WJ, Rota PA. Subacute sclerosing panencephalitis: more cases of this fatal disease are prevented by measles immunization than was previously recognized. *J Infect Dis* 2005; 192:1686–1693.
76. Mustafa MM, Weitman SD, Winick NJ, Bellini WJ, Timmons CF, Siegel JD. Subacute measles encephalitis in the young immunocompromised host: report of two cases diagnosed by polymerase chain reaction and treated with ribavirin and review of the literature. *Clin Infect Dis* 1993; 16:654–660.
77. Hamilton PM, Hanna RJ. Encephalitis complicating measles: report on 241 cases from the literature and on 44 additional cases. *Am J Dis Child* 1941; 61:483–493.
78. Tyler HR. Neurological complications of rubeola (measles). *Medicine (Baltimore)* 1957; 36:147–167.
79. Applebaum E, Dolgopol V, Dolgin J. Measles Encephalitis. *Am J Dis Child* 1949; 77:25–48.
80. Aicardi J, Goutieres F, Arsenio-Nunes ML, Lebon P. Acute measles encephalitis in children with immunosuppression. *Pediatrics* 1977; 59:232–239.
81. Ford F. Nervous complications of measles, with a summary of the literature and publication of 12 additional case reports. *Bull Johns Hopkins Hosp* 1928; 43:140–184.
82. Litvak AM, Sands IJ, Gibel H. Encephalitis complicating measles: report of 56 cases with follow-up studies in 32. *Am J Dis Child* 1943; 65:265–295.
83. Griffin DE. Measles Virus. *Fields Virology*. 2001. Knipe DN, Howley PM (eds). 4th ed. Lippincott, Williams and Wilkins, Philadelphia, pp 1401–1441.
84. Gendelman HE, Wolinsky JS, Johnson RT, Pressman NJ, Pezeshkpour GH, Boisset GF. Measles encephalomyelitis: lack of evidence of viral invasion of the central nervous system and quantitative study of the nature of demyelination. *Ann Neurol* 1984; 15:353–360.
85. Johnson RT, Griffin DE, Hirsch RL, Wolinsky JS, Roedenbeck S, Lindo de Soriano I, Vaisberg A. Measles encephalomyelitis—clinical and immunologic studies. *N Engl J Med* 1984; 310:137–141.
86. Dawson JR, Jr. Cellular inclusions in cerebral lesions of lethargic encephalitis. *Am J Pathol* 1933; 9:7–16.
87. Garg RK. Subacute sclerosing panencephalitis. *Postgrad Med J* 2002; 78:63–70.
88. Greenfield JG. Encephalitis and encephalomyelitis in England and Wales during last decade. *Brain* 1950; 73:141–166.
89. Connolly JH, Allen IV, Hurwitz LJ, Millar JH. Measles-virus antibody and antigen in subacute sclerosing panencephalitis. *Lancet* 1967; 1:542–544.
90. Horta-Barbosa L, Fuccillo DA, Sever JL, Zeman W. Subacute sclerosing panencephalitis: isolation of measles virus from a brain biopsy. *Nature* 1969; 221:974.
91. Jabbour JT, Duenas DA, Sever JL, Krebs HM, Horta-Barbosa L. Epidemiology of subacute sclerosing panencephalitis (SSPE). A report of the SSPE registry. *JAMA* 1972; 220:959–962.
92. Modlin JF, Halsey NA, Eddins DL, Conrad JL, Jabbour JT, Chien L, Robinson H. Epidemiology of subacute sclerosing panencephalitis. *J Pediatr* 1979; 94:231–236.
93. Chao D. Subacute inclusion body encephalitis. Report of 3 cases. *J Pediatr* 1962; 61:501–510.
94. Foley J, Williams D. Inclusion encephalitis and its relation to subacute sclerosing leucoencephalitis; a report of five cases. *Q J Med* 1953; 22:157–194.
95. Green SH, Wirtschafter JD. Ophthalmoscopic findings in subacute sclerosing panencephalitis. *Br J Ophthalmol* 1973; 57:780–787.
96. Dyken PR. Subacute sclerosing panencephalitis. Current status. *Neurol Clin* 1985; 3:179–196.

97. Santoshkumar B, Radhakrishnan K. Substantial spontaneous long-term remission in subacute sclerosing panencephalitis (SSPE). *J Neurol Sci* 1998; 154:83–88.
98. Billeter MA, Cattaneo R, Spielhofer P, Kaelin K, Huber M, Schmid A, Baczko K, ter Meulen V. Generation and properties of measles virus mutations typically associated with subacute sclerosing panencephalitis. *Ann N Y Acad Sci* 1994; 724:367–377.
99. Bitnun A, Shannon P, Durward A, Rota PA, Bellini WJ, Graham C, Wang E, Ford-Jones EL, Cox P, Becker L, Fearon M, Petric M, Tellier R. Measles inclusion-body encephalitis caused by the vaccine strain of measles virus. *Clin Infect Dis* 1999; 29:855–861.
100. ter Meulen V, Muller D, Kackell Y, Katz M, Meyermann R. Isolation of infectious measles virus in measles encephalitis. *Lancet* 1972; 2:1172–1175.
101. Nakayama T, Mori T, Yamaguchi S, Sonoda S, Asamura S, Yamashita R, Takeuchi Y, Urano T. Detection of measles virus genome directly from clinical samples by reverse transcriptase-polymerase chain reaction and genetic variability. *Virus Res* 1995; 35:1–16.
102. Esolen LM, Takahashi K, Johnson RT, Vaisberg A, Moench TR, Wesselingh SL, Griffin DE. Brain endothelial cell infection in children with acute fatal measles. *J Clin Invest* 1995; 96:2478–2481.
103. Gibbs FA, Gibbs EL, Carpenter PR, Spies HW. Electroencephalographic abnormality in "uncomplicated" childhood diseases. *JAMA* 1959; 171:1050–1055.
104. Aarli JA. Nervous complications of measles. Clinical manifestations and prognosis. *Eur Neurol* 1974; 12:79–93.
105. Lee KY, Cho WH, Kim SH, Kim HD, Kim IO. Acute encephalitis associated with measles: MRI features. *Neuroradiology* 2003; 45:100–106.
106. Kim SJ, Kim JS, Lee DY. Neurologic outcome of acute measles encephalitis according to the MRI patterns. *Pediatr Neurol* 2003; 28:281–284.
107. Sever JL, Zeman W. Serological studies of measles and subacute sclerosing panencephalitis. *Neurology* 1968; 18:95–97.
108. Horta-Barbosa L, Krebs H, Ley A, Chen TC, Gilkeson MR, Sever JL. Progressive increase in cerebrospinal fluid measles antibody levels in subacute sclerosing panencephalitis. *Pediatrics* 1971; 47:782–783.
109. Yaqub BA. Subacute sclerosing panencephalitis (SSPE): early diagnosis, prognostic factors and natural history. *J Neurol Sci* 1996; 139:227–234.
110. Brismar J, Gascon GG, von Steyern KV, Bohlega S. Subacute sclerosing panencephalitis: evaluation with CT and MR. *Am J Neuroradiol* 1996; 17:761–772.
111. Tuncay R, Akman-Demir G, Gokyigit A, Eraksoy M, Barlas M, Tolun R, Gursoy G. MRI in subacute sclerosing panencephalitis. *Neuroradiology* 1996; 38:636–640.
112. Ozturk A, Gurses C, Baykan B, Gokyigit A, Eraksoy M. Subacute sclerosing panencephalitis: clinical and magnetic resonance imaging evaluation of 36 patients. *J Child Neurol* 2002; 17:25–29.
113. Katz SL. Measles—its complications, treatment and prophylaxis. *Med Clin North Am* 1962; 46:1163–1175.
114. DuRant RH, Dyken PR, Swift AV. The influence of inosiplex treatment on the neurological disability of patients with subacute sclerosing panencephalitis. *J Pediatr* 1982; 101:288–293.
115. Jones CE, Dyken PR, Huttenlocher PR, Jabbour JT, Maxwell KW. Inosiplex therapy in subacute sclerosing panencephalitis. A multicentre, non-randomised study in 98 patients. *Lancet* 1982; 1:1034–1037.
116. Dyken PR, Swift A, DuRant RH. Long-term follow-up of patients with subacute sclerosing panencephalitis treated with inosiplex. *Ann Neurol* 1982; 11:359–364.
117. Gascon GG. Randomized treatment study of inosiplex versus combined inosiplex and intraventricular interferon-alpha in subacute sclerosing panencephalitis (SSPE): international multicenter study. *J Child Neurol* 2003; 18:819–827.
118. Freeman AF, Jacobsohn DA, Shulman ST, Bellini WJ, Jaggi P, de Leon G, Keating GF, Kim F, Pachman LM, Kletzel M, Duerst RE. A new complication of stem cell transplantation: measles inclusion body encephalitis. *Pediatrics* 2004; 114:e657–660.

119. Thorner AR, Dolin R. Zoonotic Paramyxoviruses: Hendra, Nipah, and Menangle Viruses. *Principles and Practice of Infectious Diseases*. 2005. Mandell GL, Bennett JE, Dolin R (eds). 6th ed. Churchill Livingstone, London, pp 2038–2044.
120. Murray K, Rogers R, Selvey L, Selleck P, Hyatt A, Gould A, Gleeson L, Hooper P, Westbury H. A novel Morbillivirus pneumonia of horses and its transmission to humans. *Emerg Infect Dis* 1995; 1:31–33.
121. O'Sullivan JD, Allworth AM, Paterson DL, Snow TM, Boots R, Gleeson LJ, Gould AR, Hyatt AD, Bradfield J. Fatal encephalitis due to novel paramyxovirus transmitted from horses. *Lancet* 1997; 349:93–95.
122. Goh KJ, Tan CT, Chew NK, Tan PS, Kamarulzaman A, Sarji SA, Wong KT, Abdullah BJ, Chua KB, Lam SK. Clinical features of Nipah virus encephalitis among pig farmers in Malaysia. *N Engl J Med* 2000; 342:1229–1235.
123. Selvey LA, Wells RM, McCormack JG, Ansford AJ, Murray K, Rogers RJ, Lavercombe PS, Selleck P, Sheridan JW. Infection of humans and horses by a newly described Morbillivirus. *Med J Aust* 1995; 162:642–645.
124. Tan CT, Goh KJ, Wong KT, Sarji SA, Chua KB, Chew NK, Murugasu P, Loh YL, Chong HT, Tan KS, Thayaparan T, Kumar S, Jusoh MR. Relapsed and late-onset Nipah encephalitis. *Ann Neurol* 2002; 51:703–708.
125. Chua KB. Nipah virus outbreak in Malaysia. *J Clin Virol* 2003; 26:265–275.
126. Wong KT, Shieh WJ, Kumar S, Norain K, Abdullah W, Guarner J, Goldsmith CS, Chua KB, Lam SK, Tan CT, Goh KJ, Chong HT, Jusoh R, Rollin PE, Ksiazek TG, Zaki SR. Nipah virus infection: pathology and pathogenesis of an emerging paramyxoviral zoonosis. *Am J Pathol* 2002; 161:2153–2167.
127. Chua KB, Lam SK, Goh KJ, Hooi PS, Ksiazek TG, Kamarulzaman A, Olson J, Tan CT. The presence of Nipah virus in respiratory secretions and urine of patients during an outbreak of Nipah virus encephalitis in Malaysia. *J Infect* 2001; 42:40–43.
128. Chong HT, Kamarulzaman A, Tan CT, Goh KJ, Thayaparan T, Kunjapan SR, Chew NK, Chua KB, Lam SK. Treatment of acute Nipah encephalitis with ribavirin. *Ann Neurol* 2001; 49:810–813.
129. Treanor JJ. Influenza Virus. *Principles and Practice of Infectious Diseases*. 2005. Mandell GL, Bennett JE, Dolin R (eds). 6th ed. Churchill Livingstone, Philadelphia, pp 2060–2085.
130. Glezen WP. Influenza Viruses. *Textbook of Pediatric Infectious Diseases*. 2004. Feigin RD, Cherry JD, Demmler GJ, Kaplan SL (eds). 5th ed. Saunders, Philadelphia, pp 2252–2269.
131. Chiu SS, Tse CY, Lau YL, Peiris M. Influenza A infection is an important cause of febrile seizures. *Pediatrics* 2001; 108:E63.
132. Haber P, DeStefano F, Angulo FJ, Iskander J, Shadomy SV, Weintraub E, Chen RT. Guillain-Barré syndrome following influenza vaccination. *JAMA* 2004; 292:2478–2481.
133. Nakamura N, Nokura K, Zettsu T, Koga H, Tachi M, Terada M, Katoh H, Itoh Y, Osawa H, Ozeki T, Yamamoto H. Neurologic complications associated with influenza vaccination: two adult cases. *Intern Med* 2003; 42:191–194.
134. Migita M, Matsumoto T, Fujino O, Takaishi Y, Yuki N, Fukunaga Y. Two cases of influenza with impaired ocular movement. *Eur J Paediatr Neurol* 2001; 5:83–85.
135. Belay ED, Bresee JS, Holman RC, Khan AS, Shahriari A, Schonberger LB. Reye's syndrome in the United States from 1981 through 1997. *N Engl J Med* 1999; 340:1377–1382.
136. Wilkins RH, Brody IA. Neurological classics IV. Encephalitis lethargica. *Arch Neurol* 1968; 18:324–328.
137. Flewett TH, Hoult JG. Influenzal encephalopathy and postinfluenzal encephalitis. *Lancet* 1958; 2:11–15.
138. Taylor JC, Ross C, Stott EJ. Influenza in the west of Scotland, 1966. *British Medical Journal* 1967; 3:406–408.
139. de Jong MD, Bach VC, Phan TQ, Vo MH, Tran TT, Nguyen BH, Beld M, Le TP, Truong HK, Nguyen VV, Tran TH, Do QH, Farrar J. Fatal avian influenza A (H5N1) in a child presenting with diarrhea followed by coma. *N Engl J Med* 2005; 352:686–691.

140. Togashi T, Matsuzono Y, Narita M. Epidemiology of influenza-associated encephalitis-encephalopathy in Hokkaido, the northernmost island of Japan. *Pediatr Int* 2000; 42:192–196.
141. Yoshikawa H, Yamazaki S, Watanabe T, Abe T. Study of influenza-associated encephalitis/encephalopathy in children during the 1997 to 2001 influenza seasons. *J Child Neurol* 2001; 16:885–890.
142. Newland JG, Romero JR, Varman M, Drake C, Holst A, Safranek T, Subbarao K. Encephalitis associated with influenza B virus infection in 2 children and a review of the literature. *Clin Infect Dis* 2003; 36:e87–95.
143. Morishima T, Togashi T, Yokota S, Okuno Y, Miyazaki C, Tashiro M, Okabe N. Encephalitis and encephalopathy associated with an influenza epidemic in Japan. *Clin Infect Dis* 2002; 35:512–517.
144. Maricich SM, Neul JL, Lotze TE, Cazacu AC, Uyeki TM, Demmler GJ, Clark GD. Neurologic complications associated with influenza A in children during the 2003–2004 influenza season in Houston, Texas. *Pediatrics* 2004; 114:e626–633.
145. Steininger C, Popow-Kraupp T, Laferl H, Seiser A, Godl I, Djamshidian S, Puchhammer-Stockl E. Acute encephalopathy associated with influenza A virus infection. *Clin Infect Dis* 2003; 36:567–574.
146. Sazgar M, Robinson JL, Chan AK, Sinclair DB. Influenza B acute necrotizing encephalopathy: a case report and literature review. *Pediatr Neurol* 2003; 28:396–399.
147. Togashi T, Matsuzono Y, Narita M, Morishima T. Influenza-associated acute encephalopathy in Japanese children in 1994–2002. *Virus Res* 2004; 103:75–78.
148. Sugaya N. Influenza-associated encephalopathy in Japan: pathogenesis and treatment. *Pediatr Int* 2000; 42:215–218.
149. Takahashi M, Yamada T, Nakashita Y, Saikusa H, Deguchi M, Kida H, Tashiro M, Toyoda T. Influenza virus-induced encephalopathy: clinicopathologic study of an autopsied case. *Pediatr Int* 2000; 42:204–214.
150. Fujimoto S, Kobayashi M, Uemura O, Iwasa M, Ando T, Katoh T, Nakamura C, Maki N, Togari H, Wada Y. PCR on cerebrospinal fluid to show influenza-associated acute encephalopathy or encephalitis. *Lancet* 1998; 352:873–875.
151. McCullers JA, Facchini S, Chesney PJ, Webster RG. Influenza B virus encephalitis. *Clin Infect Dis* 1999; 28:898–900.
152. Mori I, Nagafuji H, Matsumoto K, Kimura Y. Use of the polymerase chain reaction for demonstration of influenza virus dissemination in children. *Clin Infect Dis* 1997; 24:736–737.
153. Kurita A, Furushima H, Yamada H, Inoue K. Periodic lateralized epileptiform discharges in influenza B-associated encephalopathy. *Intern Med* 2001; 40:813–816.
154. Mizuguchi M. Acute necrotizing encephalopathy of childhood: a novel form of acute encephalopathy prevalent in Japan and Taiwan. *Brain Dev* 1997; 19:81–92.
155. Takanashi J, Barkovich AJ, Yamaguchi K, Kohno Y. Influenza-associated encephalitis/encephalopathy with a reversible lesion in the splenium of the corpus callosum: a case report and literature review. *Am J Neuroradiol* 2004; 25:798–802.
156. Straumanis JP, Tapia MD, King JC. Influenza B infection associated with encephalitis: treatment with oseltamivir. *Pediatr Infect Dis J* 2002; 21:173–175.

# Chapter 3
# Picornaviruses

**Motasem A. Abuelreish, M.D. and Mobeen H. Rathore, M.D., C.P.E., F.A.A.P.**

## Poliomyelitis

### *Introduction*

Poliomyelitis was the first enteroviral disease to be clinically recognized. Although outbreaks in Europe and the United States were reported in the early 19th century as clusters of "infantile paralysis," it was not until 1908 that the virus was isolated in monkeys by Landsteiner and Popper [1]. Successful propagation in tissue by Enders et al. in 1949 resulted in the development of effective vaccines [1]. Global eradication of poliomyelitis, although targeted for 2005 by the World Health Organization (WHO), was not achieved [2].

### *Epidemiology*

Humans are the only reservoir for polioviruses. Children younger than the age of 5 years are primarily affected. However, susceptible individuals of any age, especially those who are immunocompromised, may also develop the disease. The incubation period is 7 to 21 days, and the period of communicability is 4 to 6 weeks after infection. Poliovirus infection is highly contagious in susceptible populations. After household exposure to wild poliovirus, more than 90% of susceptible contacts become infected. Poliovirus infection results in lifelong immunity specific to the infecting viral serotype. Acute poliomyelitis peaks in the months of July to September in temperate climates and throughout the year in tropical climates.

The virus is transmitted from person to person primarily by direct fecal–oral contact. It may also be transmitted by indirect contact with infectious saliva or feces, or by contaminated sewage or water.

Long-term carrier states (i.e., excretion of virus by asymptomatic persons longer than 6 months after infection) are rare and have been reported only in immunodeficient persons.

L.L. Barton and N.R. Friedman (eds.), *The Neurological Manifestations of Pediatric Infectious Diseases and Immunodeficiency Syndromes.*

In the United States the annual number of reported cases of paralytic disease declined from a peak of more than 21,000 cases in 1952 to an average of 8 to 9 primarily vaccine-associated paralytic poliomyelitis (VAPP) cases annually during 1980 to 1994 [3]. The last indigenously acquired cases of poliomyelitis caused by wild poliovirus were detected in 1979. The shift from oral polio vaccine (OPV) to inactivated polio vaccine (IPV) in the US (in 2000) ended the occurrence of new cases of VAPP until 2005, when an imported case of VAPP was reported in Phoenix, Arizona [4]. In the Americas, the last case of poliomyelitis associated with isolation of wild poliovirus was detected in Peru in 1991 [5]. The Western Hemisphere was certified to be free of indigenous wild poliovirus in 1994, an accomplishment achieved by the exclusive use of oral poliovirus vaccine [5]. Since the initiation of the global poliomyelitis eradication initiative in 1988, the number of endemic countries in 2006 has decreased to four: Pakistan, India, Afghanistan, and Nigeria [6].

## *Pathogenesis*

Poliomyelitis is a systemic infectious disease of disparate severity that affects the central nervous system (CNS). It is a disease of the motor neurons of the anterior horn of the spinal cord and brainstem. Flaccid asymmetric weakness and muscle atrophy are the clinical hallmarks, caused by loss of motor neurons and denervation of their associated skeletal muscles. Poliomyelitis is caused by three antigenically distinct strains or serotypes of RNA viruses of the picornavirus family.

Virus enters through the mouth, and primary multiplication of the virus occurs at the site of implantation in the pharynx, gastrointestinal tract, and adjacent lymphoid tissue. Virus is usually present in the throat and in the stool before the onset of illness. One week after onset, there is little virus in the throat, but virus continues to be excreted in the stool for several weeks. The virus invades deep lymphoid tissue, and enters the blood stream causing "minor viremia" and seeding susceptible reticuloendothelial tissue. In asymptomatic infection, the virus is contained at this point and elicits the formation of type-specific antibodies. In a few persons, however, replication in the reticuloendothelial system gives rise to "major viremia," which corresponds with the "minor illness" also known as abortive poliomyelitis.

The route by which the poliovirus reaches the CNS remains uncertain and controversial. From the blood stream, the virus may invade the cells of the CNS. A study in transgenic mice expressing the human poliovirus receptor suggests that poliovirus spreads from muscles to CNS via peripheral nerves fibers, rather than directly from the blood stream [7]. Neuropathologic studies and animal studies indicate that spread is neural once the virus reaches the CNS.

Neuronal damage is caused directly by virus multiplication, but not all affected neurons are destroyed, and function may occasionally be restored within 3 to 4 weeks after onset. The regions in which neuronal lesions occur are the 1) spinal cord (anterior horn cells chiefly and, to a lesser degree, the intermediate and dorsal horn and dorsal root ganglia), 2) medulla (vestibular nuclei, cranial nerve nuclei, and the reticular formation that contains the vital centers), 3) cerebellum (nuclei in the roof and vermis only), 4) midbrain (chiefly the gray matter, but also the substantia nigra and occasionally the red nucleus), 5) thalamus and hypothalamus, 6) pallidum, and 7) cerebral cortex (motor cortex).

## *Clinical Manifestations*

The response to poliovirus infection is highly variable and has been categorized based on the severity of clinical presentation, into four responses (Table 3.1): 1) inapparent infection, 2) minor illness (abortive poliomyelitis), 3) nonparalytic poliomyelitis (aseptic meningitis), and 4) paralytic poliomyelitis. The latter two responses together are also described as the major illness, which basically reflects CNS involvement.

**Table 3.1** Poliomyelitis clinical response: frequency, features and complications

| | Clinical response | Frequency | Clinical features |
|---|---|---|---|
| | Asymptomatic | Approximately 90–95% | |
| Minor | Abortive poliomyelitis | Approximately 4–8% | Fever, malaise, anorexia, headache, sore throat |
| Major | Nonparalytic poliomyelitis | Approximately 1–5% | Aseptic meningitis (headache, vomiting, meningismus) |
| | | | Prodromal myalgias of involved muscles |
| | | | Paresthesias |
| | Paralytic poliomyelitis | Less than 2% | |
| | Spinal polio | 79% of paralytic polio | Asymmetric motor weakness |
| | | | Loss of deep tendon reflexes |
| | | | Muscular atrophy |
| | Bulbar polio | 2% of paralytic polio | Dysphagia |
| | | | Ineffective coughing |
| | | | Hoarseness, aphonia, asphyxia |
| | | | Irregular respirations |
| | | | Temperature instability |
| | | | Cardiovascular abnormalities |
| | Spino-bulbar polio | 19% of paralytic polio | Combination of spinal and bulbar polio |
| Complications | | | Respiratory failure |
| | | | Paralytic ileus and gastric dilatation |
| | | | Bladder ileus |
| | | | Polioencephalitis |
| | | | Post Polio Syndrome |

The factors that determine the type of clinical response are poorly understood. Risk factors for paralytic disease include larger inocula of virus, increasing age, and pregnancy. In the presence of inapparent poliovirus infection, tonsillectomy can precipitate bulbar poliomyelitis. Strenuous exercise during the early stages of the major illness increases the risk of paralytic disease. Paralytic poliomyelitis tends to localize in a limb that has been the site of a recent intramuscular injection or muscular injury. Persons with B-cell immunodeficiency, primarily young children with X-linked immunodeficiency syndromes, have an increased risk for CNS disease. These individuals may develop acute paralysis, or they may have an atypical course with an incubation period of several months, prolonged febrile illness, chronic meningitis, and progressive neurological dysfunction that involves both upper and lower limbs.

Up to 95% of all poliovirus infections are inapparent or asymptomatic. Infected persons without symptoms shed virus in the stool, and are able to transmit the virus to others.

"Minor illness" (abortive poliomyelitis), which coincides with viremia, has an incubation period of 3 to 7 days. Approximately 4 to 8% of polio infections consist of a minor, nonspecific illness without clinical or laboratory evidence of CNS invasion. This clinical presentation is known as abortive poliomyelitis, and is characterized by complete recovery in less than a week. Three syndromes observed with this form of poliovirus infection are: 1) upper respiratory tract infection (sore throat and low grade fever), 2) gastrointestinal disturbances (nausea, vomiting, abdominal pain, constipation, or, rarely, diarrhea), and 3) influenza-like illness. These syndromes are indistinguishable from other viral illnesses.

## *Neurological Manifestations*

"Major illness" (CNS involvement) begins 9 to 12 days after exposure, and can be nonparalytic or paralytic in nature. Approximately one third of young children who develop major illness experience a biphasic illness (the so called "dromedary" pattern), with symptoms of the minor illness preceding onset of CNS disease, followed by a short symptom-free interval.

Nonparalytic poliomyelitis (aseptic meningitis) is associated with vague malaise, fever, headache, muscle aches, and occasional paresthesias. Anorexia, nausea, vomiting, constipation, or diarrhea may be present. The temperature rises to 37.8 °C to 39.5 °C; and stiffness of the neck, back, and hamstrings soon appears. Physical examination reveals nuchal-spinal signs with changes in superficial and deep reflexes. Nuchal rigidity precedes spinal rigidity and is demonstrable by positive Kernig and Brudzinski signs. In the early stages, the reflexes normally are active. Changes in reflexes may precede weakness by 12 to 24 hours. Deep tendon reflexes become depressed or exaggerated, generally 8 to 24 hours after depression of the superficial reflexes. If there is no further progression, the temperature falls to normal, and signs of meningeal irritation gradually disappear. Complete recovery takes place in 3 to 10 days.

The symptoms of paralytic poliomyelitis are usually those of nonparalytic illness, plus weakness of one or more muscle groups. These patients appear acutely ill, with high fevers and intense muscle pain and spasms of the back and limbs. Initially, there may be increased deep tendon reflexes, but shortly before actual muscle weakness is detected, superficial and deep tendon reflexes diminish or disappear on the affected side. The onset of paralysis may be very sudden, progressing in a few hours to complete loss of motion of one or more extremities. More gradual spread of weakness also occurs and may continue during a period of 3 to 5 days. Generally, no further paralysis occurs after the temperature returns to normal.

Paralytic polio is classified into three types, depending on the level of involvement. Spinal polio is most common, and characterized by flaccid, asymmetric paralysis. Lower limbs are affected more commonly than upper limbs, but, in severe cases, there may be quadriplegia and loss of function of intercostal, abdominal, and trunk muscles. Muscles fasciculations may be seen transiently. Sensory abnormalities are rare. Changes in cognition are not related directly to the infectious process unless polioencephalitis occurs; rather, these changes are related to respiratory compromise and hypoxic or hypercapnic encephalopathy. Bladder paralysis of 1 to 3 days duration occurs in approximately 30% of patients. Bowel atony is common, occasionally to the extent of paralytic ileus. The illness reaches a plateau without change for days to weeks. Strength then begins to return and some estimate of the eventual outcome can be made after 1 month, when most reversible damage has disappeared. Very little additional recovery of strength can be expected after a period of 9 months. A variable degree of permanent weakness is observed in approximately two thirds of patients with paralytic poliomyelitis, ranging from minor debility to permanent flaccid paralysis. Patients with severe acute poliomyelitis, patients requiring mechanical ventilation because of spinal respiratory paralysis, and patients with weakness or paralysis 12 months after onset will usually be left with permanent residua. Muscular atrophy is related to denervation, as well as to disuse, of the muscles. Musculoskeletal deformities may develop if proper body alignment is not maintained and/or if adequate physical therapy is not initiated early.

Bulbar polio leads to weakness of muscles innervated by cranial nerves. Patients are extremely agitated, even delirious, or they may become stuporous. When the cranial nerves IX and X nuclei are involved, patients develop paralysis of pharyngeal and laryngeal musculature, leading to dysphagia, hoarseness, aphonia, ineffective coughing, nasal regurgitation of saliva and fluids, and deviation of the palate, uvula, and tongue. The facial muscles, as well as the tongue and mastication muscles, may also become paralyzed. External oculomotor weakness with pupil sparing may occur in rare cases. Direct infection of the brainstem reticular system can cause breathing and swallowing disruption, as well as cardiovascular abnormalities and temperature instability. Recovery from pharyngeal paralysis is evident by 10 days and is eventually complete. Although bulbar poliomyelitis causes the greatest threat to life in the first weak of illness, it is rarely responsible for permanent damage in surviving patients. Bulbospinal polio is a combination of bulbar and spinal paralysis.

### Other Complications

The most important complication of paralytic poliomyelitis is respiratory compromise. Hypertension, sometimes causing hypertensive encephalopathy, can also develop. Bladder paralysis, if not recognized and managed promptly, can lead to urinary retention, acute renal failure, and uremic encephalopathy. Rarely, polioencephalitis, manifested primarily by irritability, confusion, disturbances of consciousness, and coarse tremors occurs, primarily in infants. Seizures are common and there may be spastic paralysis, in contrast to the usual flaccid paralysis associated with poliomyelitis, which reflects the presence of upper motor neuron involvement. The illness is not distinguishable from other forms of infectious encephalitis.

The postpoliomyelitis syndrome (PPS) is a late-onset complication of paralytic poliomyelitis. Some patients who partially or fully recover from paralysis experience a new onset of muscle weakness associated with pain, atrophy, and fatigue, many years after the acute illness [8–10]. Typically, the involved muscles are the same as those affected during the original illness, but weakness may also occur in previously unaffected limb muscles. Progression of symptoms is gradual, and, as a result, affected individuals are seldom severely disabled. Population-based studies suggest that the syndrome affects 20 to 30% of previously paralyzed patients, with a peak between 25 and 35 years after acute poliomyelitis [9,10].

Although the specific cause of PPS is unknown, it is postulated that late progression of muscle weakness is a result of exhaustion of motor units previously overstressed by recovery from the acute denervation during acute poliomyelitis [11]. After the acute infection, there are fewer anterior horn cells innervating a larger number of myofibrils, thereby exaggerating the physiologic effects of aging at a later age. Other possible mechanisms include immunologic factors and other host–virus interactions [11].

## *Neuropathology*

Early in polio infection, the nervous tissue shows inflammation, neuronophagia and microglial nodules. The initial mixed pattern of inflammation is followed by chronic inflammation and subsequent loss of nerve cells. These infected nerve cells undergo eosinophilic necrosis. In the late stages of the disease, there is evidence of neuronal dropout and reactive astrogliosis [12]. Viral particles are rarely seen in nervous tissue [13,14]. Paralytic poliovirus infection causes destruction of the anterior horn motor neurons of the spinal cord [15].

## *Diagnosis*

Routine laboratory studies are generally not diagnostic. Cerebrospinal fluid (CSF) examination demonstrates changes consistent with aseptic meningitis and is not distinguishable from those of other viral diseases that cause aseptic meningitis: approximately 20 to 300 cells, predominately lymphocytes; a normal glucose level; and a normal or slightly elevated protein level. Poliovirus can be isolated by tissue culture from throat and stool specimens but very rarely from the CSF of infected individuals. In areas with a low incidence of disease, it is important to characterize virus isolates as either wild type (naturally occurring strains) or vaccine like. This characterization is accomplished via oligonucleotide mapping (finger printing) or genomic sequencing, and can be performed only at public health reference laboratories.

In the absence of viral isolates, the diagnosis of poliovirus infection can be accomplished by demonstrating a fourfold increase in neutralizing antibody titers. Neutralizing antibodies to specific serotypes can be detected in the serum as early as 1 week after infection. Serologic testing cannot distinguish between wild-type and vaccine-type infections.

The differential diagnosis of nonparalytic poliomyelitis (aseptic meningitis) encompasses a vast array of infectious etiologies, including the nonpolio enteroviruses (NPEV), herpes viruses, lymphocytic choriomeningitis virus, mycobacteria, and fungi. NPEV can cause sporadic cases of paralytic illness. The Guillain-Barré syndrome and infant botulism more often cause symmetric weakness. West Nile Virus is also an increasingly important consideration.

## *Treatment*

Specific antiviral agents for the treatment of poliomyelitis are not available. Therefore, treatment is supportive and symptomatic. The principles of management are to relieve pain and discomfort, minimize potential skeletal deformities, anticipate and meet complications, and prepare the child and family for a prolonged treatment course and for the possibility of permanent disability. Hot moist packs, hot tub baths, and physical therapy are useful ancillary measures. Follow-up neuromuscular examinations should be performed to detect minor involvement in both abortive and nonparalytic poliomyelitis. Patients with paralytic disease require hospitalization with multidisciplinary care to minimize muscular deformity and problems arising from intestinal ileus, bladder paresis, and, most importantly, from paresis or paralysis of respiratory muscles.

## *Prevention*

OPV is recommended for the global eradication of polio. It is, however, no longer distributed in the United States, where only (high potency) IPV is recommended [16–18]. Both OPV and IPV are highly immunogenic and produce, probably lifelong, immunity in virtually 100% of vaccine recipients.

# Nonpolio Enteroviruses (NPEV)

## *Introduction*

The NPEV include the coxsackieviruses, the echoviruses, and the newer numbered enteroviruses. They cause a wide variety of clinical syndromes, most of the syndromes are benign and self-limited (Table 3.2). Nevertheless, the same viruses are also associated with severe and life-threatening infections, such as aseptic meningitis, encephalitis, myocarditis, paralytic and nonparalytic poliomyelitis, and neonatal sepsis syndromes. A major burden imposed by enterovirus infections is a consequence of their ability to mimic bacterial infections. Antibiotics are frequently unnecessarily used until a bacterial etiology has been excluded. With control of poliovirus infections in much of the world, more attention has been focused on understanding the NPEV.

## *Epidemiology*

NPEV infections occur worldwide, but the exact numbers are unknown. In the tropics, infections occur throughout the year. In temperate climates in the northern hemisphere, infections are more prevalent during the summer and autumn. All races and both sexes are equally affected, but male patients are more likely to be symptomatic [19,20].

In the United States, NPEVs cause an estimated 10 to 15 million symptomatic infections and approximately 75,000 cases of enteroviral meningitis annually [21]. NPEV are the most common cause of aseptic meningitis, accounting for 85 to 95% of all cases for which an etiologic agent is identified [21,22]. Enteroviruses also account for 10 to 20% of identifiable cases of viral encephalitis [23].

Serologic surveys encompassing all enteroviral serotypes are not feasible. Antibody prevalence rates measured for a few serotypes indicate that subsequent to decline of passively acquired maternal antibodies after the age of 6 months, the

**Table 3.2** Major syndromes associated with nonpolio enteroviruses

| |
|---|
| Nonspecific febrile illness |
| Viral exanthems |
| Hand, foot, and mouth syndrome |
| Herpangina |
| Pleurodynia |
| Pericarditis/myocarditis |
| Aseptic meningitis |
| Myelitis |
| Encephalitis |

fraction of immune persons in the population rises progressively with age. Between 15 and 90% of the adult population have type-specific neutralizing antibodies for the serotype tested, depending on the serotype and the socioeconomic class of the population surveyed [20]. During epidemics, infants younger than 1 year of age, and, particularly, younger than 3 months of age, become infected at rates that exceed those of older children and adults by several fold, in part, because lumbar puncture is performed more frequently as part of the diagnostic evaluation for fever [20,24].The disease course tends to be benign in older children and more serious in neonates.

The incubation period for illness caused by enteroviral infections can rarely be determined precisely, and ranges from 2 days to 2 weeks. Patients with enteroviral illnesses typically excrete virus in throat secretions or feces for several days before the onset of symptoms and continue to excrete virus in feces for several weeks thereafter. The period of maximal communicability seems to be early in illness, when viral shedding is greatest.

## *Pathogenesis*

The NPEV are small, non-enveloped RNA viruses. Coxsackieviruses are divided into group A and group B viruses based on early observations of their pathogenicity in mice. At least 23 serotypes (serotypes 1–22, 24) of group A and 6 serotypes (serotypes 1–6) of group B are recognized. In general, group A coxsackieviruses tend to infect the skin and mucous membranes, causing herpangina, acute hemorrhagic conjunctivitis (AHC), and hand, foot, and mouth (HFM) disease. Group B coxsackieviruses tend to infect the heart, pleura, pancreas, and liver; causing pleurodynia, myocarditis, pericarditis, and hepatitis. Both group A and group B coxsackieviruses can cause nonspecific febrile illnesses, rashes, upper respiratory tract disease, and aseptic meningitis.

The enteric cytopathic human orphan (ECHO) viruses comprise 31 serotypes (serotypes 1–9, 11–27, and 29–33). They have been associated with human diseases, ranging from minor gastrointestinal to significant CNS infection. The numbered enteroviruses, types 68 to 71 and 73, have also been associated with a wide spectrum of diseases from conjunctivitis to encephalitis.

The majority of infected individuals develop subclinical infection with only a brief period of viral replication. In a minority of infected individuals, further viral replication occurs productive of a major viremia and a nonspecific febrile illness. It is during this major viremia that the NPEV seed target tissues and cause specific clinical syndromes.

## *Clinical Manifestations*

Approximately 50 to 80% of patients with NPEV infections are completely asymptomatic [20]. Patients who are symptomatic usually have undifferentiated febrile illnesses lasting only a few days, often accompanied by pharyngitis and other upper respiratory tract symptoms. Rash is also common but varies with the specific viral agent. These illnesses may be caused by virtually any enteroviral serotype and are indistinguishable clinically from infection with many other viral agents. Visceral and neurological infection and disease, as noted above, occur subsequent to viremia, but remain uncommon.

## *Neurological Manifestations*

The spectrum of neurological manifestations of NPEV infections ranges from acute uncomplicated, self-limited aseptic meningitis to more severe meningoencephalitis, or chronic meningoencephalitis in patients with altered immunity, paralytic myelitis, cerebellar ataxia, Guillain-Barré syndrome, and transverse myelitis.

Aseptic meningitis caused by enteroviruses is not clinically different from aseptic meningitis caused by other viruses. The illness may be biphasic; fever and myalgia are present for a few days, followed by defervescence and absence of symptoms for 2 to 10 days before the reappearance of fever in association with meningeal signs. Onset is usually abrupt, and fever of 38 °C to 40 °C is the most consistent clinical finding, occurring in 76 to 100% of patients [19,21]. Pharyngitis and other symptoms of upper respiratory tract infection are often present. Nuchal rigidity is found in one half of the patients, especially children older than 2 years of age. Headache is a major complaint, especially in older children and adults. The headache is usually diffuse and severe, although adolescents and adults may also experience retrobulbar pain [25]. Photophobia, nausea, and vomiting are also frequently present. Neck, back, and leg pain is common. Abdominal pain occurs in approximately one fifth of patients. The duration of clinically apparent NPEV meningitis is usually less than 1 week. Many patients report decrease in symptoms after lumbar puncture, presumably caused by CSF removal.

Less than 10% of patients with aseptic meningitis have symptoms suggestive of neurological disease [21]. Focal signs, febrile seizures, and profound lethargy are rarely a part of this syndrome. Occasionally, patients may exhibit altered levels of consciousness, including confusion and visual hallucinations, or develop complex seizures. These cases are usually defined as meningoencephalitis or encephalitis.

NPEV account for approximately 10 to 20% of cases of encephalitis of proven viral etiology [21,23]. NPEV generally cause global, nonfocal encephalitis, and, less commonly, focal disease. Clinical manifestations of enterovirus encephalitis range from mental status changes to coma. Patients with focal encephalitis may present with partial motor seizures, hemichorea, or acute cerebellar ataxia [20].

A syndrome of brainstem encephalitis (or rhombencephalitis) has been associated with enterovirus 71, most recently in Taiwan and Malaysia [26]. Grade I disease was characterized by myoclonic jerks and tremor, ataxia or both. Grade II was characterized by myoclonus and cranial nerve involvement. Grade III was characterized by transient myoclonus followed by the rapid onset of respiratory distress, cyanosis, poor peripheral perfusion, loss of the doll's eye reflex, and apnea. The fatality rate was 14% [26]. Permanent neurological deficits were noted in 16% of survivors [27].

That host age has a major impact on clinical manifestations, and outcome of infection is illustrated by the entity disseminated neonatal enterovirus infection. It is acquired primarily during the birth process and usually manifests within the first 2 weeks of life. Early manifestations are nonspecific; fever, vomiting, rash, and respiratory findings [24]. CNS involvement develops in 75% of these infants and manifests as lethargy, seizures, hemiparesis, flaccid paralysis, and coma. The disease progresses to involve major systems, causing hepatic necrosis, myocarditis, necrotizing enterocolitis, and disseminated intravascular coagulation. The echoviruses and group B coxsackieviruses are responsible for most neonatal infections [24].

Rarely, enteroviruses cause a syndrome of acute motor weakness and flaccid paralysis similar to poliomyelitis. Myelitis caused by NPEV tends to be less severe than that caused by polioviruses, because muscle weakness is less likely to persist and bulbar involvement is less common.

Coxsackievirus A9, Coxsackievirus B4 and echovirus 4 have been isolated from the CSF of a few patients with acute transverse myelitis [28]. Depending on the level of involvement, patients experience a combination of sensory (paresthesias), motor (weakness, paralysis, loss of reflexes), and/or autonomic (loss of sphincter control) symptoms [24].

The Guillain-Barré syndrome has been reported in a small number of patients infected with group A coxsackievirus types 2, 5, and 9 and echovirus types 6 and 22 [24,25].

## *Neuropathology*

There are no specific pathologic characteristics of NPEV neurological disease. Macrophage infiltration is seen in the affected neurological tissue. Enteroviruses can be identified by molecular techniques and special stains [29,30].

## *Diagnosis*

With a few exceptions, the clinical and laboratory findings accompanying acute viral meningitis are insufficiently distinct to allow an etiologic diagnosis. The epidemiologic setting (e.g., time of year) and associated systemic manifestations may be helpful in making a presumptive diagnosis.

The typical CSF profile in enterovirus meningitis is a mononuclear pleocytosis, with 100 to 300 white blood cells/$mm^3$, a normal or moderately elevated protein content, and a normal glucose concentration. Early in the disease, the CSF white blood count may exceed 1000 cells/$mm^3$, and have a predominance of neutrophils. The CSF findings in enterovirus encephalitis are similar to the findings in meningitis.

Brain imaging and the electroencephalogram in patients with encephalitis usually reflect the extent and the severity of the disease.

The definitive diagnosis of enteroviral infection is accomplished by cell culture, polymerase chain reaction (PCR), or retrospectively by serology. Isolation of enterovirus in cell culture remains the gold standard for diagnosis. A presumptive isolation of enterovirus is reported within a few days (usually <7 d). The etiologic diagnosis can be confirmed by the isolation of virus from CSF or stool specimen (in the presence of an appropriate clinical syndrome). PCR detects enteroviral RNA in the CSF of 66 to 86% of patients with enterovirus aseptic meningitis, compared with viral isolation rates of approximately 30% [20]. Serology is of limited value in the diagnosis of acute enterovirus infections.

Enterovirus-associated aseptic meningitis must be differentiated from aseptic meningitis caused by other infectious agents, including lymphocytic choriomeningitis virus, herpes simplex virus, mycobacteria, fungi, and spirochetes, as well as by CNS primary and metastatic neoplasms.

## *Treatment*

The mainstay of therapy for NPEV infections is supportive and symptomatic. Pleconaril, an antiviral previously obtainable for compassionate use in cases of severe enteroviral infections, is no longer available [20,31]. Intravenous immune globulin has been used in patients with chronic enteroviral meningoencephalitis and in neonates and older children with severe cardiac and CNS disease [32].

## *Prognosis*

Most patients with enterovirus aseptic meningitis have a benign self-limited course. Fever and signs of meningeal irritation resolve in 2 to 7 days; however, CSF pleocytosis may persist for a longer period of time [25]. The short-term prognosis of children who develop NPEV meningitis is generally excellent. However, controversy continues regarding the long-term outcome of those who incurred disease in early infancy. Early reports suggested a moderately increased risk of long-term neurological and cognitive sequelae for these infants, but recent prospective studies have indicated no measurable effects, including those with neurological findings during the acute phase [24].

The morbidity and mortality attributable to perinatal enterovirus infection may be as high as 74% and 10%, respectively, depending on the infecting serotypes. Death is seldom, if ever, the result of CNS involvement, rather, it is the result of hepatic failure or myocarditis. The prognosis of meningoencephalitis in older infants and children is generally excellent. Neurological sequelae and deaths are rare.

## References


1. Modlin JF, Coffey DJ. Poliomyelitis, poliovaccine and the post-poliomyelitis syndrome. In: Scheld WM, Whitley RJ, Durack DT, eds. *Infections of The Central Nervous System.* Lippincott-Raven. 1997; 57–72
2. World Health Organization. Fact Sheet No 114. April 2003. (http://www.who.int/mediacentre/factsheets/fs114/en/).
3. Centers for Disease control and Prevention (CDC). Paralytic poliomyelitis—United States, 1980–1994. *MMWR* 1997; 46:79–83.
4. Centers for Disease control and Prevention (CDC). Imported vaccine-associated paralytic poliomyelitis—United States, 2005. *MMWR* 2005; 55:97–99.
5. Centers for Disease control and Prevention (CDC). International Notes. Certification of Poliomyelitis Eradication—The Americas, 1994. *MMWR* 1994; 43:720–722.
6. Centers for Disease control and Prevention (CDC). Progress toward interruption of wild poliovirus transmission—worldwide, January 2005-March 2006. *MMWR* 2006; 55:458–462.
7. Ren R, Racaniello VR. Poliovirus spreads from muscle to the central nervous system by neural pathways. *J Infect Dis.* 1992; 166:747–752.
8. Rekand T, Karlsen B, Langeland N, Aarli JA. Long-term follow-up of patients with nonparalytic poliomyelitis. *Arch Phys Med Rehabil.* 2002; 83:533–537.
9. Johnson RT. Late progression of poliomyelitis paralysis: discussion of pathogenesis. *Rev Infect Dis.* 1984; 6:S568–570.
10. Trojan DA, Cashman NR, Shapiro S, Tansey CM, Esdaile JM. Predictive factors for post-poliomyelitis syndrome. *Arch Phys Med Rehabil.* 1994; 75:770–777.
11. Dalakas MC, Elder G, Hallett M, et al. A long-term follow-up study of patients with post-poliomyelitis neuromuscular symptoms. *N Engl J Med.* 1986; 314:959–963.
12. Finkelstein SD. Polioviruses. In: Connor DH, Chandler FW, Schwartz DA, Manz HJ, Lack EE, eds. *Pathology of Infectious Diseases.* Stamford, CT: Appleton & Lange. 1997; 259–263.
13. Petitjean J, Quibriac M, Freymuth F, Fuchs F. Specific detection of enteroviruses in clinical samples of molecular hybridization using poliovirus subgenomic riboprobes. *J Clin Microbiol.* 1990; 28:307–311.
14. Yang CF, De L, Holloway BP, Pallansch MA, Kew OM. Detection and identification of vaccine-related polioviruses by the polymerase chain reaction. *Virus Res.* 1991; 20:157–159.
15. Nagata N, Iwasaki T, Ami Y, et al. Differential localization of neurons susceptible to enterovirus 71 and poliovirus type 1 in the central nervous system of cynomolgus monkeys and intravenous inoculation. *J Gen Virol.* 2004; 85:2981–2989.
16. Atkinson WL, Pickering LK, Schwartz B, et al. General recommendations on immunization. Recommendations of the Advisory Committee on Immunization Practices (ACIP) and the American Academy of Family Physicians (AAFP). *MMWR* 2002; 51:1–35.
17. Centers for Disease control and Prevention (CDC). Recommendations of the Advisory Committee on Immunization Practices: revised recommendations for routine poliomyelitis vaccination. *MMWR* 1999; 48:590.
18. Centers for Disease control and Prevention (CDC). Progress towards global eradication of poliomyelitis, 2001. *MMWR* 2002; 51:253–256.
19. Rotbart HA. Viral meningitis and the aseptic meningitis syndrome. In: Scheld WM, Whitley RJ, Durack DT, eds. *Infections of the Central Nervous System.* Philadelphia, PA: Lippincott-Raven. 1997; 23–33.
20. Modlin JF. Coxsackieviruses, echoviruses, and newer enteroviruses. In: Mandell GL, Bennett JE, Dolin R, eds. *Mandell, Douglas, & Bennett's Principles and Practices of Infectious Diseases.* Churchill Livingston. 2005; 2149–2161.
21. Rotbart HA. Enteroviral infections of the central nervous system. *Clin Infect Dis.* 1995; 20:971–981.
22. Rotbart HA, Viral meningitis. *Semin Neurol.* 2000; 20:277–292.

23. Modlin JF, Degan R, Berlin LE, et al. Focal encephalitis with enterovirus infections. *Pediatrics* 1991; 88:841–845.
24. Modlin JF. Enteroviruses: coxsackieviruses, echoviruses, and newer enteroviruses. In: Long SS, Pickering LK, Prober CG. eds. *Principles and Practices of Pediatric Infectious Diseases*. Churchill Livingston. 2003; 1179–1188.
25. Cherry JD. Enteroviruses and Parechoviruses. In: Feigin RD, Cherry JD, Demmeler GJ, Kaplan SL, eds. *Textbook of Pediatric Infectious Diseases*. Saunders. 2004; 1984–2041.
26. Huang C, Liu C, Chang Y, Chen C, Wang S, Yeh T, Neurologic complications in children with enterovirus 71 infection. *N Engl J Med*. 1999; 341:936–942.
27. Romero JR, Newland JG. Viral meningitis and encephalitis: Traditional and emerging viral agents. *Semin Pediatr Infect Dis*. 2003; 14:72–82.
28. Graber D. Acute transverse myelitis and Coxsackie A9 virus infection. *Pediatr Infect Dis J*. 1994; 13:77.
29. Kandolf R, Hofschneider PH. Molecular cloning of the genome of a cardiotropic Coxsackie B3 virus: full length, reverse transcribed recombinant cDNA generates infectious virus in mammalian cells. *Proc Natl Acad Sci USA*. 1985; 82:4818–4822.
30. Cova L, Kopecka H, Aymard M, Girard M. Use of cRNA probes for the detection of enteroviruses by molecular hybridization. *J Med Virol*. 1988; 24:11–18.
31. Abzug MJ, Cloud G, Bradley J. Double blind placebo-controlled trial of Pleconaril in infants with enterovirus meningitis. *Pediatr Infect Dis J*. 2003; 22:335–340.
32. *Red Book. Report of the Committee on Infectious Diseases*. Enterovirus (Nonpoliovirus) Infections. American Academy of Pediatrics. Elk Groove, IL. 2006; 284–285.

# Chapter 4
# Arboviruses

José R. Romero, M.D., F.A.A.P.

## Arboviral Infections

### *Introduction*

The arboviruses are a heterogeneous collection of more than 500 viruses in distinct viral families linked by a common mode of transmission to humans: the bite of an insect or arthropod [1]. Approximately 150 arboviruses are capable of causing disease (including neuroinvasive disease) in humans. This chapter will focus primarily on the major North American arboviruses that have been associated with central nervous system (CNS) infections.

The enzootic cycle of the arboviruses requires replicative phases in their respective avian or mammalian vertebrate hosts as well as in their insect or arthropod vectors. Infections of humans (i.e., epizootic infection) by the arboviruses are incidental to the enzootic life cycle of the viruses and, with rare exceptions, result in a "dead-end" infection without subsequent human-to-human transmission. Arboviral infections occur during the summer months and coincide with periods of increased activity of their insect and arthropod vectors. With the exception of Colorado tick fever (CTF) and Powassan (POW) viruses, which are transmitted by ticks, all other North American arboviruses are transmitted by mosquito vectors.

The majority of human arboviral infections result in subclinical disease or febrile syndromes that do not involve the CNS. When the CNS is involved, meningitis or encephalitis commonly result. However, clinical overlap between these two syndromes (i.e., meningoencephalitis) frequently occurs [2]. Viral meningitis can be described as a febrile illness associated with clinical signs of meningeal irritation (neck stiffness, Kernig and/or Brudzinski signs) but without the presence of neurological dysfunction that arises as a result of a viral infection. Viral encephalitis may be defined as a febrile illness with evidence of brain parenchymal dysfunction as manifested by an altered state of consciousness and/or objective signs of neurological dysfunction (e.g., seizures, cranial nerve palsies, dysarthria, abnormal reflexes, and paralysis) that is usually the result of viral replication within brain parenchyma.

L.L. Barton and N.R. Friedman (eds.), *The Neurological Manifestations of Pediatric Infectious Diseases and Immunodeficiency Syndromes.*

# The Flaviviridae

The *Flaviviridae* family of RNA viruses is comprised of three genera: Flavivirus, Pestivirus, and Hepacivirus [3]. Members of this family associated with CNS infections in humans reside within two complexes of the genus Flavivirus: Japanese encephalitis complex (Japanese encephalitis, West Nile, St. Louis encephalitis (SLE), and Murray Valley encephalitis viruses) and tick-borne encephalitis complex (including POW, tick-borne encephalitis, Kyasanur forest disease, and Omsk hemorrhagic fever viruses).

## *St. Louis Encephalitis*

### Epidemiology

SLE was first recognized as a distinct clinical entity in the early 1930s after studies of brain tissue from fatal cases of encephalitis, obtained from a large outbreak of encephalitis in St. Louis, Missouri, revealed the presence of a virus distinct from that of other viruses known at the time [4–9].

The virus is widely distributed throughout the American continent [10,11]; virtually every state in the United States has reported outbreaks or sporadic cases of SLE. Biologic differences between SLE virus strains seem to exist. Epidemic strains from the eastern and southern United States associated with high attack rates and high mortality rates in humans have been demonstrated to exhibit greater neurovirulence in animal models. In contrast, endemic western strains, which are associated with lower mortality rates in humans, exhibit intermediate or low virulence in animal models [12–14].

SLE virus is maintained enzootically in the western and central states by transmission between birds and mosquitos. The principle mosquito vector in the western and central United States is *Culex tarsalis*. Infections in humans occur sporadically. In the eastern states, SLE virus is transmitted as temporally separated sporadic cases or localized outbreaks by *C. pipiens*, *C. quinquefasciatus*, and *C. nigripalpus*.

Until the introduction of West Nile virus (WNV) in 1999, SLE virus was the single major cause of epidemic encephalitis in the United States [15,16]. From 1955 to 1975, 4624 cases of SLE were reported to the Centers for Disease Control and Prevention. For the period spanning 1976 to 2000, the number of reported cases fell to 1432. In 2003, only 37 cases were reported. Recent human seroprevalence studies indicate that, in certain areas of the western United States, SLE may no longer be endemic [17].

### Clinical and Neurological Manifestations

The clinical presentation of SLE virus infection varies from subclinical infection to severe, fatal encephalitis, and is age related [2,7,11]. The overwhelming majority of SLE virus infections in humans are asymptomatic. The ratio of clinical to subclinical infections varies from 1:800 in children younger than 10 years of age to 1:85 in adults [11].

Three neurological syndromes associated with SLE virus infection have been reported (listed in order of decreasing frequency of occurrence in children): 1) encephalitis (fever with significant neurological dysfunction); 2) aseptic meningitis (fever and evidence of meningeal irritation in the absence of neurological dysfunction); and 3) febrile headache alone [2]. In infants, children, and adolescents, encephalitis, aseptic meningitis, and febrile headache occur in 56%, 38%, and 6% of cases, respectively [2]. With advancing age, encephalitis becomes more prevalent, such that, in individuals of at least 60 years of age, encephalitis occurs in 87% and aseptic meningitis in only 2% [20].

Although almost every report of the clinical features of SLE includes children, specific reports of the clinical findings in children are limited [6,7,18–23]. The incubation period of SLE ranges from 4 to 21 days [2,24]. The onset of neurological illness may be heralded by nonspecific symptoms of malaise, fever, headache, somnolence, myalgias, abdominal and back pain, and, occasionally conjunctivitis, photophobia, and upper respiratory tract symptoms (i.e., sore throat) [6]. This prodrome may be absent or of very brief duration [18]. Fever is nearly universal, and ranges between 38.9 °C and 40 °C in more than half of the affected children. Headache is almost always present in most children who are able to report it. Nausea and vomiting occur in approximately three quarters of children in reported series [18,19]. Abdominal pain is also more frequently reported in children [23,25]. Seizures have been more common in children, as have been vomiting and diarrhea. Abnormal neurological signs and symptoms include altered sensorium, including coma (42%); evidence of meningeal irritation (nuchal rigidity, Kernig sign, and Brudzinski sign) (85%); seizures (24%); and cranial nerve palsies (12%) [18,19]. Other reported findings include paresis, tremors, ataxia (27%), and Babinski sign (30%).

The principal neurological complications are neurasthenic in nature and include headache, insomnia, lethargy, drowsiness, nervousness, personality changes, difficulty concentrating, memory impairment, vertigo, and fatigability [6,7,18,26,27]. In many patients, neurological sequelae improve and resolve over time [28]. Specific neurological residua include tremor, disturbances of gait, and cranial nerve involvement.

Children seem to have significantly better outcomes than adults. Intellectual impairment in children rarely, if ever, occurs [28]. In the only report specifically focusing on children, Barrett et al. [18] noted that, although 14 (54%) of 26 children still exhibited neurological abnormalities at follow-up examinations conducted 3 to 17 weeks after discharge, all demonstrated improvement from initial examination. Abnormalities included Babinski sign (50%), behavioral problems (43%), ankle clonus (29%), hyperactive deep tendon reflexes (21%), generalized hypertonicity (7%), generalized hypotonicity (7%), or ataxia (7%). Among five patients found to have electroencephalogram (EEG) abnormalities during the acute phase of the illness, all showed improvement when reevaluated during convalescence. Tremors occur infrequently as sequelae in children. The mortality rate from SLE ranges from 1 to 20% [7,25,29] and is directly related to increasing age.

## Pathogenesis and Neuropathology [7,11,30–33]

After inoculation of SLE virus, replication takes place in regional lymph nodes with subsequent viral dissemination to multiple organs, including, in some cases, the CNS [32]. The exact mechanism through which SLE virus gains entry into the CNS is presently unknown. Animal data suggest that some flaviviruses may gain access to the CNS via active transport through cerebral microvascular endothelial cells [33]. Intrathecal production of virus-specific antibodies as well as viral clearance by activated microglial cells and macrophages is essential to patient recovery from encephalitis caused by flaviviruses. The mechanism of injury to infected cells may be through activation of an apoptotic pathway leading to cell death [34].

In humans, only the CNS has demonstrated pathologic changes after SLE virus infections. Gross examination of the brains of patients who have died from SLE reveals varying degrees of congestion of the meninges and parenchyma. A lymphocytic infiltrate is seen on microscopic examination of the meninges and perivascular lymphocytic cuffing occurs around the arterial and venous vessels of the brain. Within the parenchyma of the brain, nodules made up of monocytes, lymphocytes, and microglial cells can be seen. Degenerating neurons are seen in nearly every case. The most severely affected area of the brain is the substantia nigra, followed by the thalamic nuclei. Melanin released from lysed neurons of the substantia nigra can be seen within macrophages.

## Diagnosis

The cerebrospinal fluid (CSF) opening pressure is generally increased [7]. The CSF glucose concentration is usually normal. Elevation of CSF protein is seen in the majority of cases, but concentrations above 200 mg/dl are unusual. CSF leukocyte counts are usually less than 200 cells/$mm^3$ and lymphocytic in nature [2,6,7,18–21,24,33]. Early in the course of the illness, no pleocytosis or a predominance of polymorphonuclear leukocytes may be seen [2,6,23].

The EEG is frequently abnormal in children and adults with encephalitis, and demonstrates diffuse generalized slowing and delta wave activity [2,18,22,35,36]. Focal discharges and spike activity have been described that mimic herpes simplex virus (HSV) encephalitis [18,36].

Two reports document the finding of edema of the substantia nigra on T2-weighted magnetic resonance imaging (MRI) scans in some patients with SLE. Enhancement did not occur with gadolinium infusion [36,37].

Successful isolation of SLE virus from serum is possible but is limited by the brevity of the viremia that precedes the onset of neurological disease [1,38]. The yield by viral culture from the CSF is significantly lower. SLE virus has successfully been isolated from brain tissue. *In situ* tissue viral antigen detection in the brain has a low sensitivity because of the sparse number of cells infected. Nucleic acid amplification detection of SLE virus in CSF has met with limited success [38].

The major diagnostic modality is still serology [1,11,39]. IgM capture enzyme-linked immunosorbent assay (ELISA) is the most commonly used test for the diagnosis of SLE. Virus-specific IgM is present in the CSF and or serum of 40% of infected individuals by the fourth day after onset of illness, and in virtually all individuals by day 10 of illness [1]. The finding of SLE IgM in the CSF is diagnostic of acute infection with SLE. However, the same may not be true of finding SLE IgM in serum, because virus-specific IgM may persist for up to a year after infection [1,39]. Viruses within the Japanese encephalitis serogroup share antigenic cross-reactivity with other members of the serogroup. In North America, serologic cross-reactions between SLE, WNV, and POW virus can occur [1]. Determination of the specific etiology of the disease is accomplished with viral neutralization assays.

### Treatment

Treatment is supportive, with close monitoring of respiratory as well as fluid and electrolyte status. A recent study suggests that early initiation of intravenous, followed by subcutaneous interferon-α2b may reduce the severity and duration of complications of SLE [40].

### Prevention

Prevention of SLE virus infection requires public health and personal measures. The former include control of mosquito breeding habitats, judicious use of mosquito larvicides, and active surveillance for SLE virus-infected mosquitoes. Individuals should use insect repellents, protective clothing, and insecticides. Screening and mosquito bed nets may also be warranted.

## *West Nile Neuroinvasive Syndromes*

### Epidemiology

WNV, the etiologic agent of West Nile fever (WNF) and West Nile meningoencephalitis (WNME), is a virus found worldwide [3,41–46]. It made its American debut in 1999 as the causative agent of an epidemic of aseptic meningitis and encephalitis in New York City [43]. The virus derives its named from the geographic location where it was first isolated from an infected individual in 1937: the West Nile district of Uganda [41].

After WNV's North American introduction, cases of WNME remained at relatively low levels though 2001 and then exploded in 2002 and 2003 when there were 2143 and 2866 cases of neuroinvasive WNV infection, respectively. During 2004 and 2005, 2611 cases in patients younger than 19 years of age were reported (54 with meningitis, 50 with encephalitis, and 136 with WNF; 21 had other or unknown manifestations) [47]. Currently, WNV has superseded all indigenous North American arboviruses as the single most important cause of arboviral CNS disease in the United States. The enzootic cycle of WNV in North America is maintained primarily by *Culex* mosquitoes and birds of the family *Corvidae*. However, with each year since its introduction, a growing number of mosquito species have been found that can harbor WNV. The virus has been found in 43 of the 173 North American species of mosquitoes [48].

The overwhelming majority of infections in humans result in dead end transmission of WNV. However, human-to-human transmission through blood transfusion, organ transplantation, transplacentally, and, possibly, breast feeding has been documented [47,49–55].

## Clinical Manifestations

The incubation period of WNV infection ranges from 2 to 14 days, but usually is 2 to 6 days [56,57]. In immunosuppressed patients, incubation periods up to 21 days have been reported [52,54]. The majority of WNV infections in humans result in subclinical disease. Approximately 20% of those infected develop WNF, a mild febrile illness characterized by an abrupt onset of fever accompanied by malaise, anorexia, nausea, vomiting, headache, and myalgias [56,58–60]. A macular, papular or morbilliform exanthem and diffuse lymphadenopathy may also be seen. Because of its mild nature, only approximately half of individuals with WNF seek medical attention. Nonneurological complications reported include rhabdomyolysis, myocarditis, orchitis, pancreatitis, hepatitis, and vitritis [43,59,61].

## Neurological Manifestations

More severe forms of disease (encephalitis, meningitis, meningoencephalitis, and acute flaccid paralysis) develop in fewer than 1% (1 in 140 to 320) of persons infected with the WNV [46,59,60]. Although cases of WNV CNS infection have been reported in children, the vast majority (>90%) of reported cases have occurred in adults [16,59,62]. Multiple reports have documented that the single most significant risk factor for the development of neuroinvasive disease as well as adverse outcome is increasing age [59,60]. Chronic illness (hypertension, diabetes mellitus, and coronary artery disease) and immunosuppressive conditions (transplantation) have also been identified as risk factors for severe disease.

In adults, encephalitis and meningoencephalitis account for approximately 63% of WNV neuroinvasive infections [43,46,59,63–65]. Meningitis has been reported to occur in between 42% and 16% of those with WNV neuroinvasive disease. WNV has also been linked to the development of the acute flaccid paralysis syndrome [65–67].

The symptoms of neuroinvasive WNV infections (i.e., encephalitis or meningitis), primarily described in adults, include fever (91%), headache (58%), altered mental status (51%), weakness (52%), neck stiffness (24%), seizures (7%), gastrointestinal symptoms (i.e., nausea, vomiting, and diarrhea) (53%), rash (15%) [59,63,65,68]. Other reported findings include coma, myalgias, arthralgias, anorexia, sore throat, photophobia, tremors, and dyskinesias [43,48,68].

Patients with the acute flaccid paralysis syndrome exhibit asymmetric weakness, hypotonia, absent or diminished or absent deep tendon reflexes, without pain or sensory loss in the affected limb(s) [43,66,67]. In severe cases, changes in bowel or bladder function may occur as well as acute respiratory distress requiring assisted mechanical ventilation. This syndrome may occur in the absence of meningitis or encephalitis.

Limited reports of the clinical presentations of WNV-associated encephalitis, meningoencephalitis, acute flaccid paralysis, and meningitis in children exist [59,61,62,65,69–77]. Initially, case reports focused on cases of WNV encephalitis. In a case of encephalitis, the presentation of fever, headache, vomiting, and left-sided hemiparesis suggested HSV encephalitis [71]. Another child with WNV-associated encephalitis reportedly lapsed into a coma but, ultimately, regained consciousness [71]. In a report of an atypical presentation of meningoencephalitis, the child presented with fever, sore throat, headache, a macular rash on the face and trunk, meningismus, and generalized weakness [72]. His clinical course was complicated by the development of focal seizures.

More recently, larger case series of WNV neuroinvasive disease in children have appeared [61,65,75,77]. The presentation of WNV meningitis in children is similar to that typically described in adults. The reported clinical findings of WNV encephalitis in children have included fever, headache, vomiting, diarrhea, abdominal pain, myalgia, rash, seizures, confusion, paralysis, tremor, facial palsy, photophobia, ataxia, and dysphasia.

In the only reported pediatric case of acute flaccid paralysis, fever, vomiting, and diarrhea, as well as facial and truncal rash were present on admission [73]. The child subsequently developed flaccid paralysis of the left arm in association with neck, shoulder, and back pain. Deep tendon reflexes were absent in the left arm but sensory function was intact.

Chorioretinitis, reported in adults and a congenitally infected infant, has not been noted in other children.

Sequelae of WNV neuroinvasive disease include fatigue, fever, weakness, difficulty concentrating, memory loss, depression, paresis, tremor, myoclonus, and parkinsonism [56,58,62,63,68]. Between 50% and 65% of individuals will have evidence of neuropsychiatric dysfunction at the time of discharge [63,78]. Persistent symptoms have been noted in nearly two thirds of patients 1 month after discharge [58]. and in one half to two thirds at 1-year follow-up [56].

Sejvar et al. documented that the neuropsychiatric outcome at 8 months for patients with meningitis and encephalitis was generally favorable [68]. All patients with meningitis had returned to work and reported normal or nearly normal function. In cases of severe encephalitis, achievement of premorbid function levels without evidence of residual disability was observed in the majority of patients. In contrast, patients recovering from acute flaccid paralysis fared the poorest. No patient had improvement of weakness or in electromyographic findings.

The mortality rate in WNV neuroinvasive syndromes in adults has been linked to advanced age and underlying illness [43,59,64]. Case fatality rates in hospitalized patients have ranged from 4 to 14% [46,56,59,60,63–65,68,78]. Hospitalized persons 75 years or older are nine times more likely to die than younger patients. Other reported independent risk factors for death have been change in level of consciousness and anemia at presentation [64].

Reported neurological residua in pediatric cases of WNV neuroinvasive disease have been limited to cases of encephalitis and have consisted of unilateral facial palsy, and difficulties with memory and comprehension [69,71,74,79]. Although reports of fatalities in children exist [70], reviews of reported cases from 1999, 2000, and 2002 failed to document any deaths among children [62,65,74].

## Pathogenesis and Neuropathology

The pathogenesis of WNV encephalitis has been explored in several animal model systems [80–83]. Infection in mice and hamsters results in meningoencephalitis and an acute flaccid paralysis-like syndrome similar to that observed in humans [81]. Subcutaneous inoculation of WNV in mice produces peak viremia by the second day after infection, which clears by the sixth day. Virus can subsequently be detected in regional lymph nodes, spleen, brain, and spinal cord. Because of the simultaneous of appearance of virus at both sites within the CNS, a hematogenous route for the CNS infection has been postulated. Similar to human infections, in the animal models, neurons are the principal target in the CNS. Preferential involvement of Purkinje cells, anterior horn cells in the spinal cord, and neurons of the thalamus and basal ganglia is seen [82,84]. Three mechanisms have been postulated for the neuronal injury seen in WNV infection [85]: 1) viral injury to infected neurons via apoptosis; 2) targeting of infected neurons by cytotoxic T lymphocytes; and 3) neuronal death as a result of bystander injury.

Clearance of virus from the blood and CSF is dependent on humoral immunity. WNV-specific antibodies are detectable in the majority of individuals during the second week of infection [1,48].

Gross examination of the brain, spinal cord, and meninges may be unremarkable or may demonstrate evidence of edema. In severe cases, the leptomeninges may show a perivascular monocytic infiltrate [48,79]. Parenchymal findings of WNV encephalitis can be seen in the deep nuclei (thalamus, caudate, lentiform nuclei), medulla, the substantia nigra, and other regions of the brainstem as well as the proximal spinal cord [48,56,59,79]. Histologic features of fatal cases of WNV encephalitis include perivascular mononuclear inflammatory infiltrates, microglial nodules in the brain parenchyma, and focal mononuclear inflammation along the cranial nerve roots of the medulla [43,48,59,86]. Neuronal necrosis or neuronophagia may be seen. In the cerebellum, the Purkinje cell layer demonstrates inflammation, neuronal loss, and gliosis [48]. The microglial nodules are composed of lymphocytes and histiocytes. The CNS pathologic changes are the result of direct viral replication in neuronal and glial cells as well as the cytotoxic immune response to infected cells [56]. Viral antigen is detectable in neurons of fatal cases [43,56,79].

In fatal cases associated with acute flaccid paralysis, the anterior horns of cervical and lumbar regions are the most severely involved [86]. Evidence of neuronophagia, neuronal loss, and perivascular monocytic infiltrates have been found [48,86]. Loss of ganglionic neurons, nodules of Nageotte and perivascular lymphocytic aggregates have been seen in the dorsal roots and sympathetic ganglia [86].

## Diagnosis

The CSF generally shows a predominantly lymphocytic pleocytosis with fewer than 200 cells/mm$^3$ [43,59,60,63,65,67,68,71–73]. Cell counts as high as 2600 cells/mm$^3$ have been recorded [56,63,64,67]. Increased protein concentration (up to 900 mg/dl) and a normal glucose concentration are generally observed [43,59,60,63,65,67,68,71–73].

In the majority of patients with WNV encephalitis, the EEG is abnormal [65,68]. Electroencephalographic abnormalities have included diffuse irregular slow waves, focal sharp waves, and subclinical electroencephalographic seizures. In patients with acute flaccid paralysis, electromyography and nerve conduction studies document evidence of denervation consisting of reduced compound muscle action potentials in association with normal sensory nerve action potentials consistent with anterior horn cell disease [59,66–68,73].

MRI scanning is considerably more sensitive than computed tomographic (CT) scanning in identifying CNS abnormalities in patients with WNV neuroinvasive disease. MRI scan findings include inflammation of the basal ganglia and, in particular, the thalamus and substantia nigra, leptomeningeal enhancement, and enhancement of the periventricular areas [59,60,63,68,86,87]. In a child with encephalitis, focal enhancement of the right temporal lobe was noted [78]. In a child with acute flaccid paralysis, MRI scan of the spine documented edema of the anterior horns of the cervical spinal cord [73].

The diagnosis of WNV infections is serologic [1,48]. The IgM capture ELISA is the most commonly used test. Virus-specific IgM antibody is present in the CSF and or serum of 40% of infected individuals by the fourth day after onset of illness and in virtually all individuals by day 10 of illness [1]. The finding of WNV-specific IgM in the CSF is diagnostic of acute infection. However, the same may not be said to be true of finding WNV IgM antibodies in serum. Virus-specific IgM has been shown to persist in serum for nearly a year and a half after primary infections [1,88]. When only serum is used for diagnosis, a second serum sample should be obtained at least 2 weeks later to document a four fold increase in specific antibody titers [62]. Because cross-reactions between SLE, WNV, and POW virus can occur [1], viral neutralization assays are required to determine the specific etiologic agent.

Viral culture is of limited use in the diagnosis of WNV infection because of its lack of sensitivity [60]. Nucleic amplification for diagnosis of WNV infection has met with similar limitations [38,60].

## Treatment

Treatment of WNV neuroinvasive syndromes is primarily supportive, with close attention to the monitoring of respiratory status. Patients with severe muscle weakness or paralysis may require mechanical ventilation. No specific antiviral therapy is currently available for the treatment of WNV neuroinvasive syndromes. Work in animal models suggests that intravenous immunoglobulin and interferon-α may be therapeutically efficacious [89,90]. An anecdotal report in humans suggests that the use of interferon-α2b may improve recovery from WNV encephalitis [91].

### Prevention

Prevention of WNV infection entails measures similar to those used for the prevention of SLE.

## *Powassan Encephalitis*

### Epidemiology

Powassan encephalitis is a rare CNS infection caused by POW virus, a tick-borne flavivirus first isolated from a 5-year-old Canadian boy [92] with fatal encephalitis. Approximately 30 cases of POW encephalitis were reported in North America between 1958 and 2002 [92–113]. The detection of recent cases is undoubtedly the result of increased testing for WNV-related neuroinvasive syndromes [112]. Approximately two thirds of all reported cases have occurred in children younger than 15 years of age; the majority of cases have occurred in male patients.

POW virus or a variant is endemic in Canada, the Eastern United States, Colorado, South Dakota [101,114] and Far Eastern Russia [114–116]. North American POW virus has been found in four species of *Ixotid* ticks and *Dermanacentor andersoni* [112,114]. Evidence of POW virus infection has been found in 38 species of mammals [112]. The principle vertebrate host is thought to be the groundhog (*Marmota monax*). The American red squirrel (*Tamiasciurus hudsonicus*) and the white-footed mouse (Peromyscus leucopus) may also be significant hosts [115].

### Clinical and Neurological Manifestations

Because of the diminutive size of *Ixodes* ticks, they are frequently overlooked and many patients fail to give a history of a tick bite. The reported incubation period of POW virus infection ranges from 8 to 34 days [94,95]. The onset of frank encephalitis may be heralded by a 1- to 3-day period of nonspecific symptoms such as fever, malaise, sore throat, lethargy, somnolence, myalgia, emesis, and headache. A fine macular erythematous rash has been described in some cases [101,103].

In both children and adults, infection with POW virus more commonly results in encephalitis or meningoencephalitis than in meningitis alone. All patients have evidence of an altered sensorium ranging from confusion or stupor to frank coma.

Evidence of meningeal irritation may be found in only a minority of cases. Seizures have been more commonly reported in children. The presence of pyramidal tract signs is common and focal palsies or pareses may occur.

Less frequently reported findings include nystagmus [92], facial palsy [95], ophthalmoplegia [112], and olfactory hallucinations [105]. Acute flaccid paralysis with permanent residua has also been reported [106].

The case fatality rate in POW encephalitis ranges from 10 to 15%. For cases with known outcome, approximately 60% have demonstrated significant short and long-term neurological sequelae. Reported short-term sequelae include apnea, psychosis, dysarthria, and spasticity.

Convalescence may be prolonged and long-term sequelae are common. These sequelae include spastic quadriplegia, headaches, hemiparesis, mental retardation, spastic aphasia, muscle weakness, ophthalmoplegia, cognitive difficulties, and memory dysfunction.

## Pathogenesis and Neuropathology

Only two reports contain information regarding the neuropathology of Powassan encephalitis [92,111]. Inflammatory changes were distributed diffusely throughout the brain. In one case, the cerebellum and spinal cord seemed to be less involved than other regions of the CNS [92]. In the other case, the mediotemporal lobes, ventral midbrain, and basal ganglia were the most involved areas [111]. Perivascular, mononuclear cell infiltrates and parenchymal infiltrates composed of macrophages, microglia, and rare polymorphonuclear cells have been noted. Neuronophagia and eosinophilic, neuronal inclusions were also observed.

## Diagnosis

Examination of the CSF reveals a lymphocytic pleocytosis of generally less than 200 cells/$mm^3$. In some cases, the initial CSF cell count may be normal, only to show a lymphocytic pleocytosis at repeat examination [92,111]. The CSF glucose level is normal and the protein level is generally mildly elevated (67–96 mg/dl).

EEG in patients with encephalitis has revealed generalized slow wave activity. In one report, localization of delta wave activity, in addition to focal neurological findings, suggested HSV encephalitis [105].

MRI scans in patients with POW encephalitis has revealed changes consistent with microvascular ischemia or demyelinating disease located in the parietal lobe in one case and temporal lobes in another [112]. CT scanning of the brain has not been useful.

Successful isolation of POW virus from postmortem brain tissue has been reported [92,100]. The principle diagnostic modality remains serology by documentation of POW specific IgM and neutralizing antibodies in CSF or serum. Virus-specific antibody detection is important to exclude other cross-reacting flaviviruses [117].

### Treatment

No antiviral therapy is currently available for the treatment of POW encephalitis. Treatment is supportive. Mechanical ventilation may be required because of apnea or failure to protect the airway. Anticonvulsant therapy has been used in patients *with seizures*.

### Prevention

Because transmission of POW virus to humans can only occur via a tick bite, prevention focuses on protection from tick bites using measures previously discussed.

# Bunyaviridae

The *Bunyaviridae* family is comprised of five genera: *Bunyavirus*, *Phebovirus*, *Nairoviurus*, *Hantavirus*, and *Tospovirus* [118]. The most important human CNS pathogens reside within the California serogroup of the *Bunyavirus* genus. These include La Crosse (LAC), California encephalitis, Jamestown Canyon, snowshoe hare (SH), trivittatus, and Keystone viruses.

## *La Crosse Encephalitis*

### Epidemiology

The etiology of LAC encephalitis is an RNA virus of the same name. The principal vector and reservoir of LAC virus is the eastern tree hole mosquito, *Ochlerotatus triseriatus* [119–121]. *Ae. Ablopicutus*, the tiger mosquito, may also be an accessory vector [122] in southeastern United States. Enzootic viral amplification occurs in various small mammal hosts: eastern chipmunk (*Tamias striatus*), grey squirrel (*Sciurus carolinensis*), and red fox (*Vulpes fulva*). Epizootic infections of humans are incidental and do not result in transmission to other humans. Most of the reported cases occur from July through September or early October.

In the United States, for the period spanning 1964 through 2002, an average of 76 LAC encephalitis cases were reported per year [119,120]. In 2002, a record 167 cases were reported from 16 states. This apparent increase may have been the result of increased human case surveillance for WNV infections [119,120]. Although cases of LAC encephalitis have predominately been reported from the northern midwestern states, 30 states reported at least one case from 1964 to 1996 [123,124]. Most recently, West Virginia has become the state reporting the highest number of LAC encephalitis cases per year.

In endemic areas, the annual incidence of the disease is approximately 10 to 30 per 100,000 in individuals younger than 15 years of age [125]. Approximately 98% of cases of LAC encephalitis occur in children and adolescents ≤14 years of age [124–128]. Male patients overwhelmingly account for the majority of cases in all reported series [125,128–131]. Factors associated with an increased risk of acquisition of LAC infection include residence in close proximity to the edge of a forest or within 100m of one or more tree holes [131], presence of artificial containers and discarded tires [124], and outdoor exposure.

## Clinical and Neurological Manifestations [125–127,129–133]

The incubation period for LAC encephalitis ranges from 5 to 15 days [124]. Only 0.3 to 4% of LAC virus infections result in symptomatic disease [124]. In the largest reported series of hospitalized children with LAC CNS disease, aseptic meningitis and meningoencephalitis each accounted for 13% of cases, whereas encephalitis accounted for the remaining 74% [124].

Typically, the onset of illness is characterized by a prodrome of 2- to 3-days duration comprised of fever (86–100%), headache (75–91%), malaise, and gastrointestinal symptoms (i.e., nausea, vomiting, and anorexia) (56–100%) [125–127, 129–132]. Lethargy or an altered sensorium follow in 42 to 100% of reported cases. Six to 33% of children will progress to frank coma. Seizures have been reported in between 46% and 62% of children. These may be generalized, focal, partial, partial complex, or status epilepticus. Balfour et al. described a subset of patients whose presentation was that of a sudden onset of fever and headache, followed 12 to 24 hours later by the abrupt onset of focal or generalized seizures that were prolonged and difficult to control [127].

Between 24% and 60% of children have signs of meningeal irritation. Focal neurological findings occur in 16 to 25% of cases. Other less frequently encountered neurological abnormalities include photophobia, cranial nerve pareses, hemiparesis, aphasia, dysarthria, chorea, ataxia, and altered deep tendon reflexes.

In the largest and most recently reported series of children with LAC encephalitis, 11% of children had clinical deterioration within 4 days of admission to the hospital [125]. Factors associated with clinical deterioration included a history of vomiting and a lower Glasgow Coma Scale score on admission. Nearly 60% of hospitalized children required admission to the intensive care unit. One quarter required mechanical ventilation and 17% received mannitol for control of intracranial hypertension.

The overall case fatality rate in LAC infection is less than 1%, but may approach 1% in hospitalized patients [124]. Neurological sequelae have been reported in 12 to 46% of children [125,127,129]. The early convalescent period may be complicated by emotional lability, irritability, personality problems, and headaches [126,132]. In addition to recurrent seizures and hemiparesis, long-term sequelae, such as cognitive and neurobehavioral abnormalities (i.e., attention-deficit–hyperactivity disorder) have been reported [125,127,130]. Neurological findings reported at follow-up have included extraneous movements, poor fine-finger coordination, and mild reflex asymmetries [129]. Long-term EEG abnormalities have been reported in up to one third of children with LAC encephalitis [134].

## Pathogenesis and Neuropathology

The G1 glycoprotein of the viral envelope serves as the viral attachment protein to mammalian cells [135]. Animal data suggest that the M RNA segment that encodes this protein may be a determinant of neurovirulence, as may be the L RNA segment of LAC virus that encodes the viral RNA-dependent RNA polymerase [136]. Death of infected neurons may be the result of apoptosis [137].

Information regarding the neuropathologic findings of LAC encephalitis is based on postmortem specimens from two fatal cases and a brain biopsy specimen [127,138–140]. On gross examination, the brain is swollen, with congested leptomeninges. Histologic changes are confined to the cerebral cortex and basal ganglia. Involvement of the brainstem is present, particularly in the pons. Perivascular mononuclear cell cuffing is observed within the cerebrum and meninges. Degenerating neurons and neuronophagia are also observed, surrounded by polymorphonuclear, mononuclear, and microglial cells. Confluent patches of inflammatory cells and perivascular edema are widely distributed. The spinal cord is grossly congested. Petechial hemorrhages may be present in the cervical cord.

## Diagnosis

CSF analysis generally reveals a lymphocytic pleocytosis, usually less than 200 cells/mm$^3$ [125–127,129–133]. The CSF glucose level was normal and protein level mildly increased in the minority of all reported cases [125–127,129–133]. The peripheral white cell count may reveal a leukocytosis in association with predominance of polymorphonuclear cells, but it is not useful in differentiating LAC encephalitis from other CNS infections.

EEG abnormalities are seen in the majority of cases of LAC encephalitis [125–127,129–133]. In one report, nearly half of those with abnormal EEGs had findings suggestive of HSV encephalitis; focality or periodic lateralizing epileptiform discharges, which were usually localized to the temporal lobe [125].

CT scanning of the brain may be less sensitive than MRI scanning for the detection of focal lesions in the brain [124]. In one study, only 11 (12%) of 92 children had changes on CT scan in comparison with 4 of 10 children who had abnormalities identified using MRI scanning with gadolinium enhancement. It is important to note that in three of the children in whom abnormalities were seen, these were only detected after cerebral herniation. Abnormal findings on CT scan include generalized, focal, or multifocal edema. MRI scans with enhancement reveals focal areas of enhancement predominantly located in the cortical areas.

LAC virus has been difficult to isolate from CSF and brain tissue of human cases. The diagnosis of LAC encephalitis is established though serologic methods seeking the presence of viral-specific IgM in the CSF or serum. Ninety-three percent of patients have detectable IgM virus specific antibodies by the 5th day of illness [141]. As with WNV, IgM in serum may persist for more than 6 months.

### Treatment

Because of the risk of progressive worsening of neurological status in 5 to 15% of cases, close observation with frequent neurological monitoring is a key component of the management of children with LAC encephalitis [125,141]. Deterioration of the Glasgow Coma score should warrant transfer to an intensive care setting, if the child in not already there. Attention to airway patency is critical. In one report, 25% of children with LAC encephalitis required mechanical ventilation [125]. In severe cases, monitoring of intracranial pressure may be warranted. Close attention to fluid and electrolyte status is important because the development of hyponatremia and the syndrome of inappropriate antidiuretic hormone (SIADH) have been documented [125,142]. Seizures should be treated with anticonvulsants.

Although no proven therapy exists, one case report has suggested that ribavirin may be a therapeutic consideration in patients with confirmed LAC encephalitis [140].

### Prevention

Prevention of LAC encephalitis focuses on eliminating mosquito breeding sites and use of personal protective measures delineated for SLE.

## *CNS Infections Caused by Minor Members of the California Serogroup*

Other members of the California serogroup that have been associated with CNS infections include California encephalitis, Jamestown Canyon, SH, trivittatus, and Keystone viruses [142]. Only four cases of California encephalitis have been reported, of which two occurred in children, and all have been in California [143,144]. Both children had diagnoses of encephalitis that resulted in significant neurological sequelae in one.

Jamestown Canyon virus (JCV) has been identified in enzootic cycles in at least 13 states in the United States and six provinces in Canada and may be under diagnosed [145,146]. In contrast to LAC encephalitis, JCV encephalitis occurs primarily in adults; only a handful of cases have been reported in children or adolescents [145–148]. In adults, a respiratory prodrome may precede the onset of CNS symptoms [146].

SH virus, a virus closely related to LAC virus, is widely distributed across Canada and has been reported in several states in the United States that border Canada [149]. The majority of the reported cases of SH CNS infections have occurred in children and resulted in mild encephalitis [149–152].

CNS infections caused by trivittatus and Keystone viruses seem to be very rare events and occur even less frequently than California virus encephalitis [148,152].

## References


1. Tsai TF, Chandler. Arboviruses. *Manual of Clinical Microbiology*. 2003. Murray PR, Baron J, Jorgensen JH, Pfaller MA, Yolken RH (eds). 8th ed. American Society for Microbiology Press, Washington, DC, pp 1553–1569.
2. Brinker KR, Monath TP. The acute disease. *St. Louis Encephalitis*. 1980. Monath TP (ed). American Public Health Association, Washington, DC, pp 503–534.
3. Heinz FX, Collett MS. Purcell RH, Gould EA, Howard CR, Houghton M, Moorman RJM, Rice CM, Thiel HJ. Family Flaviviridae. Virus Taxonomy. *Seventh Report of the International Committee on Taxonomy of Viruses*. 2000. van Regenmortel, Fauquet CM, Bishop HL, Carstens EB, Estes MK, Lemon SM, Maniloff J, Mayo MA, McGeoch DJ, Pringle CR, Wickner RB (eds). Academic Press, San Diego, CA, pp 859–878.
4. Muckenfuss RS, Armstrong C, McCordock HA. Encephalitis: Studies on experimental transmission. *Public Health Reports* 1933; 48:1341–1343.
5. Webster LT, Fite GL. A virus encountered in the study of material from cases of encephalitis in the St. Louis and Kansas City Epidemics of 1933. *Science* 1933; 78:463–465.
6. Muckenfuss RS. Clinical observations and laboratory investigations of the 1933 epidemic of encephalitis in St. Louis. *Bulletin of the New York Academy of Medicine* 1934; 10:444–453.
7. Report on the St. Louis outbreak of encephalitis. 1935. Public Health Bulletin No. 214, U.S. Government Printing Office, Washington, D.C.
8. Hammon WM, Reeves WC, Brookman B, Izumi EM. Isolation of viruses of Western and St. Louis encephalitis from Culex tarsalis mosquitos. *Science* 1941; 94:328–330.
9. Reeves WC, Hammon WM, Izumi EM. Experimental transmission of St. Louis encephalitis virus by Culex pipien Linnaeus. *Proc Soc Exper Biol & Med* 1942; 50:125–128.
10. Karabatsos N. General characteristics and antigenic relationships. *St. Louis Encephalitis*. 1980. Monath TP (ed). American Public Health Association, Washington, DC, pp 105–158.
11. Monath TP, Tsai T. Flaviviruses. *Clinical Virology*. 2002. Richman DD, Whitley RJ, Hayden FG (eds). 2nd Edition. American Society for Microbiology, Washington, DC, pp 1097–1151.
12. Monath TP. Epidemiology. *St. Louis Encephalitis*. 1980. Monath TP (ed). American Public Health Association, Washington, DC, pp 239–312.
13. Monath TP, Cropp CB, Bowen GS, Kemp GE, Mitchell CJ, Gardner JJ. Variation in virulence for mice and rhesus monkeys among St. Louis encephalitis virus strains of different origin. *Am J Trop Med Hyg* 1980; 29:948–962.
14. Trent DW, Monath TP, Bowen GS, Vorndam AV, Cropp CB, Kemp GE. Variation among strains of St. Louis encephalitis virus: basis for a genetic, pathogenetic, and epidemiologic classification. *Ann N Y Acad Sci* 1980; 354:219–237.
15. Centers for Disease Control and Prevention: Summary of Notifiable Diseases-United States, 2001. *MMWR* 2003; 50:1–110.
16. Centers for Disease Control and Prevention: Summary of Notifiable Diseases-United States, 2002. *MMWR* 2004; 51:1–84.
17. Reisen WK. Epidemiology of St. Louis Encephalitis virus. *Advances in Viral Research: The Flavivirus: Detection, Diagnosis and Vaccine Development* 2003; 61:139–183.

18. Barret FF, Yow MD, Phillips CA. St. Louis encephalitis in children during the 1964 epidemic. *JAMA* 1965; 193:381–385.
19. Blattner RJ, Heys FM. St. Louis encephalitis: occurrence in children in the St. Louis area during nonepidemic years 1939-1944. *JAMA* 1945; 129:854–857.
20. Kaplan AM, Longhurst WL, Randall DL. Saint Louis encephalitis in children. *West J Med* 1978; 128:279–281.
21. Brady MT, Romelia M. Premortem isolation of Saint Louis encephalitis virus: case report and implications for hospital and laboratory personnel. *Pediatr Infect Dis* 1985; 4:548–550.
22. Southern PM, Jr., Smith JW, Luby JP, Barnett JA, Sanford JP. Clinical and laboratory features of epidemic St. Louis encephalitis. *Ann Intern Med* 1969; 71:681–689.
23. Quick DT, Thompson JM, Bond JO. The 1962 epidemic of St. Louis Encephalitis in Florida. IV. Clinical features of cases occurring in the Tampa Bay Area. *Am J Epidemiol* 1965; 681:415–427.
24. Leake JP, Musson EK, Chope HD. Epidemiology of epidemic encephalitis, St. Louis type. *JAMA* 1934; 103:728–731.
25. Beckman JW. Neurologic aspects of the epidemic of encephalitis in St. Louis. *Arch Neurol Psychiatry* 1935; 33:732–751.
26. Bredeck JF, Broun GO, Hempelmann TC, McFadden JF, Spector HI. Follow up studies of the 1933 St. Louis epidemic of encephalitis. *JAMA* 1938; 111:15–17.
27. Azar GJ, Bond JO, Chappell GL, Lawton AH. Follow-up studies of St. Louis encephalitis in Florida: Health questionnaire findings. *Ann Intern Med* 1965; 63:212–220.
28. Finley KH, Riggs N. Convalescence and Sequelae. *St. Louis Encephalitis*. 1980. Monath TP (ed). American Public Health Association, Washington, DC, pp 535–550.
29. Townsend TE, Bishop TP, Higdem BD et al. St. Louis encephalitis outbreak- Arkansas. *MMWR* 1991; 40:605–607.
30. Gardner JJ, Reyes MG. Pathology. *St. Louis Encephalitis*. 1980. Monath TP (ed). American Public Health Association, Washington, DC, pp 551–559.
31. Suzuki M, Phillips CA. St. Louis encephalitis. A histopathologic study of the fatal cases from the Houston epidemic in 1964. *Arch Pathol* 1966; 81:47–54.
32. Tsai TF. Flaviviruses. *Textbook of Pediatric Infectious Diseases*. Feigin RD, Cherry JD, Demmler GJ, Kaplan SL (eds). 5th ed. Saunders, Philadelphia, PA, 2003. pp 2189–2231.
33. Dropolic B, Masters CL. Entry of neurotropic arboviruses into the central nervous system: an in vitro study using mouse brain endothelium. *J Infect Dis* 1990; 16:685–691.
34. Parquet MC, Kumatori A, Hasebe F, Mathenge EG, Morita K. St. Louis encephalitis virus induced pathology in cultured cells. *Arch Virol* 2002; 147:1105–1119.
35. Brinker KR, Paulson G, Monath TP, Wise G, Fass RJ. St Louis encephalitis in Ohio, September 1975: clinical and EEG studies in 16 cases. *Arch Intern Med*; 139:561–566.
36. Wasay M, Diaz-Arrastia R, Suss RA, Kojan S, Haq A, Burns D, Van Ness P. St Louis Encephalitis: A review of 11 cases in a 1995 Dallas, Tex, epidemic. *Arch Neurol* 2000; 57:114–118.
37. Cerna F, Mehrad B, Luby JP, Burns D, Fleckenstein JL. St. Louis encephalitis and the substantia nigra: MR imaging evaluation. *AJNR Am J Neuroradiol* 1999; 20:1281–1283.
38. Lanciotti RS. Molecular amplification assays for the detection of flaviviruses. *Advances in Viral Research: The Flavivirus: Detection, Diagnosis and Vaccine Development* 2003; 61:67–99.
39. Kuno G. Serodiagnosis of flaviviral infections and vaccinations in humans. *Advances in Viral Research: The Flavivirus: Detection, Diagnosis and Vaccine Development* 2003; 61:3–65.
40. Rahal JJ, Anderson J, Rosenberg C, Reagan T, Thompson LL. Effect of Interferon-α2b therapy on St. Louis viral meningoencephalitis: clinical and laboratory results of a pilot study. *J Infect Dis* 2004; 190:1084–1087.
41. Smithburn KC, Hughes TP, Burke AW, Paul JH. A neurotropic virus isolated from the blood of a native of Uganda. *Am J Trop Med* 1940; 20:471–492.
42. Smithburn KC. Differentiation of the West Nile virus from the viruses of St. Louis and Japanese B encephalitis. *J Immunol* 1942; 44:25–31.

43. Asnis DS, Conetta R, Teixeira AA, Waldman G, Sampson BA. The West Nile Virus outbreak of 1999 in New York: the Flushing Hospital experience. *Clin Infect Dis* 2000; 30:413–418.
44. Hayes CG. West Nile virus: Uganda, 1937, to New York City, 1999. *Ann N Y Acad Sci*. 2001; 951:25–37.
45. Spigland I, Jasinska-Klingberg W, Hofsbi E, Goldblum N. Clinical and laboratory observations in an outbreak of West Nile fever in Israel. *Harefuah* 1958; 54:275–281.
46. Tsai TF, Popovici F, Cernescu C, Campbell GL, Nedelcu NI. West Nile encephalitis epidemic in southeastern Romania. *Lancet* 1998; 352:767–771.
47. Hayes EB. West Nile virus disease in children. *Pediatr Infect Dis J*. 2006; 2511:1065–1066.
48. Granwehr BP, Lillibridge KM, Higgs S, Mason PW, Aronson JF, Campbell GA, Barrett AD. West Nile virus: Where are we now? *Lancet Infect Dis* 2004; 4:547–556.
49. Centers for Disease Control and Prevention. Possible West Nile virus transmission to an infant through breast-feeding-Michigan, 2002. *MMWR*. 2002; 51:877–878.
50. Centers for Disease Control and Prevention. Investigations of West Nile virus infections in recipients of blood transfusion and organ transplantation. *MMWR* 2002; 51:884–895.
51. Centers for Disease Control and Prevention. Intrauterine West Nile virus infection—New York, 2002. *MMWR* 2002; 51:1135–1136.
52. Iwamoto M, Jernigan DB, Guasch A, Trepka MJ, Blackmore CG, Hellinger WC, Pham SM, Zaki S, Lanciotti RS, Lance-Parker SE, DiazGranados CA, Winquist AG, Perlino CA, Wiersma S, Hillyer KL, Goodman JL, Marfin AA, Chamberland ME, Petersen LR. Transmission of West Nile virus from an organ donor to four transplant recipients. *N Engl J Med* 2003; 348:2196–2203.
53. Harrington T, Kuehnert MJ, Kamel H, Lanciotti RS, Hands S, Currier M, Chamberland ME, Petersen LR, Marfin AA. West Nile virus infection transmitted by blood transfusion. *Transfusion* 2003; 43:1018–1022.
54. Pealer LN, Marfin AA, Petersen LR, Lanciotti RS, Page PL, Stramer SL, Stobierski MG, Signs K, Newman B, Kapoor H, Goodman JL, Chamberland ME; West Nile Virus Transmission Investigation Team. Transmission of West Nile virus through blood transfusion in the United States in 2002. *N Engl J Med* 2003; 349:1236–1245.
55. Alpert SG, Fergerson J, Noel LP. Intrauterine West Nile virus: ocular and systemic findings. *Am J Ophthalmol* 2003; 136:733–735.
56. Campbell GL, Marfin AA, Lanciotti, RS, Gubler DJ. West Nile virus. *Lancet Infect Dis* 2002; 2:519–529.
57. Komar N. West Nile virus: Epidemiology and ecology in North America. *Advances in Viral Research: The Flavivirus: Detection, Diagnosis and Vaccine Development* 2003; 61:185–234.
58. Watson JT, Pertel PE, Jones RC, Siston AM, Paul WS, Austin CC, Gerber SI. Clinical characteristics and functional outcomes of West Nile Fever. *Ann Intern Med* 2004; 141:360–365.
59. Nash D, Mostashari F, Fine A, Miller J, O'Leary D, Murray K, Huang A, Rosenberg A, Greenberg A, Sherman M, Wong S, Layton M; 1999 West Nile Outbreak Response Working Group. The outbreak of West Nile virus infection in the New York City area in 1999. *N Engl J Med* 2001; 344:1807–1814.
60. Petersen LR, Marfin AA. West Nile virus: a primer for the clinician. *Ann Intern Med* 2002; 137:173–179.
61. Yim R, Posfay-Barbe KM, Holt D, Fatula G, Wald ER. Spectrum of clinical manifestations of West Nile virus infection in children. *Pediatrics* 2004; 4:1673–1675.
62. Hayes EB, O'Leary DR. West Nile virus infection: a pediatric perspective. *Pediatrics* 2004; 113:1375–1381.
63. Weiss D, Carr D, Kellachan J, Tan C, Phillips M, Bresnitz E, Layton M, West Nile Virus Outbreak Response Working Group. Clinical findings of West Nile virus infection in hospitalized patients, New York and New Jersey, 2000. *Emerg Infect Dis* 2001; 7:654–658.
64. Chowers MY, Lang R, Nassar F, Ben-David D, Giladi M, Rubinshtein E, Itzhaki A, Mishal J, Siegman-Igra Y, Kitzes R, Pick N, Landau Z, Wolf D, Bin H, Mendelson E, Pitlik SD,

Weinberger M. Clinical characteristics of the West Nile fever outbreak, Israel, 2000. *Emerg Infect Dis* 2001; 7:675–678.
65. Klein C, Kimiagar I, Pollak L, Gandelman-Marton R, Itzhaki A, Milo R, Rabey JM. Neurological features of West Nile virus infection during the 2000 outbreak in a regional hospital in Israel. *J Neurol Sci* 2002; 200:63–66.
66. Centers for Disease Control and Prevention. Acute flaccid paralysis syndrome associated with West Nile virus infection–Mississippi and Louisiana, July–August 2002. *MMWR* 2002; 51:825–828.
67. Sejvar JJ, Leis AA, Stokic DS, Van Gerpen JA, Marfin AA, Webb R, Haddad MB, Tierney BC, Slavinski SA, Polk JL, Dostrow V, Winkelmann M, Petersen LR. Acute flaccid paralysis and West Nile virus infection. *Emerg Infect Dis* 2003; 9:788–793.
68. Sejvar JJ, Haddad MB, Tierney BC, Campbell GL, Marfin AA, Van Gerpen JA, Fleischauer A, Leis AA, Stokic DS, Petersen LR. Neurologic manifestations and outcome of West Nile virus infection. *JAMA* 2003; 290:511–515.
69. Carey DE, Rodrigues FM, Myers RM, Webb JK. Arthropod-borne viral infections in children in Vellore, South India, with particular reference to dengue and West Nile viruses. *Indian Pediatr* 1968; 5:285–296.
70. George S, Gourie-Devi M, Rao JA, Prasad SR, Pavri KM. Isolation of West Nile virus from the brains of children who had died of encephalitis. *Bull World Health Organ* 1984; 62:879–882.
71. Vidwan G, Bryant KK, Puri V, Stover BH, Rabalais GP. West Nile virus encephalitis in a child with left-side weakness. *Clin Infect Dis* 2003; 37:91–94.
72. Weinstein M. Atypical West Nile virus infection in a child. *Pediatr Infect Dis J* 2003; 22:842–844.
73. Heresi GP, Mancias P, Mazur LJ, Butler IJ, Murphy JR, Cleary TG. Poliomyelitis-like syndrome in a child with West Nile virus infection. *Pediatr Infect Dis J* 2004; 23:788–789.
74. Horga MA, Fine A. West Nile virus. *Pediatr Infect Dis J* 2001; 20:801–802.
75. Francisco AM, Glaser C, Frykman E, et al. 2004 California pediatric West Nile virus case series. *Pediatr Infect Dis J*. 2006; 25:81–84.
76. Civen R, Villacorte F, Robles DT, et al. West Nile virus infection in the pediatric population. *Pediatr Infect Dis J*. 2006; 25:75–78.
77. LaBeaud AD, Lisgaris MV, King CH, Mandalakas AM. Pediatric West Nile virus infection: neurologic disease presentations during the 2002 epidemic in Cuyahoga County, Ohio. *Pediatr Infect Dis J* 2006; 25:751–753.
78. Fratkin JD, Leis AA, Stokic DS, Slavinski SA, Geiss RW. Spinal cord neuropathology in human West Nile virus infection. *Arch Pathol Lab Med* 2004; 128:533–537.
79. Spiegel R, Miron D, Gavriel H, Horovitz Y. West Nile virus meningoencephalitis complicated by motor aphasia in Hodgkin's lymphoma. *Arch Dis Child* 2002; 86:441–442.
80. Eldadah AH, Nathanson N. Pathogenesis of West Nice virus encephalitis in mice and rats: II, virus multiplication, evolution of immunofluorescence, and development of histological lesions in the brain. *Am J Epidemiol* 1967; 86:776–790.
81. Diamond MS, Shrestha B, Marri A, Mahan D, Engle M. B cells and antibody play critical roles in the immediate defense of disseminated infection by West Nile encephalitis virus. *J Virol* 2003; 77:2578–2586.
82. Xiao SY, Guzman H, Zhang H, Travassos da Rosa AP, Tesh RB. West Nile virus infection in the golden hamster *(Mesocricetusauratus)*: a model for West Nile encephalitis. *Emerg Infect Dis* 2001; 7:714–721.
83. Ratterree MS, Gutierrez RA, Travassos da Rosa AP, Dille BJ, Beasley DW, Bohm RP, Desai SM, Didier PJ, Bikenmeyer LG, Dawson GJ, Leary TP, Schochetman G, Phillippi-Falkenstein K, Arroyo J, Barrett AD, Tesh RB. Experimental infection of rhesus macaques with West Nile virus: level and duration of viremia and kinetics of the antibody response after infection. *J Infect Dis* 2004; 189:669–676.
84. Omalu BI, Ghakir AA, Wang G, Lipkin WI, Wiley CA. Fatal fulminant pan-meningopolioencephalitis due to West Nile virus. *Brain Pathol* 2003; 13:465–472.

85. Shrestha B, Gottlieb D, Diamond MS. Infection and injury of neurons by West Nile encephalitis virus. *J Virol* 2003; 77:13203–13213.
86. Bosanko CM, Gilroy J, Wang AM, Sanders W, Dulai M, Wilson J, Blum K. West Nile virus encephalitis involving the substantia nigra: neuroimaging and pathologic findings with literature review. *Arch Neurol* 2003; 60:1448–1452.
87. Solomon T. Flavivirus encephalitis. *N Engl J Med* 2004; 351:370–378.
88. Roehrig JT, Nash D, Maldin B, Labowitz A, Martin DA, Lanciotti RS, Campbell GL. Persistence of virus-reactive serum immunoglobulin M antibody in confirmed West Nile virus encephalitis cases. *Emerg Infect Dis* 2003; 9:376–379.
89. Morrey JD, Day CW, Julander JG, Blatt LM, Smee DF, Sidwell RW. Effect of interferon-alpha and interferon-inducers on West Nile virus in mouse and hamster animal models. *Antivir Chem Chemother* 2004; 15:101–109.
90. Ben-Nathan D, Lustig S, Tam G, Robinzon S, Segal S, Rager-Zisman B. Prophylactic and therapeutic efficacy of human intravenous immunoglobulin in treating West Nile virus infection in mice. *J Infect Dis* 2003; 188:5–12.
91. Sayao AL, Suchowersky O, Al-Khathaami A, Klassen B, Katz NR, Sevick R, Tilley P, Fox J, Patry D. Calgary experience with West Nile virus neurological syndrome during the late summer of 2003. *Can J Neurol Sci* 2004; 31:194–203.
92. McLean DM, Donahue WL. Powassan virus: isolation of virus from a fatal case of encephalitis. *CMAJ* 1959; 80:708–711.
93. Goldfield M, Austin SM, Black HC, Taylor BF, Altman R. A non-fatal human case of Powassan virus encephalitis. *Am J Trop Med Hyg* 1973; 22:78–81.
94. Smith R, Woodall JP, Whitney E, Deibel R, Gross MA, Smith V, Bast TF. Powassan virus infection. A report of three human cases of encephalitis. *Am J Dis Child* 1974; 127: 691–693.
95. Rossier E, Harrison RJ, Lemieux B. A case of Powassan virus encephalitis. *CMAJ* 1974; 110:1173–1174.
96. Deibel R, Flanagan TD, Smith V. Central nervous system infections in New York State. Etiologic and epidemiologic observations, 1974. *N Y State J Med* 1975; 75:2337–2342.
97. Conway D, Rossier E. A case report: Powassan virus encephalitis with shoulder girdle involvement. *Can Dis Wkly Rep* 1976; 2-22:85–87.
98. Rossier E. Thyphoid—New Brunswick. *Can Dis Wkly Rep* 1976; 2:202–203.
99. Deibel R, Flanagan TD, Smith V. Central nervous system infections. Etiologic and epidemiologic observations in New York State, 1975. *NY State J Med* 1977; 77:1398–1404.
100. Deibel R, Srihongse S, Woodall JP. Arboviruses in New York State: An attempt to determine the role of arboviruses in patients with viral encephalitis and meningitis. *Am J Trop Med Hyg* 1979; 28:577–582.
101. Mahdy MS, Wilson M, Wherrett B, Dorland R. Powassan virus (POWV) encephalitis in Ontario: A case of meningoencephalitis attributed to infection with POWV in eastern Ontario. *Arboviral Encephalitides in Ontario with Special Reference to St. Louis Encephalitis.* 1979. Mahdy MS, Spence L, Joshua JM (eds). Ministry of Health, Ontario, Canada.
102. Joshua JM. A case of Powassan virus encephalitis-Ontario. *Can Dis Wkly Rep* 1979; 5-30:129–130.
103. Partington MW, Thomson V, O'Shaughnessy MV. Powassan virus encephalitis in southeastern Ontario. *CMAJ* 1980; 123:603–606.
104. Mahdy MS, Bansen E, McLaughlin B. California and Powassan virus disease in Ontario, 1977-1980. *Can Dis Wkly Rep* 1982; 8-38:185–191.
105. Embil JA, Camfield P, Artsob H, Chase DP. Powassan virus encephalitis resembling herpes simplex encephalitis. *Arch Intern Med* 1983; 143:341–343.
106. Jackson AC. Leg weakness associated with Powassan virus infection—Ontario. *Can Dis Wkly Rep* 1989; 15:123–124.
107. Artsob H. Powassan Encephalitits. *The Arboviruses: Epidemiology and Ecology.* 1989. Monath TP (ed). Volume IV. CRC Press, Inc., Boca Raton, FL, pp 30–49.

108. Fitch WM, Artsob H. Powassan encephalitis in New Brunswick. *Can Fam Physician* 1990; 36:1289–1990.
109. Arboviral disease—United States, 1994. *MMWR* 1995; 44:641–644.
110. Kolski H, Ford-Jones EL, Richardson S, Petric M, Nelson S, Jamieson F, Blaser S, Gold R, Otsubo H, Heurter H, MacGregor D. Etiology of acute childhood encephalitis at The Hospital for Sick Children, Toronto, 1994-1995. *Clin Infect Dis* 1998; 26:398–409.
111. Gholam BI, Puksa S, Provias JP. Powassan encephalitis: A case report with neuropathology and literature review. *CMAJ* 1999; 161:1419–1422.
112. Outbreak of Powassan encephalitis—Maine and Vermont, 1999-2001. *MMWR* 2001; 50:761–764.
113. Ford-Jones EL, Fearon M, Leber C, Dwight P, Myszak M, Cole B, Greene PB, Artes S, McGeer A, D'Cunha C, Naus M. Ontario West Nile Virus Working Group. Human surveillance for West Nile virus infection in Ontario in 2000. *CMAJ* 2002; 166:29–35.
114. Gritsun TS, Nuttall PA, Gould EA. Tick-Borne Flaviviruses. *Advances in Viral Research: The Flavivirus: Detection, Diagnosis and Vaccine Development* 2003; 61:318–324.
115. Shope RE. Epidemiology of other arthropod-borne flaviviruses infecting humans. *Advances in Viral Research: The Flavivirus: Detection, Diagnosis and Vaccine Development* 2003; 82:1657–1665.
116. Ebel GD, Spielman A, Telford SR 3rd. Phylogeny of North American Powassan virus. *J Gen Virol* 2001; 82:1657–1665.
117. Ralph ED. Powassan encephalitis. *CMAJ*. 1999; 161:1416–1417.
118. Mertz GJ. Bunyaviridae: Bunyaviruses, Phleboviruses, Nairoviruses, and Hantaviruses. *Clinical Virology*. 2002. Richman DD, Whitley RJ, Hayden FG (eds). 2nd Ed. American Society for Microbiology Press, Washington DC, pp 921–947.
119. Pantuwatana S, Thompson WH, Watts DM, Yuill TM, Hanson RP. Isolation of La Crosse virus from field collected Aedes triseriatus larvae. *Am J Trop Med Hyg*. 1974; 23:246–250.
120. Watts DM, Thompson WH, Yuill TM, DeFoliart GR, Hanson RP. Overwintering of La Crosse virus in Aedes triseriatus. *Am J Trop Med Hyg*. 1974; 23:694–700.
121. Thompson WH, Beaty BJ. Venereal transmission of La Crosse (California encephalitis) arbovirus in Aedes triseriatus mosquitoes. *Science* 1977; 196:530–531.
122. Gerhardt RR, Gottfried KL, Apperson CS, et al: First isolation of La Crosse virus from naturally infected Aedes albopictus. *Emerg Infect Dis* 2001; 7:807–811.
123. LeDuc JW. Epidemiology and ecology of the California serogroup viruses. *Am J Trop Med Hyg* 1987; 37:60S–68S.
124. McJunkin JE, Khan RR, Tsai TF. California-La Crosse encephalitis. *Infect Dis Clin North Am* 1998; 12:83–93.
125. McJunkin JE, de los Reyes EC, Irazuzta JE, et al: La Crosse encephalitis in children. *N Engl J Med* 2001; 344:801–807.
126. Cramblett HG, Stegmiller H, Spencer C: California encephalitis virus infections in children. Clinical and laboratory studies. *JAMA* 1966; 198:108–112.
127. Balfour HH Jr, Siem RA, Bauer H, et al: California arbovirus (La Crosse) infections. I. Clinical and laboratory findings in 66 children with meningoencephalitis. *Pediatrics* 1973; 52:680–691.
128. Srihongse S, Grayson MA, Deibel R: California serogroup viruses in New York State: the role of subtypes in human infections. *Am J Trop Med Hyg* 1984; 33:1218–1227.
129. Chun RW, Thompson WH, Grabow JD, et al: California arbovirus encephalitis in children. *Neurology* 1968; 18:369–375.
130. Balkhy HH, Schreiber JR. Severe La Crosse encephalitis with significant neurologic sequelae. *Pediatr Infect Dis J* 2000; 19:77–80.
131. Erwin PC, Jones TF, Gerhardt RR, Halford SK, Smith AB, Patterson LER, Gottfried KL, Burkhalter KL, Nasci RS, Schaffner W. La Crosse encephalitis in Eastern Tennessee: Clinical, environmental, and entomologic characteristics from a blinded cohort study. *Am J Epidemiol* 2002; 155, 1060–1065.

132. Hilty MD, Haynes RE, Azimi PH, Cramblett HG. California encephalitis in children. *Amer J Dis Child* 1972; 124:530–533.
133. Hardin SG, Erwin PC, Patterson L, New D, Graber C, Halford SK. Clinical comparisons of La Crosse encephalitis and enteroviral central nervous system infections in a pediatric population: 2001 surveillance in East Tennessee. *Am J Infect Control* 2003; 31: 508–510.
134. Grabow JD, Matthews CG, Chun RWM, Thompson WH. The electroencephalogram and clinical sequelae of California arbovirus encephalitis. *Neurology* 1969; 19:394–404.
135. Ludwig GV, Israel BA, Christensen BM, Yuill TM, Schultz KT. Role of La Crosse virus glycoproteins in attachment of virus to host cells. *Virology* 1991; 181:564–571.
136. Griot C, Pekosz A, Lukac D, Scherer SS, Stilmock K, Schmeidler D, Endres MJ, Gonzalez-Scarano F, Nathanson N. Polygenic control of neuroinvasiveness in California serogroup bunyaviruses. *J Virol* 1993; 67:3861–3867.
137. Pekosz A, Griot C, Stillmock, Nathanson N, Gonzalez-Scarano F. Protection from La Crosse virus encephalitis with recombinant glycoproteins: role of neutralizing anti-G1 antibodies. *J Virol* 1995; 69:3475–3481.
138. Thompson WH, Kalfayan B, Anslow RO: Isolation of California encephalitis group virus from a fatal human illlness. *Amer J Epidemiol* 1965; 81:245.
139. Kalfayan B. Pathology of La Crosse virus infection in humans. *California Serogroup Viruses*. 1983. Calisher CH, Thompson WH (eds). Alan R. Liss, Inc., New York, NY, pp 179–186.
140. McJunkin JE, Khan R, de los Reyes EC et al: Treatment of severe La Crosse encephalitis with intravenous ribavirin following diagnosis by brain biopsy. *Pediatrics* 1997; 99:261–267.
141. Rust RS, Thompson WH, Matthews CG, Beaty BJ, Chun RW. La Crosse and other forms of California encephalitis. *J Child Neurol* 1999; 14:1–14.
142. Hammon WM, Reeves WC. California encephalitis virus, a newly described agent. *Calif Med* 1952; 77:303–309.
143. Eldridge BF, Glaser C, Pedrin RE, Chiles RE. The first reported case of California encephalitis in more than 50 years. *Emerg Infect Dis* 2001; 7:451–452.
144. Calisher CH. Taxonomy, classification, and geographic distribution of California serogroup bunyaviruses. *Prog Clin Biol Res* 1983; 123:1–16.
145. Grimstad PR, Shabino CL, Calisher CH, Waldman RJ. A case of encephalitis in a human associated with a serologic rise to Jamestown Canyon virus. *Am J Trop Med Hyg* 1982; 31:1238–1244.
146. Deibel R, Srihongse S, Grayson MA, Grimstad PR, Mahdy MS, Artsob H, Calisher CH. Jamestown Canyon virus: the etiologic agent of an emerging human disease? *Prog Clin Biol Res* 1983; 123:313–325.
147. Srihongse S, Grayson MA, Deibel R. California serogroup viruses in New York State: the role of subtypes in human infections. *Am J Trop Med Hyg* 1984; 33:1218–1227.
148. Artsob H. Distribution of California serogroup viruses and virus infections in Canada. *Prog Clin Biol Res* 1983; 123:277–290.
149. Fauvel M, Artsob H, Calisher CH, Davignon L, Chagnon A, Skvorc-Ranko R, Belloncik S. California group virus encephalitis in three children from Quebec: clinical and serologic findings. *CMAJ* 1980; 122:60–64.
150. Artsob H, Spence L, Caughey WC, Wherrett JR. Aseptic meningitis in Ontario. *Can Med Assoc J* 1981; 125:958, 962.
151. Artsob H, Spence L, Surgeoner G, Helson B, Thorsen J, Grant L, Th'ng C. Snowshoe hare virus activity in Southern Ontario. *Can J Public Health* 1982; 73:345–349.
152. Gates EH, Bond JO, Lewis AL. California group arbovirus encephalitis in Florida children. *J Florida M A* 1968; 55:37–40.

# Chapter 5
# Togaviruses

**José R. Romero, M.D., F.A.A.P., Meera Varman, M.D., F.A.A.P., and Leslie L. Barton, M.D.**

## Eastern Equine Encephalitis

### *Introduction*

Eastern equine encephalitis (EEE) is a severe and devastating, insect-borne, arboviral neurological infection caused by eastern equine encephalitis virus (EEEV) [1–4]. Human infections (i.e., epizootic infection) by the arboviruses are incidental to the enzootic life cycle of the viruses and, with extremely rare exceptions, result in a "dead-end" infection without subsequent human-to-human transmission (Table 5.1).

### *Epidemiology*

EEEV is a member of the Alphavirus genus in the *Togaviridae* family of RNA viruses [5]. Recent evaluation of the EEEV complex indicates that it is composed of four antigenic subtypes [6]. Antigenic subtypes II to IV, distributed throughout Central and South America, do not seem to cause human disease. In contrast, antigenic subtype I, which is found in Canada, the eastern United States, and the Caribbean islands, has been clearly linked to serious central nervous system (CNS) infections in humans. The remainder of this section will focus on the North American subtype of EEEV.

The principal mosquito vector for avian enzootic EEEV transmission is *Culiseta melanura*. This species of mosquito is ornithophagic, feeding on wading and passerine birds that inhabit hardwood habitats of coastal and inland swamps. The geographic distribution of EEEV in North America coincides with its vector. Several mosquito species (*Aedes sollicitans, Aedes vexans, Aedes canadensis, and Coquillitidea perturbans*) serve for epizootic transmission of EEEV to horses, humans, and swine [6,7].

L.L. Barton and N.R. Friedman (eds.), *The Neurological Manifestations of Pediatric Infectious Diseases and Immunodeficiency Syndromes.*

**Table 5.1** Summary of Togaviridae associated with encephalitis

| | Geographic distribution | Mosquito vectors | Common signs and symptoms | Mortality in cases of encephalitis | Sequelae |
|---|---|---|---|---|---|
| Eastern equine encephalitis | Eastern and Gulf coasts and selected inland areas of the United States, Southern Mexico, Caribbean, and Central and South America | Culiseta<br>Aedes | Fever, headache, altered mental status, abdominal pain, seizures, periorbital and facial edema in infants, Brudzinski and Kernig signs | 30% to >80%, highest in infants and children | 1/3 to 1/2 of survivors |
| Western equine encephalitis | Western United States, Canada, endemic to the Western hemisphere | Culiseta<br>Culex | Fever, headache, seizures, nuchal rigidity, full fontanelle, tremulousness | Rare | 40% of infants |
| Venezuelan equine encephalitis | South and Central America, Mexico, Florida, and Southwestern United States | Aedes<br>Culex<br>Psorophora<br>Mansonia<br>Deinocerites | Fever, headache, chills, pharyngitis, myalgias, meningismus, cervical lymphadenitis | 10–15%, higher in children younger than 4 yr | |
| Sindbis | Europe, Africa, Asia, and Australia | Culex | Rash, polyarthritis, fever, myalgia; encephalitis (rare) | | Residual joint symptoms in up to 1/3 |

In the United States, EEE is a seasonal disease that occurs during the summer and early fall, primarily on the Atlantic and the Gulf coasts [7–9]. From 2000 to 2005, 62 cases of probable or confirmed EEE or meningitis were reported to the Centers for Disease Control and Prevention (CDC) [8,9]. Of these, approximately one third occurred in 2005. Early reports of EEE indicated that more than 80% of the cases were in children, 42% in infants at most 1 year of age [2,10]. Infants, children, and adolescents account for approximately 20% of the more recent cases [9,11,12]. These differences most likely are the result of lifestyle changes that have occurred during the latter half of the 20th century.

## *Clinical and Neurological Manifestations*

CNS disease is a relatively uncommon consequence of EEEV infection but seems to be age related. In one report, the overall ratio of clinical to subclinical EEEV infection was 1:23 [13]. For children younger than 4 years of age, the ratio of clinical to subclinical EEEV infection was 1:8. For individuals aged 5 to 14 years, the ratio was 1:26. Between the ages of 15 and 54 years, the ratio ranged from 1:>17 to 1:>47. Finally, for those individuals aged 55 years and older, the ratio was 1:16. Thus, in this study, young children and the elderly were at greatest risk to develop symptomatic disease if infected with EEEV.

The incubation period of EEE ranges from 3 to 10 days. The onset of neurological symptoms is preceded by a prodrome consisting of fever, headache, confusion, lethargy, myalgias, vomiting, and abdominal pain. In older children, adolescents, and adults, the prodrome generally lasts 5 to 7 days but has been reported to be as prolonged as 3 to 4 weeks [9,12,14]. In infants and young children, the prodromal period may be short or totally absent [2,9,11,14]. The onset of illness in these age groups is rapid and characterized by fever, altered mental status, seizures, vomiting, and cyanosis.

Fever is seen in more than 80% of cases and ranges from 39 °C to greater than 41 °C. Headache is almost always present in those old enough to report it. An unusual and interesting finding described in early reports of the illness in infants is the finding of periorbital, facial, and upper extremity edema [3,10]. This seemed to occur from 2 to 4 days after the onset of illness.

As the illness progresses, frank neurological findings become readily apparent. Signs of meningeal irritation, such as a positive Brudzinski or Kernig sign are present in up to 60% of patients. A bulging fontanelle is seen in infants. Fibrillation of muscle groups, twitching, spasticity, and rigidity are also frequent findings. Focal weakness, hemiplegia, hemiparesis, or flaccid or spastic paralysis may occur [7,11,12,14,15].

At least 90% of patients with encephalitis will progress to stupor or coma [2,9,10,12]. Seizures occur in 50 to 75% of patients [9,10,12]. These may be generalized, focal, or, rarely, partial complex in nature [12]. Cranial nerve palsies, in particular, cranial nerve VII, and oculomotor phenomena have been reported to also occur [12]. The loss of normal or the presence of abnormal spinal reflexes has been reported.

Of all North American causes of arboviral encephalitis, EEEV results in the most severe disease and has the highest case fatality rate. Several clinical and laboratory findings have been found to portend a poor outcome. The absence of a prodrome or the presence of an abbreviated prodrome as well as a rapid onset of deep coma have been reported to be associated with poor outcome [2,11]. The finding of burst suppression or disorganized background with delta slowing on electroencephalographic (EEG) evaluation also predicts poor outcome [11]. In more recent reports, elevated cerebrospinal fluid (CSF) white blood cell counts and the development of hyponatremia have been shown to be predictive of poor outcome [11].

Approximately one third to one half of survivors will have moderate to severe neurological sequelae. These sequelae include vegetative state, profound cognitive impairment, emotional lability, seizure disorders, spasticity, paralysis, motor weakness, cranial nerve palsy, blindness, deafness, and aphasia [2,3,7,9–11].

The reported mortality rates from larger series range from 36 to 68%, with infants and children having the highest rates [9,10,12,13]. In smaller series, mortality rates have exceeded 80% [14]. The lower mortality rates associated with EEE in the more recent literature may be a reflection of the inclusion of small numbers of pediatric patients and improvements in supportive care.

### *Neuropathology*

A composite summary [2,3,11,12,16] of the pathologic CNS findings of patients (mostly children) who have succumbed to EEE reveals that the brain may be edematous with meningeal congestion and an absence of pyogenic exudates. Microscopic examination of the meninges reveals infiltration with polymorphonuclear cells and large mononuclear cells. Microscopic examination of the brain documents perivascular cuffing. Polymorphonuclear cells, lymphocytes, and large mononuclear cells predominate early. As the disease progresses, the infiltrate becomes primarily lymphocytic and monocytic in nature. The spinal cord is spared in the majority of cases. Focal necrotic lesions consisting of polymorphonuclear cells and microglia are seen diffusely distributed in the brain. In severe cases, the lesions are noted in the basal ganglia, brainstem, and cerebral cortex.

## Western Equine Encephalitis

### *Introduction*

Western equine encephalitis (WEE) is caused by western equine encephalitis virus (WEEV), one of the 17 arboviruses known to cause CNS infections in humans in North America [17–20].

## *Epidemiology*

WEEV is a member of the Alphavirus genus in the *Togaviridae* family of RNA viruses [5]. The principal mosquito vector for avian enzootic WEEV transmission, *Culex tarsalis*, feeds on passerine birds (e.g., sparrows and house finches). As is the case with all arboviruses, WEE is a seasonal disease that parallels the activity of its vector and is seen during the summer and early fall.

In North America, WEEV is found in the western United States and Canada. Today, it is an extremely rare cause of encephalitis in humans [7,8,21]. From 1988 to 2004, only four cases were reported to the CDC. The last major outbreak of WEE in the United States occurred in 1987 in Colorado, during which, 41 cases were reported [7].

## *Clinical and Neurological Manifestations*

Children and the elderly are more likely to develop clinically apparent disease if infected with WEE [7,22]. The clinical to subclinical case ratio has been found to be 1:58 and 1:1150 for children younger than 4 years and for adults, respectively.

The incubation period of WEE ranges from 2 to 10 days. In newborns and infants, the onset of illness is typically abrupt [23–29]. Fever is almost universally present and may be as high as 41.7 °C. Seizures occur in 70 to 80% of infants and tend to be generalized and intractable. Physical examination generally reveals a lethargic or irritable infant with a full, tense fontanelle. Nuchal rigidity may be present in up to one third of cases. Increased muscle tone with generalized rigidity, hyperreflexia, and, at times, frank opisthotonus is noted.

In older children and adolescents, a prodromal period of 2 to 5 days consisting of fever, intense headache, nausea, vomiting, somnolence, and irritability may precede the onset of CNS manifestations [16,28]. Signs of meningeal irritation are present in 50 to 90% of children 2 years or older. Although seizures are common in infants, they tend to be less common in older patients, occurring in 10 to 15% of children older than the age of 5 years and adolescents. Seizures may be focal in nature. Focal neurological findings may mimic herpes simplex encephalitis. Paresis, palsy, spasticity, tremulousness, and decreased deep-tendon reflexes may be seen.

Transplacental transmission has been documented in three infants and suspected in two other infants [26,30,31]. These reports indicate that the mothers became ill 2 days before or on the day of delivery. All infants were healthy at birth and all became ill within the first week of life, with fever, seizures, bulging fontanelle, and nuchal rigidity.

Although the overall mortality associated with WEE has been reported to range from 3 to 15% [32,33], the sequelae are significant and seen more frequently in infants and children. In one report, 44% of infants younger than 3 months of age had extensive brain damage [7]. Reported sequelae have included severe mental retardation, persistent muscle weakness, persistent spasticity, cerebral atrophy, visual impairment, deafness, intracranial calcifications, and paralysis [25,26,28,29,34].

## *Neuropathology*

In one report of an infant with virologically confirmed WEE, brain biopsy revealed acute degeneration with infiltration of lymphocytes, microglia, and macrophages. No evidence of perivascular cuffing or glial proliferation was observed [29].

Postmortem examination, primarily of adult patients, reveals minimal gross findings [30,35,36]. The appearance of the brain and spinal cord may range from normal to minimally edematous with congestion of the vessels, or may show extreme vascular congestion. Microscopic examination reveals edema and mild mononuclear cell infiltration of the meninges and perivascular accumulation of cells throughout the vessels of the brain. One report indicated that polymorphonuclear perivascular cuffing was more common in the gray matter, whereas the vessels in the white matter exhibited more mononuclear perivascular cuffing [35]. Petechiae may be seen and are usually perivascular in location. Focal lesions consisting of polymorphonuclear cells are diffusely distributed throughout the brain. In the more severe lesions, there is tissue destruction with invasion of microglia.

## *Diagnosis*

### Eastern Equine Encephalitis

Examination of the CSF reveals increased pressure, protein levels, and white blood cells [2,3,11,12]. The CSF leukocyte count generally ranges from 200 cells/mm$^3$ to 2000 cells/mm$^3$, but may be as high as 4000 cells/mm$^3$. Polymorphonuclear cells predominate earlier and mononuclear cells later in the disease course.

EEG evaluation of patients demonstrates diffuse slowing consistent with a generalized encephalitis [11,12]. Focal slowing and periodic lateralizing epileptiform discharges have also been reported.

Neuroimaging documents abnormalities in the majority of patients. Magnetic resonance imaging (MRI) scanning is the modality of choice because it is more sensitive than computed tomographic (CT) scanning [12,37]. Focal lesions have been found in the basal ganglia (71%), thalami (71%), and brainstem (43%). Less commonly reported findings include cortical lesions, enhancement of the leptomeninges, and periventricular white matter changes.

### Western Equine Encephalitis

The CSF white cell count has been reported to be as high as 2000 cells/mm$^3$ but generally is less than 500 cells/mm$^3$. Interestingly, in infants, the CSF pleocytosis typically has a polymorphonuclear predominance whereas a lymphocytic pleocytosis predominates in older children and adolescents [25–28]. This may be a reflection of a more abrupt presentation in infants and, consequently, earlier examination of the CSF. The CSF glucose level is normal and the protein level may be normal or moderately increased.

Limited reports of EEG or modern neuroimaging findings in children exist. The EEG findings were markedly abnormal in one case and demonstrated multifocal spikes, polyspikes, and slow waves [29]. In that case, the results of a CT scan of the brain was normal on two occasions. In another case of neonatal WEE, a CT scan obtained at the onset of illness revealed diffuse low-density signals in the white matter. Four months after the acute episode, multiple, symmetrically distributed, intracranial calcifications were seen in both cerebral hemispheres, in the insular cortex, and in the thalamus [36].

EEEV can be isolated both in cell culture and after intracerebral inoculation of suckling mice [17]. In contrast, WEEV is extremely difficult to isolate from blood or CSF. However, WEEV can be isolated from cerebral tissue obtained either by brain biopsy or on postmortem examination. Newer molecular diagnostic approaches have been reported for both EEE and WEE and include reverse-transcriptase (RT) polymerase chain reaction (PCR) assays [38]. These are not widely available nor have they been fully validated for use in humans.

The mainstay for confirmatory diagnosis of EEEV and WEEV infection remains serology [17]. In most diagnostic virology laboratories, enzyme-linked immunosorbent assay (ELISA) IgM capture assays are used to establish the diagnosis. Forty percent of patients with arbovirus infection will have detectable IgM in CSF and/or serum by day 4 of illness. This increases to nearly 100% of patients by day 10 of illness. It is essential that the presence of virus-specific IgM antibodies be sought in both CSF and serum specimens. A single positive IgM result from CSF is sufficient to confirm acute EEEV infection. However, because of persistence for up to 1 year, IgM detection from serum alone should be considered to be presumptive evidence of recent infection.

### *Treatment*

Treatment for EEE and WEE is supportive, because no specific antiviral agent is available.

## Rubella

### *Introduction*

Rubella is one of the six classic childhood exanthems. Its major clinical significance went unnoticed until 1941, when an Australian ophthalmologist, Norman McAlister Gregg, reported a series of congenital defects (congenital cataract, heart defect, and deafness) in neonates born to mothers who had rubella during pregnancy

[39,40]. This initial report alerted the world to the teratogenic potential of rubella infection during pregnancy. The rubella pandemic of 1964 provided the opportunity to study the devastating results of congenital rubella infection on a worldwide scale. Unfortunately, however, congenital rubella syndrome (CRS) was not a reportable disease in the United States until 1966.

## *Epidemiology*

Rubella virus is a small, enveloped RNA virus, a member of the *Rubivirus* genus in the *Togaviridae* family [5]. Unlike all other *Togaviridae*, rubella virus does not require an arthropod vector for transmission. Humans are the only host for rubella virus.

Rubella virus is spread via the respiratory route by contact with infected respiratory droplets [41,42]. The incubation period ranges from 14 to 21 days [41]. After inoculation, rubella virus replicates in the epithelium of the nasopharynx and upper respiratory tract, then spreads via the lymphatic system to the regional lymph nodes. This results in viremia in 1 to 3 weeks, in association with viral shedding in nasopharyngeal secretions. Rubella virus has been isolated from patients 7 days before to 14 days after the onset of rash.

Rubella virus has a worldwide distribution [43,44]. Before the implementation of routine rubella vaccination in 1969 and until 2000, rubella infections peaked in the spring and trended downward in late summer and autumn [45,46]. Epidemics of rubella occurred in 5- to 9-year cycles [44,45].

In the United States, the incidence of rubella and CRS decreased to near nonexistence after the institution of rubella vaccination in 1969 [46]. From 2001 to 2004, only a single outbreak of rubella occurred in 2002 and involved only five individuals. In 2004, nine cases of rubella were reported nationwide [48]. Only five infants with CRS, three of whose mother were foreign-born, were reported to the CDC between 2001 and 2004 [46]. By comparison, of the 122 cases of CRS reported to the National Congenital Rubella Syndrome Registry in the United States between 1985 and 1996, approximately 44% were in Hispanics; 22% of the latter were imported [47]. Thus, the current epidemiologic surveillance data suggests that rubella is no longer endemic in the United States [46].

## *Clinical Manifestations*

In adults and older children, infection with rubella virus is a mild, self-limited febrile illness characterized by a discrete, erythematous, maculopapular rash [41,42,48,49]. The rash begins on the face and spreads downward to involve the entire body. The average duration of the exanthem is 3 days, but may be as short as 1 day and as long as 5 days.

Additional clinical findings include lymphadenopathy (most pronounced in the suboccipital and posterior auricular lymph nodes), malaise, or conjunctivitis. Arthralgia and arthritis occur in up to 70% of infected adult and adolescent females and may be immunologically mediated [50]. Rare complications include thrombocytopenia, encephalitis, neuritis, myopericarditis, and orchitis. Twenty to 50% of rubella infections are asymptomatic.

Fetal rubella infection may result in miscarriage or a wide array of congenital defects in the newborn infant, referred to as the CRS [49]. In the pregnant, rubella-naïve woman, the severity of the teratogenic effects of rubella virus infection on the fetus depends on the gestational time of infection [51]. Maternal rubella infection during first 12 weeks of pregnancy can result in congenital infection in 80% of neonates, compared with 54% if infection occurs at 13 to 14 weeks and 25% if infection occurs at the end of second trimester [52]. Infection beyond 12 weeks of gestation generally results in neonatal sequelae that are less severe. CRS comprises a multitude of clinical features, including low birth weight, microcephaly, sensorineural deafness, microphthalmos, cataracts, retinopathy, cardiovascular defects (most commonly patent ductus arteriosus), thrombocytopenia, and, rarely, hepatitis and pneumonitis. Endocrinopathies resulting in hypothyroidism and diabetes as well as immunologic abnormalities may also develop beyond the neonatal period.

Infants with congenital rubella infection may be contagious for 1 year or longer [53]. Rubella virus persists in infants infected in utero, and the virus has been recovered from multiple body sites [53].

## *Neurological Manifestations*

### Postnatal Rubella Infection of the CNS

#### Encephalitis [54–68]

Neurological complications after postnatally acquired rubella infection are relatively rare in children. The incidence of rubella encephalitis has been reported to range from 1:4300 to 1:24,000, with a median of 1:5000 to 1:6000 cases [58–61,68]. The onset of neurological symptoms generally occurs 2 to 4 days after the appearance of the rash, rarely as early as day 1 and as late as day 21 [61,63,65,68]. Presenting signs and symptoms include fever, headache, lethargy or somnolence, vomiting, ataxia, aphasia, confusion, disorientation, and nystagmus. Approximately 40% of patients present with or develop seizures during the course of the illness. Paraplegia, hemiplegia, and cranial nerve palsies have been reported. Nuchal rigidity, frank meningeal signs, and abnormal reflexes (i.e., absence of abdominal or cremasteric reflexes, Babinski, or hyperreflexia) may be found on physical examination. Somnolence or lethargy may progress to frank coma in some children.

Additional neurological manifestations of postnatal rubella infection include transverse myelitis and polyradiculopathy [56,67–69], optic neuritis [64], carotid arteritis [64], Guillain-Barré syndrome [70], and a clinical entity similar to subacute sclerosing panencephalitis (SSPE) [71,72].

Reported persistent sequelae in patients with rubella encephalitis include quadriplegia, hemiparesis, residual bulbar disturbances, ataxia, aphasia, and hyperreflexia [55,58,59,64,68]. In the only study to explore the impact of rubella encephalitis on intellectual function, no significant loss of intellectual function was found [59]. One patient was found to have reading difficulty in association with a visual disturbance. No defects in social adjustment were detected on testing. Interestingly, results of follow-up EEGs in five of seven patients were found to be borderline or definitely abnormal. Reported mortality rates have ranged from 0 to 37.5% [58,60,61,68].

## Congenital Rubella Syndrome

### Congenital Rubella Encephalitis

Neurological involvement is a cardinal feature of congenital rubella infection. In addition to its teratogenic effects on the CNS, rubella virus can also cause congenital encephalitis. In their comprehensive review of 100 infants with proven congenital rubella infection, Desmond et al. documented that 93% had evidence of congenital rubella encephalitis during the first 18 months of life (Table 5.2) [7].

Three neurological patterns emerged from this group of infants with congenital rubella encephalitis. In 74% of infants, the pattern was that of lethargy and hypotonicity in association with a full anterior fontanelle. In these infants, irritability overshadowed the early lethargy. The infants were restless, in constant motion and cried frequently. They exhibited sweating, vasomotor instability and excessive sucking. Despite adequate caloric intake, these infants failed

**Table 5.2** Clinical findings in congenital rubella encephalitis [62]

| Clinical finding | Percent (N = 100 patients) |
|---|---|
| Disturbances in muscle tone | 86% |
| Head retraction or back arching | 49% |
| Bulging anterior fontanelle | 45% |
| Irritability | 45% |
| Vasomotor instability | 33% |
| Lethargy | 28% |
| Seizures | 27% |
| Asymmetry of tone or reflexes | 22% |
| Incoordination of suck or swallow | 15% |
| Abnormal cry | 8% |

to gain weight appropriately. Evidence of variable reflexes, intense photophobia, and overreaction to stimuli was noted. They tended to have extensor posturing of the head and lower extremities when crying. Opisthotonic posturing or true opisthotonus was present. Those with the most severe manifestations had marked developmental delay. Approximately half of the infants in this group improved between 6 and 12 months of age.

A second pattern (16%) consisted of hypotonic infants who exhibited poor feeding, weight gain, motor activity, and socialization. Difficulties in feeding, such as poor suck, poor swallow, vomiting, or hyperperistalsis, were common. As with the first group of infants, intermittent opisthotonus, irritability, hyperactivity and increased tone were also present but did not appear until after 6 months of age. Improvement was generally observed at 9 to 12 months.

In the final pattern, seen in only 10% of infants, the onset of neurological symptoms was abrupt, with the appearance of seizures or a meningitis-like picture. In more than half, the onset of seizures was in the first week of life.

The outcome of infants with congenital rubella encephalitis is generally poor, with up to a 20% mortality rate. Among infants who survived and were followed for 18 months, only 6% were found to be free of neuromotor, speech, hearing, and visual problems [73]. Microcephaly was noted in 81% of the surviving children. Some authors report a 15 to 30% reduction in the anticipated size of the brain in these children [74].

Sensorineural hearing loss is commonly encountered in congenital rubella. The severity of hearing deficits secondary to rubella infection may vary from patient to patient and between a patient's two ears [75].

## Progressive Rubella Panencephalitis

A late-onset neurological consequence of congenital rubella infection is progressive rubella panencephalitis [76,77]. Progressive rubella panencephalitis was initially described in 1975. It has significant similarities with SSPE of measles. Progressive rubella panencephalitis may present initially with learning disorder, ataxia, spasticity, speech difficulty, and seizures. Neurological deterioration occurs during the second decade of life, and progresses inexorably during a period of 8 to 10 years, terminating in death [76,77]. No or a very minimal CSF pleocytosis may be present. The CSF protein level is elevated. In particular, the globulin levels are increased. Serum and CSF rubella titers are markedly elevated [76,77].

Long-term neurological sequelae after congenital rubella encephalitis includes hyperactivity, autism, pes valgus secondary to opisthotonic posturing, growth retardation, motor in coordination, speech delay, developmental delay, hearing loss, visual impairment, and cerebral palsy [73,78]. Other commonly observed behavioral manifestations [73,79] include short attention span, emotional lability, and easy distractibility. Microcephaly occurs in approximately 70 to 80% of patients with CRS; these children may be of normal intelligence [80].

## *Neuropathology*

Histopathologic examination [56,58,62] of the brains of patients who have succumbed to postnatal rubella encephalitis revealed round cell infiltration of the meninges and lymphocytic perivascular infiltration in the brain parenchyma. Small areas of focal hemorrhage were distributed throughout the brain. Perivascular demyelinization has also been reported [56].

Significant changes have been observed in the brains of infants with CRS. One series of 89 affected infants revealed cerebral vasculitic lesions in 52% [74]. Brain abnormalities included: 1) destruction of arteries and veins along with granular deposits, 2) defects of internal elastic lamina with proliferation of subintimal fibrous tissue, 3) deposition of granular material around capillaries, and 4) endothelial proliferation and thickening of vessel walls. The subendothelial metachromatic deposits of vessel walls project into the lumen, with subsequent narrowing of vessels.

Evaluation of the temporal bones from infants diagnosed with hearing loss have demonstrated partial collapse and adherence of Reissner's membrane to the striae vascularis and organ of Corti [75]. Hair cells were reported to be in abundance within the organ of Corti. Perivascular infiltrates were observed in the middle ear.

Rubella virus causes chromosomal breakage and inhibition of cell multiplication [81], a finding that may explain the intrauterine and postnatal growth retardation as well as subnormal number of cells in body organs observed in the infected fetus.

Postmortem examination of children who have died of progressive rubella encephalitis has revealed ventricular dilation and alteration of white matter on gross examination of the brain. Microscopic analysis has revealed perivascular aggregation of lymphocytes and plasma cells, granular deposits in the vessel walls, microglial nodules, destruction of Purkinje cells, and demyelination. In contrast to SSPE, inclusion bodies are absent.

## *Diagnosis*

On exposure to rubella during pregnancy, maternal rubella immunity must be promptly ascertained [82]. If maternal antibody is present, the fetus is considered to be protected. If no rubella antibody is detected, subsequent serologic testing at 2 and 6 weeks is necessary to determine whether infection has occurred. If maternal symptoms of rubella develop, a nasal culture and a serum IgM should be obtained. The diagnosis of acute maternal rubella, whether symptomatic or asymptomatic, necessitates maternal counseling regarding the risk to the fetus.

In children with postnatal rubella encephalitis, the CSF analysis generally reveals a lymphocytic pleocytosis, with less than 200 cells/$mm^3$, elevated protein levels, and normal glucose levels. Rubella virus antigens have been detected and the virus has been isolated from the brain tissue or CSF of patients with rubella encephalitis. Results of EEG examination may be normal or may reveal slow delta waves, diffuse spikes, and focal abnormalities [59,62–64,66–68,79]. CT or MRI scan of the brain may be normal or demonstrate areas of low density or cerebral edema [67,68].

Examination of the CSF of infants with congenital rubella encephalitis reveals moderately increased protein with a mild to moderate pleocytosis. Rubella virus was cultured from the CSF of 37% of cases tested. Persistence of virus in CSF throughout the first year of life occurred in 32% of those in whom it was possible to detect virus in CSF. EEG abnormalities are seen in 36%. Intracranial calcifications occur rarely and are detected by CT scan of the brain.

### *Treatment*

No specific therapeutic measures are available for congenital rubella infection other than comprehensive supportive care. Long-term management includes monitoring of feeding, growth, and developmental milestones. Appropriate neurological therapy, psychologic, audiologic, and ophthalmologic referrals should be made. Visual deficits and language delays may be minimized with prompt attention to glaucoma, cataracts, and hearing loss.

### *Prevention*

Infants with congenital rubella infection should be considered to be contagious. Childcare centers should notify susceptible pregnant caregivers of their risk should they be exposed to CRS infants. Children diagnosed with rubella in the postnatal period should be excluded from attending school or childcare center for 7 days after onset of the rash [82].

Vaccination with live attenuated rubella vaccine is the cornerstone of disease prevention. It is recommended for all children 12 months of age or older, adolescents, and adults who are susceptible [83]. Rubella vaccine is contraindicated in pregnancy and in the immunocompromised host. However, between 1971 and 1989, the CDC followed 324 susceptible pregnant women who inadvertently received rubella vaccine. None of the infants delivered by these women had evidence of malformations consistent with CRS.

## References

1. Broeck TN, Merril MH. Serological difference between eastern and western equine encephalitis virus. *Proc Soc Exper Biol Med* 1933; 31:217–220.
2. Feemster RY. Outbreak of encephalitis in man due to the eastern virus of equine encephalitis. *Am J Publ Health* 1938; 28:1403–1410.
3. Farber S, Hill A, Connerly ML, Dingle JH. Encephalitis in infants and children cause by the virus of the eastern variety of equine encephalitis. *JAMA* 1940; 114:1725–1731.

4. Schoening HW, Giltner LT, Shahab MS. Equine encephalomyelitis produced by inoculation of human encephalitis virus. *Science* 1938; 88:409–410.
5. Weaver SC, Dalgarno L, Frey TK, Huang HV, Kinney RM, Rice CM, Roehrig JT, Shope RE, Strauss EG. Family Togaviridae. Virus Taxonomy. *Seventh Report of the International Committee on Taxonomy of Viruses*. 2000. van Regenmortel, Fauquet CM, Bishop HL, Carstens EB, Estes MK, Lemon SM, Maniloff J, Mayo MA, McGeoch DJ, Pringle CR, Wickner RB (eds). Academic Press, San Diego, CA, pp 879–889.
6. Brault AC, Powers AM, Chavez CL, Lopez RN, Cachon MF, Gutierrez LF, Kang W, Tesh RB, Shope RE, Weaver SC. Genetic and antigenic diversity among eastern equine encephalitis viruses from North, Central, and South America. *Am J Trop Med Hyg* 1999; 61:579–586.
7. Tsai TF, Weaver SC, MonathTP. Alphaviruses. *Clinical Virology*. 2002. Richman DD, Whitley RJ, Hayden FG (eds). 2nd Edition. American Society for Microbiology Washington, DC, pp 1177–1210.
8. Centers for Disease Control and Prevention: Summary of Notifiable Diseases-United States, 2004. *MMWR* 2006; 55:1–79.
9. Centers for Disease Control and Prevention. Eastern Equine Encephalitis—New Hampshire and Massachusetts, August–September 2005. *MMWR* 2006; 55:697–700.
10. Feemster RY. Equine encephalitis in Massachusetts. *N Engl J Med* 1957; 257:701–704.
11. Przelomski MM, O'Rourke E, Grady GF, Berardi VP, Markley HG. Eastern equine encephalitis in Massachusetts: a report of 16 cases, 1970–1984. *Neurology* 1988; 38:736–739.
12. Deresiewicz RL, Thaler SJ, Hsu L, Zamani AA. Clinical and neuroradiographic manifestations of eastern equine encephalitis. *N Engl J Med* 1997; 336:1867–1874.
13. Goldfield M, Welsh JN, Taylor BF. The 1959 outbreak of Eastern encephalitis in New Jersey. 5. The inapparent infection:disease ratio. *Am J Epidemiol* 1968; 87:32–33.
14. Hart KL, Keen D, Belle EA. An outbreak of eastern equine encephalitis in Jamaica West Indies. I. Description of human cases. *Am J Trop Med Hyg* 1964; 13:331–341.
15. Morse RP, Bennish ML, Darras BT. Eastern equine encephalitis presenting with a focal brain lesion. *Pediatr Neurol* 1992; 8:473–475.
16. Belle EA, Grant LS, Thorburn MJ. An outbreak of eastern equine encephalomyelitis in Jamaica. II. Laboratory diagnosis and pathology of eastern equine encephalomyelitis in Jamaica. *Am J Trop Med Hyg* 1964; 13:335–341.
17. Tsai TF, Chandler LJ. Arboviruses. *Manual of Clinical Microbiology*. 2003. Murray PR, Baron EJ, Jorgensen JH, Pfaller MA, Yolken RH, (eds). 8th ed. American Society for Microbiology Press, Washington, DC, pp 1553–1569.
18. Meyer KF, Haring CM, Howitt B. The etiology of epizootic encephalomyelitis of horses in the San Joaquin Valley, 1930. *Science* 1931; 74:227–228.
19. Meyer KF. A summary of recent studies on equine encephalomyelitis. *Ann Int Med* 1932; 6:644–645.
20. Howitt BF. Recovery of the virus of equine encephalitis from the brain of child. *Science* 1938; 88:455.
21. Centers for Disease Control and Prevention: Summary of Notifiable Diseases—United States, 2000. *MMWR* 2002; 49:1–100.
22. Buss WC, Howitt BF. Human equine encephalomyelitis in Kern County, California, 1938, 1939, and 1940. *Amer J Pub Hlth* 1941; 31:935–944.
23. Davis JH. Equine encephalitis (western type) in children. Report of case with residual atrophy of the brain. *J Pediatr* 1940; 16:591–595.
24. Platou RV. Equine encephalitis in infancy. *Amer J Dis Child* 1940; 60:1155–1169.
25. Medovy H. Western equine encephalitis in infants. *Canad Pub Hlth J* 1942; 33:307–313.
26. Medovy H. Western equine encephalitis in infants. *J Pediatr* 1943; 22:308–318.
27. Ecklund CM. Human Encephalitis of the Western Equine type in Minnesota in 1941: clinical and epidemiological study of serologically positive cases. *Am J Hyg* 1946; 43:171–193.
28. Cohen RC, O'Connor RE, Townsend TE, Webb PA, McKey RW. Western equine encephalitis. Clinical observation in infants and children. *J Pediatr* 1953; 43:26–34.
29. Englund JA, Breningstall GN, Heck LJ, Lazuick JS, Karabatsos N, Calisher CH, Tsai TF. Diagnosis of western equine encephalitis in an infant by brain biopsy. *Pediatr Infect Dis J* 1986; 5:382–384.

30. Shinefield HR, Townsend TE. Transplacental transmission of western equine encephalomyelitis. *J Pediatr* 1953; 42:21–25.
31. Copps SC, Giddings LE. Transplacental transmission of western equine encephalitis. *Pediatrics* 1959; 24:31–33.
32. Noran HH, Baker AB. Sequels of equine encephalomyelitis. *Arch Neurol Psych* 1943; 49:398–413.
33. McGowan JE Jr, Bryan JA, Gregg MB. Surveillance of arboviral encephalitis in the United States, 1955-1971. *Am J Epidemiol* 1973; 97:199–207.
34. Somekh E, Glode MP, Reiley TT, Tsai TF. Multiple intracranial calcifications after western equine encephalitis. *Pediatr Infect Dis J* 1991; 10:408–409.
35. Baker AB, Noran HH. Western variety of equine encephalitis in man. *Arch Neurol Psych* 1942; 47:565–587.
36. Quong TL. The pathology of Western equine encephalitis. *Canad Pub Hlth J* 1942; 33:300–307.
37. Piliero PJ, Brody J, Zamani A, Deresiewicz RL. Eastern equine encephalitis presenting as focal neuroradiographic abnormalities: case report and review. *Clin Infect Dis* 1994; 18:985–988.
38. Linssen B, Kinney RM, Aguilar P, Russell KL, Watts DM, Kaaden OR, Pfeffer M. Development of reverse transcription-PCR assays specific for detection of equine encephalitis viruses. *J Clin Microbiol* 2000; 38:1527–1535.
39. Cooper L. Z. The History and Medical Consequences of Rubella. *Rev Infect Dis* 1985; 7:S2–9.
40. Gregg NM. Congenital cataract following German measles in the mother. *Trans Ophthal Soc Aust* 1941; 3:35–46.
41. Green RH, Balsamo MR, Giles JP, Krugman S, Mirick GS. Studies of the natural history and prevention of rubella. *Am J Dis Child* 1965; 110:348–365.
42. Heggie AD, Robbins FC. Natural rubella acquired after birth: clinical features and complications. *Am J Dis Child* 1969; 118:12–17.
43. Cockburn WC. World aspects of epidemiology of rubella. *Am J Dis Child* 1969; 118:113–121.
44. Assaad L, Ljungars-Esteves K. Rubella-world impact. *Rev Infect Dis* 1985; 7:S29–36.
45. Witte JJ, Karchmer AW, Case G. Epidemiology of rubella. *Am J Dis Child* 1969; 118:107–111.
46. Reef SE, Redd SB, Abernathy E, Zimmerman L, Icenogle JP. The epidemiological profile of rubella and congenital rubella in the United States, 1998-2004: The evidence for absence of endemic transmission. *CID* 2006;43:S126–132.
47. Schluter WW, Reef SE, Redd SC, Dykewicz CA. Changing epidemiology of congenital rubella syndrome in the United States. *J Infect Dis* 1998; 178:636–641.
48. Cooper LZ, Ziring PR, Ockerse AB, Fedun BA, Kiely B, Krugman S. Rubella: clinical manifestations and management. *Am J of Dis Child* 1969; 118:18–29.
49. Cherry JD. Togaviridae: Rubella virus. *Textbook of Pediatric Infectious Diseases 2004*. Feigen RD (ed). 5th Edition. Saunders, Philadelphia, PA; pp 2134–2162.
50. Frey TK. Neurological aspects of rubella virus infection. *Intervirology* 1997; 40:167–75.
51. Forbes JA. Rubella: Historical aspects. *Am J of Dis Child* 1969; 118:5–11.
52. Miller E, Cradock-Watson JE, Pollock TM. Consequences of confirmed maternal rubella at successive stages of pregnancy. *Lancet* 1982; 2:781–784.
53. Phillips CA, Melnick JL, Yow MD, Bayatpour M, Burkhardt M. Persistence of virus in infants with congenital rubella and in normal infants with a history of maternal rubella. *JAMA* 1965; 193:111–113.
54. Merritt HH, Koskoff YD. Encephalomyelitis following German measles. *Am J Med Sci* 1936; 191:690–696.
55. Barraclough WW. German measles encephalomyelitis. *Canad Med Ass J* 1937; 36:511–513.
56. Davidson C, Friedfeld L. Acute encephalitis following German measles. *Amer J Dis Child* 1938; 55:496–510.
57. Bradford RIC. Two cases of rubella meningoencephalitis. *Br Med J* 1943; 1:312–313.
58. Margolis FJ, Wilson JL, Top FH. Postrubella encephalomyelitis. Report of cases in Detroit and review of literature. *J Pediatr* 1943; 23:158–165.

59. Kenny FM, Michaels RH, Davis KS. Rubella encephalopathy. *Amer J Dis Child* 1965; 110:374–380.
60. Sherman FE, Michaels RH, Kenny FM, Acute encephalopathy (encephalitis) complicating rubella. Report of cases with virologic studies, cortisol production determination, and observations at autopsy. *JAMA* 1965; 192:675–681.
61. Walker JM, Nahmia AJ. Neurologic sequelae of rubella infection. *Clin Pediatr* 1966; 5:699–702.
62. Rose HD. Fatal rubella encephalitis. *Amer J Med Sci* 1974; 268:287–290.
63. Naveh Y. Friedman A. Rubella encephalitis successfully treated with corticosteroids. *Clin Pediatr* 1975; 14:286–287.
64. Connolly JH, Hutchinson WM, Allen IV, Lyttle JA, Swallow MW, Dermott E, Thomsom D. Carotid artery thrombosis, encephalitis, myelitis and optic neuritis associated with rubella virus infections. *Brain* 1975; 98:583–594.
65. Squadrini F, Taparelli F, De Rienzo B, Giovannini G, Pagani C. Rubella virus isolation from cerebrospinal fluid in postnatal rubella encephalitis. *Br Med J* 1977; 19:1329–1330.
66. Bechar M, Davidovich S, Goldhammer G, Machtey I, Gadoth N. Neurological complications following rubella infection. *J Neurol* 1982; 226:283–287.
67. Bitzan M. Rubella myelitis and encephalitis in childhood. A report of two cases with magnetic resonance imaging. *Neuropediatrics* 1987; 18:84–87.
68. Dwyer DE, Hueston L, Field PR, Cunningham AL, North K. Acute encephalitis complicating rubella virus infection. *Pediatr Infect Dis J* 1992; 11:238–240.
69. Morris MH, Robbins A. Acute infectious myelitis following rubella. *J Pediatr* 1943; 23:365–367.
70. Saeed AA, Lange LS. Guillain-Barré syndrome after rubella. *Postgrad Med J* 1978; 54:333–334.
71. Wolinsky JS, Berg BO, Maitland CJ. Progressive rubella panencephalitis. *Arch Neurol* 1976; 33:722–723.
72. Lebon P, Lyon G. Non-congenital rubella encephalitis. *Lancet* 1974; 2; 468.
73. Desmond MM, Wilson GS, Melnick JL, Singer DB, Zion TE, Rudolph AJ, Pineda RG, Ziai M, Blattner RJ. Congenital rubella encephalitis: course and sequelae. *J Pediatr* 1967; 71:311–331.
74. Rorke LB. Nervous system lesions in the congenital rubella syndrome. *Arch Otolaryngol* 1973; 98:249–251.
75. Brookhouser PE, Bordley JE. Congenital rubella deafness. Pathology and pathogenesis. *Arch Otolaryngol* 1973; 98:252–257.
76. Weil ML, Itabashi H, Cremer NE, Oshiro L, Lennette EH, Carnay L. Chronic progressive panencephalitis due to rubella virus simulating subacute sclerosing panencephalitis. *N Engl J Med* 1975; 292:994–998.
77. Townsend JJ, Baringer JR, Wolinsky JS, Malamud N, Mednick JP, Panitch HS, Scott RA, Oshiro L, Cremer NE. Progressive rubella panencephalitis. Late onset after congenital rubella. *N Engl J Med* 1975; 292:990–993.
78. Ziring PR. Congenital rubella: the teenage years. *Pediatr Ann* 1977; 6:762–770.
79. Pampiglione G, Young SE, Ramsay AM. Neurological and electroencephalographic problems of the rubella epidemic of 1962. *Br Med J* 1963; 5368:1300–1302.
80. Munro ND, Smithells RW, Sheppard S, Holzel H, Jones G. Temporal relations between maternal rubella and congenital defects. *Lancet* 1987; 330:201–204.
81. Nusbacher J, Hirschhorn K, Cooper LZ. Chromosomal abnormalities in congenital rubella. *N Engl J Med* 1967; 276:1409–1413.
82. American Academy of Pediatrics: Rubella. *Red Book: Report of the Committee on Infectious Diseases*. 2006. Pickering LK (ed). 27th ed. Elk Grove Village, IL, American Academy of Pediatrics, 2006, pp. 574–579.
83. Centers for Disease Control. General Recommendations on Immunization. Recommendations of the Advisory Committee on Immunization Practices (ACIP) and American Academy of Family Physicians (AAFP). *MMWR* 2002; 51:1–36.

# Chapter 6
# Rhabdoviruses

**Allan D. Friedman, M.D., M.P.H. and Sean O. McKenna, M.D.**

## Rabies

### *Introduction*

Rabies is a viral infection that primarily infects the central nervous system. Recognized since antiquity, it was known as lyssa in ancient Greece, which gave rise to its genus name—lyssavirus. The Sanskrit word rabhas, meaning to do violence, is thought to be the origin of the English word rabies. As early as 1271, wolf attacks of humans were reported to lead to rabies. However, with the development of cities and proliferation of domestic dogs, rabies increasingly was associated with dog bites [1]. After the identification of the infectivity of saliva and brain tissue in the nineteenth century, Pasteur demonstrated the protective effect of immunization with nerve tissue vaccine.

Today, rabies remains a public health concern. Despite improved vaccines and better understanding of the progression and pathophysiology of the disease, rabies remains a generally fatal disease. Rabies is not cured with existing therapies once symptoms develop, with only rare exceptions of survival with supportive care.

### *Epidemiology*

In developing nations, dogs remain the major reservoir and vector for human infection. In the United States and much of the rest of North America, the bat, skunk, raccoon, and fox are the primary vectors. Although raccoons predominate on the east coast, skunks are the major reservoir in the middle of the country. Foxes and coyotes are seen in the south-central and southwest, and infected skunks are found in much of California.

The silver-haired and eastern pipistrelle bats are of particular note for several reasons: the rabies virus found in these bats may more easily penetrate human skin and, because their teeth punctures are small, many bites go unnoticed. Bats also are a source of infection via aerosol. This has been reported from exposure in bat caves and in laboratory workers [2].

L.L. Barton and N.R. Friedman (eds.), *The Neurological Manifestations of Pediatric Infectious Diseases and Immunodeficiency Syndromes.*

During the past century, the incidence of rabies in humans in the United States has dropped dramatically to single digits per year. From 1990 to 2004, there were 47 cases of human rabies in the United States; 72% were associated with bat exposure. Worldwide, it is estimated that approximately 50,000 people die from rabies each year and approximately 4 million people receive postexposure vaccination [3,4].

## *Pathogenesis*

Rabies is caused by an RNA virus belonging to the Rhabdoviridae family in the genus Lyssavirus. There are seven serotypes, of which, at least six are found in bats. All mammals are susceptible to infection with rabies virus.

Inoculation of the virus usually is via a bite into the subcutaneous tissue. The virus spreads to the central nervous system by axonal transport, and from there to other organs by way of the sympathetic and somatic systems [5]. Although effects on the nervous system are the primary source of rabies morbidity, the virus has been demonstrated in the heart, adrenal glands, gastrointestinal tract, and pancreas [6]. The incubation period for rabies is highly variable. Typically, the time from bite to first appearance of symptoms is 20 to 60 days. However, disease has appeared as early as 5 to 6 days and, occasionally, the incubation period has been longer than 6 months; confirmed rabies has occurred even 7 years after the exposure [2].

## *Clinical Manifestations*

The initial symptoms of rabies are vague and nonspecific. Anxiety, malaise, or depression may be present early, followed by fever. The first localizing findings may be tingling, itching, or pain at the bite site.

## *Neurological Manifestations*

Two distinct patterns of neurological disease can develop 2 to 10 days later. The more common form, furious rabies, is characterized by agitation, changing levels of consciousness, hyperactivity, and bizarre behavior. Nuchal rigidity with meningismus and hoarseness caused by laryngospasm may be present. Sore throat and hypersalivation may occur. A classic manifestation of the furious form of rabies is hydrophobia, a fear of water brought on by painful spasms of the laryngeal and pharyngeal muscles after consumption of liquids. Spasms can create fear and anxiety when attempting to drink and can lead to tracheal aspiration of liquids. It has been suggested that the encephalitis may produce inhibition of inspiratory motor neurons, with exaggeration of respiratory reflexes. This, in turn, may produce a conditioned response in which fear increases spasm with swallowing; in some cases, just the sight of water may induce spasm [7]. Another related clinical finding is aerophobia. In patients with this symptom, spasms may occur when air is blown across the face [8]. Meningismus is commonly present. Cranial nerves are frequently involved, typically with paralysis of the palate and vocal cords. Reflexes may be hyperactive in some patients, whereas in others they may be absent.

The second less common pattern of neurological disease is the paralytic form. It is most likely to occur in patients bitten by vampire bats and is characterized by flaccid paralysis, usually starting in proximity to the bite site. Cranial nerves can become involved, resulting in an expressionless face. These patients do not develop hydrophobia or aerophobia [8].

The final phase of rabies is marked by alteration of consciousness. Coma may be complicated by cerebral edema, evidence of inappropriate antidiuretic hormone secretion, diabetes insipidus, and hypotension. Death from rabies is usually caused by cardiac or respiratory problems. The virus has been recovered from the heart. Most cardiac events are secondary to myocarditis resulting from direct infection, leading to arrhythmias and circulatory collapse. Alternatively, death may be secondary to aspiration or laryngeal spasms [2].

## *Neuropathology*

The postmortem appearance of the brain in furious rabies generally is that of an encephalitis with Negri bodies (eosinophilic cytoplasmic inclusions). Meningeal inflammation predominates in some cases [9]. In paralytic rabies, the spinal cord demonstrates severe inflammation and necrosis. Demyelination occurs in peripheral nerves. Negri bodies are rarely noted in the cerebral cortex. These inclusions may also be seen in the heart in patients with myocarditis [10].

## *Diagnosis*

Clinical diagnosis should be confirmed by laboratory testing. Cerebrospinal fluid findings are nonspecific (moderate numbers of white blood cells with a predominance of lymphocytes and elevated protein), as are electroencephalographic and computed tomographic findings. If the suspected animal is apprehended, its brain can be stained for rabies virus using fluorescein-labeled antibody or enzyme-coupled antibodies. Polymerase chain reaction amplification or dot hybridization techniques can be used to identify rabies RNA in tissue. Viral culture techniques are also available for confirmation of the diagnosis. Human saliva, cerebrospinal fluid, urine, and respiratory secretion cultures may be positive after 2 to 3 weeks of illness. Rabies-specific antigen may be reliably and rapidly detected by direct fluorescent antibody staining of saliva, brain tissue, and, early during the illness, from samples obtained from the nape of the neck near the hairline or smears from corneal epithelial cells [4].

A history of an animal bite or close contact with an animal at risk for carrying rabies may suggest the diagnosis. When that history is not available, a variety of other diagnoses should also be considered. These include herpes simplex virus, arbovirus, enterovirus, and rickettsial infections, as well as tetanus. Noninfectious diseases with clinical presentations similar to rabies include Guillain-Barré syndrome and porphyria [11].

## *Treatment*

Postexposure prevention of rabies comprises three modalities: wound cleansing, and both passive and active immunoprophylaxis. Immediate and thorough cleansing of the bite site with soap and water is essential. Some authorities also recommend that this initial washing be followed by local instillation of ethyl alcohol (43% or greater) [12].

Passive immunoprophylaxis with rabies immunoglobulin and active immunization should begin as soon as possible after the bite has occurred. Worldwide, most rabies vaccines are produced in nerve tissue. However, these vaccines may induce autoimmune central nervous system disease, require a large number of doses to induce adequate protection, and are associated with a higher failure rate than seen with the more successful cell culture vaccine available in the United States. Human diploid cell culture vaccine is highly immunogenic, does not contain heterologous protein, and is highly efficacious, as has been demonstrated in clinical trials. Newer cell culture vaccines seem to be less expensive and equally efficacious [13]. Postexposure human rabies vaccination is administered immediately and then on days 3, 7, 14, and 28. The decision to initiate postexposure prophylaxis is based on the type, availability, and health of the attacking animal. The risk of rabies from household dogs, cats, and ferrets in the United States is extremely low. Healthy-appearing pets may be observed for 10 days and, if they remain healthy appearing, postexposure prophylaxis is obviated. In contrast, bats, skunks, raccoons, foxes, most other carnivores, and woodchucks are considered rabid, unless the area is known to be rabies free. Livestock, rodents, and lagomorphs are almost always rabies free and must be considered on an individual basis [14]. Human-to-human spread has not been reported, although spread via transplanted organs has occurred [15].

Pre-exposure prophylaxis is indicated for people whose vocation, avocation, or living situation puts them at higher risk than the general population for exposure to potentially rabies-infected animals [14].

No specific antirabies therapy is currently available. Mortality for patients who have received no pre-exposure or postexposure prophylaxis has been nearly 100%. Patients who develop disease despite partial prophylaxis have been reported to have significant neurological residua or have died. Treatment for symptomatic disease has been disappointing and remains primarily supportive. Maintenance of comfort and minimization of pain should be a priority in all patients with overt rabies. Recently, a teenager was reported to have survived rabies after "anti-excitotoxic" therapy, until her immune response matured. The therapeutic regimen included ketamine, ribavirin, and amantadine [16]. Further studies are needed to determine the efficacy of this regimen.

## References


1. Steele, JH. History of Rabies, in *The Natural History of Rabies*. Baer, GM (ed). Academic Press. New York 1975; pp 1–29.
2. Plotkin, SA. Rabies. *Clin Infect Dis* 2000; 30:4–12.
3. *Red Book-Report of the Committee on Infectious Diseases*. American Academy of Pediatrics 2006; 27:552–559.
4. Noah, DL, Drenzek, C, Smith, JS, Krebs, JW, et al. Epidemiology of human rabies in the United States, 1980-1996. *Ann Int Med* 1998; 128:922–930.
5. Jackson, AC. *Rabies in Viral Pathogenesis*. Nathanson, N. Ahmed, R., Gonzalez-Scarano, F., et al. (eds). Lippincott-Raven. Baltimore 1997; pp 575–591.
6. Jogai, S, Radotra, BD, Banerjee, AK. Rabies viral antigen in extracranial organs: a post-mortem study. *Neuropathol Appl Neurobiol* 2002; 28:334–338.
7. Warrell DA, Davidson NM, Pope HM, et al. Pathophysiologic studies in human rabies. *Am J Med* 1976; 60:190–199.
8. Warrell, DA, Warell, MJ. Human rabies and its prevention: An overview. *Rev. Infect Dis* 1988; 10:S726–S731.
9. Dupont JR, Earl, KM. Human rabies encephalitis: a study of 49 fatal cases with a review of the literature. *Neurology* 1965; 15:1023–1034.
10. Chopra JS, Banerje AK, Murthy JMK, Pal SR. Paralytic rabies: clinicopathologic study. *Brain* 1980; 103:789–802.
11. Plotkin SA, Rabies (Hydrophobia, Rage, Lyssas) in *Krugman's Infectious Diseases of Children*. Gershon A, Hotez P, Katz, S (eds.). Mosby, Philadelphia. 2004; pp 477–491.
12. Dean DJ, Baer, GM, Thompson, WR. Studies on the local treatment of rabies-infected wounds. *Bull WHO* 1963; 28:477–486.
13. Plotkin, SA, Wiktor, TJ. Rabies vaccination. *Ann Rev Med* 1978; 29:583–591.
14. Advisory Committee for Immunization Practices, Human rabies prevention-United States. *MMWR* 1999; 48:(suppl RR-D) 1–21.
15. Srinivasan A, Burton EC, Kuehnert, MJ, et al. Transmission of rabies virus from an organ donor to four transplant recipients. *N Engl J Med* 2005; 352:1103–1111.
16. Willougby, RE, Tieves KS, Hoffman GM et al. Survival after treatment of rabies with induction of coma. *N Engl J Med* 2005; 352:2508–2514.

# Chapter 7
# Adenoviruses

Allan D. Friedman, M.D., M.P.H. and Sean O. McKenna, M.D.

## Adenoviruses

### Introduction

Adenoviruses are responsible for a wide variety of clinical diseases. Although most commonly associated with illnesses of the respiratory tract, these viruses have been responsible for infections of the gastrointestinal tract, heart, eyes, skin, liver, urinary, as well as nervous systems [1].

Common clinical respiratory illnesses associated with adenoviruses include pharyngitis, tonsillitis, and pneumonia. Less often seen are the common cold, laryngotracheitis, bronchiolitis, pertussis-like syndrome, unilateral hyperlucent lung, and bronchiolitis obliterans. Eye infections caused by adenoviruses present as keratoconjunctivitis, follicular conjunctivitis, and pharyngoconjunctivitis. Dermatologic disease caused by adenovirus can present as erythema multiforme, Stevens-Johnson syndrome, roseola-like illness, or morbilliform and rubelliform exanthems. Gastroenteritis caused by adenoviruses is common. Less frequent gastrointestinal manifestations of adenoviral infection include mesenteric lymphadenitis, intussusception, appendicitis, hepatitis, and pancreatitis. The genitourinary tract is infrequently infected with adenovirus; when this does occur the clinical findings can include acute hemorrhagic cystitis, nephritis, and orchitis. Adenovirus infects the heart rarely, but can produce myocarditis or pericarditis. Thyroiditis, deafness, and arthritis have also been associated with adenovirus infection. Neurological manifestations of adenovirus infection include encephalitis and meningitis [2–4].

### Epidemiology

Adenoviruses are typically found in the throat, stool, and conjunctiva. Transmission is by aerosolized droplets, for which close contact is necessary; by fomites; or by the fecal–oral route. Infections can be sporadic or epidemic. The incubation

L.L. Barton and N.R. Friedman (eds.), *The Neurological Manifestations of Pediatric Infectious Diseases and Immunodeficiency Syndromes.*

period extends from 2 to 14 days for respiratory infections and from 3 to 10 days for gastrointestinal infections [5]. Excretion of virus can occur intermittently for months after the initial infection, but contagiousness peaks during the initial days of acute illness. Re-infections can occur and usually will result in asymptomatic disease or minimal symptoms [2,6].

Most infants are born with maternally derived protective neutralizing antibodies to adenoviruses. During the first months of life, these antibodies wane and only 14% of infants still have detectable maternal antibody at 6 months of age. Adenovirus infections typically occur during the second 6 months of life and by 1 year of age, approximately one half of babies have detectable antibodies to adenoviruses. The incidence of disease in children peaks from 6 months to 5 years of age, diminishes [1], but remains relatively common in school-age children, and decreases in high school and college [7]. Military recruits appear to be the only adults with notable rates of infection [7].

Although adenoviral disease occurs throughout the year, respiratory infection is most likely during the winter, spring, and early summer. There does not seem to be a seasonal pattern to enteric adenoviral infections. Adenoviruses are found worldwide [8].

Infection occurs approximately equally in male and female patients, but there have been reports of higher incidences of disease in male patients [8]. Disease severity is greatest in neonates and in immunocompromised patients. There is an inverse relationship between socioeconomic status and the incidence of adenoviral infection. Although a direct association with race has not been shown, there are reports of higher incidence in native populations in Canada and in New Zealand [9].

## *Etiology and Pathogenesis*

Adenoviruses are DNA viruses that may infect humans as well as animals. Nearly 50 immunologically distinct adenoviruses have been associated with human disease; many are capable of infecting more than one organ system and causing a variety of clinical manifestations [3].

Adenoviruses can be isolated from most sites, including throat, eye, stool, urine, peritoneal and pericardial fluid, as well as from specimens taken from lymph nodes, liver, kidney, and brain. In cell cultures, adenoviruses can cause cytopathic effects as early as 8 hours after inoculation [10–12].

## *Clinical Manifestations*

Most upper respiratory tract infections with adenoviruses cause febrile disease and have an associated pharyngitis. Pharyngitis caused by adenovirus may be clinically similar to that caused by group A streptococci, with tonsillar exudates and cervical adenopathy. Headaches, myalgias, chills, cough, malaise, abdominal discomfort, and nasal congestion may also be present. Most adenoviral pharyngitis is associated with adenovirus types 1, 2, 3, 5, and 7 [13]. These same serotypes are also most commonly associated with cold symptoms and may account for approximately 3% of all common colds in children [14].

The more severe or fatal adenovirus infections have been associated with types 3, 7, and 21 [15]. Younger children and infants are more likely to have severe disease. Abrupt onset of fever and cough can be followed by tachypnea and dyspnea. Wheezes and rales may be noted on physical examination. Chest radiographs may show bilateral infiltrates and hyperinflation and may mimic bacterial pneumonia. Normal or low white blood cell counts with a lymphocytosis and failure to respond to antibiotics may help differentiate adenoviral pneumonia from bacterial pneumonia. Lobar collapse can occur. Recovery in nonfatal cases may take weeks, and subsequent exacerbations have been reported [16]. Permanent pulmonary residua after adenoviral pneumonia in children are not infrequent and may include bronchiolitis obliterans, bronchiectasis, and unilateral hyperlucent lung [17].

Epidemic acute respiratory disease caused by adenoviruses has been reported from the military. Typically, it is a short-duration acute respiratory disease with fever. After a 5- to 7-day incubation period, symptoms including pharyngitis, laryngitis, tracheitis, nonproductive cough, and fever develop. Headache, malaise, myalgias, chills, abdominal pain, adenopathy, and dizziness may also occur. The disease may spread to the lower respiratory tract, producing wheezing and pneumonia. Clinical resolution is slow and symptoms may persist for up to a month [18].

Acute follicular conjunctivitis is the most common adenoviral eye infection and is, in general, unilateral and benign. Follicular lesions with erythema and lymphoid follicular hyperplasia may be seen on the conjunctiva. Symptoms include lacrimation, burning, itching, and a foreign body sensation in the eye. Pharyngoconjunctival fever is characterized by fever, sore throat, cough, sore or burning eyes, coryza and stuffiness, headache, anorexia, and malaise. Other less common findings include lacrimation, photophobia, sneezing, epistaxis, nausea, vomiting, diarrhea, and abdominal pain. The throat typically shows injection, erythema, and hypertrophied lymphatic tissue. There is injection and erythema of the conjunctiva and edema is common. Cervical and preauricular nodes are commonly enlarged [19,20]. Epidemic keratoconjunctivitis is more common in adults than children and has been associated with nosocomial transmission in ophthalmology clinics [5]. Symptoms include a sensation of a foreign body in the eye, followed by photophobia, edema, hyperemia, discharge, and lacrimation. Preauricular adenopathy is common, and pharyngitis and rhinitis may be present. The eyes may become painful, and punctate opacities may develop in the cornea. These opacities may extend subepithelially and leave infiltrates that may persist for months and may result in blurry vision [21].

Adenoviruses are also rarely associated with exanthems. Erythematous, maculopapular rashes have been mistaken for measles, Kawasaki disease, rubella, or roseola. Typically, when a rash is present, other symptoms of adenoviral infection, such as pharyngitis, conjunctivitis, or pneumonia are also present [22].

Adenovirus infections in immunocompromised patients can be serious or even life threatening. In pediatric transplant recipients, adenoviral infection occurs most commonly in the liver, lung, and gastrointestinal tract. Adenovirus serotypes 1, 2, and 5 are most frequently recovered from these patients [23]. Hepatic necrosis has been reported in patients with acquired immunodeficiency syndrome (AIDS), severe immunodeficiency states, and transplant patients [24]. In bone marrow transplant patients, symptoms most commonly involve the gastrointestinal and respiratory tracts, but central nervous system (CNS) involvement has also been noted in a few of these patients. This may include a prolonged course characterized by symptoms of meningoencephalitis [25].

## *Neurological Manifestations*

Neurological complications of adenovirus infections are uncommon, generally sporadic in nature and present with meningoencephalitis [26]. Symptoms, which include lethargy, meningismus, and headache, can occur in isolation or with fever, cough, pharyngitis, and anorexia [4]. Adenovirus types 1 to 7, 12, and 32, have been recovered from the brain as well as cerebrospinal fluid (CSF). Both transplant recipients as well as patients with immunoglobulin deficiencies may have prolonged or chronic CNS involvement. Davis et al. also described fatal subacute adenoviral meningoencephalitis in the recipient of a bone marrow transplant. The patient was noted to have "unique, bilaterally symmetrical degeneration in the inferomedial temporal cortex, amygdaloid nuclei, hippocampi, hypothalamus, and some brainstem nuclei [27]". Adenoviruses have been isolated from patients with symptoms characteristic of Reye syndrome. Edwards et al. reported three children, younger than 1 year of age, who met the criteria for Reye syndrome and had positive cultures for adenoviruses from one or more specimens, including stool, throat, urine, and liver tissue [28]. In addition, Linseen's report of a child who presented with transverse myelitis and increased myelin basic protein in the CSF added demyelination and transverse myelitis to the list of neurological sequelae of adenovirus infections [29]. Publications that are more recent have detailed additional neurological complications of adenovirus infection. Straussberg et al. described a syndrome of transient encephalopathy in seven infants who presented with a classic prodromal respiratory viral illness that progressed to lethargy and obtundation without seizures [30]. All seven patients had intercurrent catarrhal signs and hepatomegaly. In contrast, Ohtsuki et al. detailed three patients whose acute encephalopathy, secondary to adenovirus type 7 infection, led to seizures by days 8 to 10 [31]. Ooi et al. described an instance in which adenovirus seems to have exacted its neurological toll not alone, but in concert with an enterovirus during a hand, foot, and mouth disease outbreak [32]. Patients in this series of eight children in Malaysia developed acute flaccid paralysis previously not described with adenovirus. Four of the children fully recovered, three had residual flaccid paralysis, and one was lost to follow-up but had been improving at discharge. The pathophysiologic basis of the neurological disease in this report was postulated to be either direct damage of spinal anterior horn cells or neuropathic effects on the brachial or lumbosacral plexus.

## *Differential Diagnosis*

Upper and lower respiratory symptoms caused by adenoviruses are similar to those caused by other viruses, such as respiratory syncytial virus, parainfluenza viruses, influenza viruses, rhinovirus, Epstein-Barr virus, cytomegalovirus, and enteroviruses. Bacterial infections with similar respiratory presentations include *Bordetella pertussis, Mycoplasma pneumoniae, Streptococcus pneumoniae*, and *Streptococcus pyogenes*.

Gastrointestinal symptoms caused by adenoviruses may be confused with those caused by rotavirus, noroviruses, and astroviruses. Bacterial infections that may have a similar presentation include *Yersinia enterocolitica, Escherichia coli*, salmonella, shigella, and *Campylobacter*.

Neurological syndromes attributed to adenoviruses are similar to those caused by enteroviruses, herpes viruses, arboviruses, influenza viruses, poliovirus, and Epstein-Barr virus as well as *Mycoplasma pneumoniae*.

## *Diagnosis*

Laboratory confirmation of adenovirus infection can be made by culture, polymerase chain reaction, immunoassays, or serologic testing. Specimens of respiratory secretions and stool are most frequently used [33]. Polymerase chain reaction can be used to identify adenovirus DNA in formalin-fixed, paraffin-embedded tissues [34]. Adenovirus isolates can be characterized through neutralization testing, sequencing hexon and complete fiber genes, and restriction enzyme analysis [34]. CSF findings are most typical of viral infection with the presence of a normal glucose level, a normal or moderately elevated protein level, and a high white blood cell count with neutrophil predominance initially.

## *Treatment*

Immunocompetent patients generally have a self-limited disease and recover fully; treatment options are few and management is largely supportive. Ribavirin has been used in immunocompromised patients with adenovirus infections of the gastrointestinal tract, bladder, and lungs; there are no reports of its successful use in CNS infection. A recent report documents the development of hyperammonemia with the use of ribavirin in an immunocompromised patient, an adverse effect that may limit the drug's usefulness [35]. Cidofovir has been used to treat disseminated adenovirus infection in a pediatric liver transplant patient, with improvement in clinical status and viral clearance. Reported side effects are few and include hypophosphatemia, acidosis, proteinuria, uveitis, and reduced ocular pressure [36]. Therapy for adenovirus meningoencephalitis is primarily supportive, including maintenance of adequate cerebral and systemic perfusion, oxygenation, and minimizing elevations in intracranial pressure. Recent efforts to treat severe adenoviral infections have also included the empiric use of intravenous immunoglobulin (IVIG) [32,37]. Seidel et al. have described impressive improvement of symptoms of adenovirus-associated macrophage activation syndrome within 72 hours of IVIG therapy. IVIG may prove to be a beneficial, if mysterious, therapy in cases of life-threatening illness [37].

## References


1. Enders, JF, Bell, JA, Dingle, JH, et al. "Adenovirus" group name proposed for new respiratory-tract viruses. *Science* 1956; 124:119–120.
2. Brandt, CD, Kim, HW, Vargosko, AJ, et al. Infections in 18 000 infants and children in a controlled study of respiratory tract disease. I. Adenovirus pathogenicity in relation to serologic type and illness syndrome. *Am J Epidemiol* 1969; 90:484–500.
3. Brandt, CD, Kim, HW, Rodriquez, WJ, et al. Adenoviruses and pediatric gastroenteritis. *J Infect Dis* 1985: 151:437–443.
4. Kelsey, DS. Adenovirus meningoencephalitis. *Pediatrics* 1978: 61:291–293.
5. American Academy of Pediatrics. [Adenovirus]. In: Pickering LK, Baker CJ, Long SS, McMillan JA, eds. *Red Book: 2006 Report of the Committee on Infectious Diseases*. 27th ed. Elk Grove Village, IL: American Academy of Pediatrics; 2006:202–204.
6. Couch, RB, Carte, TR, Douglas, RG, et al. Effect of route of inoculation on experimental respiratory viral disease in volunteers and evidence for airborne transmission. *Bacteriol Rev* 1966; 30:517–529.
7. Van der Veen, J. The role of adenoviruses in respiratory disease. *Am Rev Respir Dis* 1963; 88: 167–180.
8. Herrmann, EC Jr. Experiences in laboratory diagnosis of adenovirus infections in routine medical practice. *Mayo Clin Proc* 1968; 43:635–644.
9. Gold, R, Wilt, JC, 8.Adhikari, PK, et al. Adenoviral pneumonia and its complications in infancy and childhood. *J Can Assoc Radiol* 1969; 20:218–224.
10. Foy, HM. *Adenoviruses in Viral Infections of Humans: Epidemiology and Control*, 1989, Evans, AS (ed), Plenum, New York, pp 77–94.
11. Grabow, WOK, Puttergill, DL, Bosch, A. Propagation of adenovirus type 40 and 41 in the PLC/PRF/5 primary liver carcinoma cell line. *J Virol Methods* 1992; 37:201–208.
12. Boyer, GS, Leuchtenberger, C, Ginsberg, HS. Cytological and cytochemical studies of HeLa cells infected with adenovirus. *J Exp Med* 1957; 105:195–214.
13. Moffet,HL, Siegel, AC, Doyle, HK. Nonstreptococcal pharyngitis. *J Pediatr* 1968; 73:51–60.
14. Pereira, MS. Adenovirus infections. *Postgrad Med J* 1973; 49:798–801.
15. Simila, S, Ylikorkala, O, Wasz-Hockert, O. Type 7 adenovirus pneumonia. *J Pediatr* 1971; 79: 605–611.
16. James, AG, Lang, WR, Liang, AY, et al. Adenovirus type 21 bronchopneumonia in infants and young children. *J Pediatr* 1979; 95:530–533.
17. Simila, S, Linna, O, Lanning, P, et al. Chronic lung damage caused by adenovirus type 7. A ten year follow-up study. *Chest* 1989; 80:127–131.

18. Sohier, R, Chardonnett, Y, Prunieras, M. Adenoviruses: Status of current knowledge. *Prog Med Virol* 1965; 7:253–255.
19. Martone, WJ, Hierholzer, JC, Keenlyside, RA, et al. An outbreak of adenovirus type 3 disease at a private recreation center swimming pool. *Am J Epidemiol* 1980; 111:229–237.
20. Kendall, EJC, Riddle, RW, Tuck, HA, et al. Pharyngoconjunctival fever: School outbreaks in England during the summer of 1955 associated with adenovirus type 3, 7, and 14. *Br Med J* 1957; 2:131–136.
21. Barnard, DL, Hart, JCO, Marmion, VJ, et al. Outbreak in Bristol of conjunctivitis caused by adenovirus type 8 and its epidemiology and control. *Br Med J* 1973; 2:165–169.
22. Cherry, JD. Newer viral exanthems, in *Advances in Pediatrics*, 1969, Schulman, I (ed), Year Book Medical Publishers, Chicago, pp. 233–286.
23. Michaels, MG, Green, M, Wald, ER, et al. Adenovirus infection in pediatric liver transplant recipients. *J Infect Dis* 1992; 165:170–174.
24. Krilov, LR, Rubin, LG, Frogel, M, et al. Disseminated adenovirus infection with hepatic necrosis in patients with human immunodeficiency virus infection and other immunodeficiency states. *Rev Infect Dis* 1990; 12:303–307.
25. Baldwin, A, Kingmen, H, Darville, et al. Outcome and clinical course of 100 patients with adenovirus infection following bone marrow transplant. *Bone Marrow Transplant* 2000; 26: 1333–1338.
26. Chou, SM, Roos, R, Burrell, R, Gutmann, L, Harley, JB. Subacute focal adenovirus encephalitis. *J Neuropathol Exp Neurol* 1973; 32:34–50.
27. Davis, D, Henslee, PJ, Markesbery, WR. Fatal adenovirus meningoencephalitis in a bone marrow transplant patient. *Annals Neurol* 1988; 23:385–389.
28. Edwards, K, Bennett, SR, William, LG, et al. Reye's Syndrome associated with adenovirus infections in infants. *Am J Dis Child* 1985; 139:343–346.
29. Linseen, WH, Gabeels, FJ, Wevers, RA. Infective acute transverse myelopathy. Report of two cases. *Neuropediat* 1991; 22: 107–109.
30. Straussberg, R, Harel, L, Levy, Y, Amir, J. A syndrome of transient encephalopathy associated with adenovirus infection. *Pediatrics* 2001; 107:69–72.
31. Ohtsuki, N, Kimura, S, Nezu, A. Three cases with acute encephalopathy related with adenovirus type 7 infection. *No To Hattatsu* 2000; 32:68–72.
32. Ooi, MH, Wong, SC, et al. Adenovirus type-21 associated acute flaccid paralysis during an outbreak of hand-foot-and-mouth disease in Sarawak, Malaysia. *CID* 2003; 35:550–559.
33. Ruuskanen, O, Meurman, O, Sarkkinen, J. Adenoviral disease in children: a study of 105 hospital cases. *Pediatrics* 1985; 76:79–83.
34. Turner, PC, Bailey AS, Cooper, RJ, et al. The polymerase chain reaction for detecting adenovirus DNA in formalin-fixed paraffin-embedded tissue obtained post mortem. *J Infect* 1993; 27:43–46.
35. Bertrand, P, Faro, A, Cantwell, P, et al. Intravenous ribavirin and hyperammonemia in an immunocompromised patient infected with adenovirus. *Pharmacotherapy* 2000; 20: 1216–1220.
36. Carter, BA, Karpen, SJ, Quiros-Tejeira, RE, et al. Intravenous Cidofovir therapy for disseminated adenovirus in a pediatric liver transplant recipient. *Transplantation* 2002; 74: 1050–1052.
37. Seidel, M, et al. IVIG treatment of adenovirus infection-associated macrophage activation syndrome in a two-year-old boy: case report and review of the literature. *Pediatric Hematology/Oncology* 2003; 20:445–451.

# Chapter 8
# Arenaviruses

**Daniel J. Bonthius, M.D., Ph.D., Leslie L. Barton, M.D., Hannah Klein de Licona, Nancy E. Bonthius, Pharm.D., and Bahri Karacay, Ph.D.**

## Lymphocytic choriomeningitis virus (LCMV)

### *Introduction*

Arenaviruses are prevalent in the environment and commonly infect humans, where they can induce both neurological and systemic disease. These enveloped single-stranded RNA viruses derive their name from the Latin word *arenosus*, meaning "sandy," because of the granular appearance of the viral ribosomes observable on electron microscopy [1,2]. All members of the arenavirus family are maintained in nature by persistent, generally asymptomatic, infection of specific species of rodent hosts. Infected animals harbor high titers of virus and excrete infectious virus in their urine, saliva, and other secretions. Humans become infected when they contact viruses excreted by these infected host animals.

Eighteen arenavirus species have been identified [3], but only seven are known to cause human disease (Table 8.1). Among the arenaviruses that are pathogenic in humans, lymphocytic choriomeningitis virus (LCMV) is the most prevalent, covers the largest geographic range, and is the best studied, both in humans and in laboratory animals. Thus, LCMV is the prototype arenavirus and will be the focus of this chapter. The diseases induced by the other arenaviruses will be discussed briefly at the chapter's end.

LCMV was initially isolated by Armstrong and Lillie in 1933 from the cerebrospinal fluid (CSF) of a woman with meningoencephalitis. This new infectious agent was named "lymphocytic choriomeningitis virus" for the pathologic changes that it induced in the choroid plexus and meninges of infected mice and monkeys [4]. Clinical and etiologic studies identified LCMV as one of the most frequent infectious causes of aseptic meningitis in humans [5].

The first recognized case of congenital infection with LCMV was reported in England in 1955 [6]. In the decades that followed, multiple cases of congenital LCMV infection were reported throughout Europe. Although LCMV has been recognized as an important cause of aseptic meningitis in the United States for decades, the first cases of congenital LCMV infection were not reported in the United States until 1993 [7,8].

L.L. Barton and N.R. Friedman (eds.), *The Neurological Manifestations of Pediatric Infectious Diseases and Immunodeficiency Syndromes.*

**Table 8.1** Arenaviruses and human diseases

| Virus | Geographic distribution | Disease in humans | Host in nature |
|---|---|---|---|
| Lymphocytic choriomeningitis virus (LCMV) | All continents except Antarctica | Acquired prenatally: congenital lymphocytic choriomeningitis<br>Acquired postnatally: lymphocytic choriomeningitis | *Mus musculus* |
| Guanarito virus | Venezuela | Venezuelan hemorrhagic fever | *Sigmidon alstoni* |
| Junia virus | Argentine pampas | Argentine hemorrhagic fever | *Calomys musculinis* |
| Lassa fever virus | Western Africa | Lassa fever | *Mastomys* |
| Machupo virus | Bolivia | Bolivian hemorrhagic fever | *Calomys callosus* |
| Sabia virus | Brazil | Sabia virus hemorrhagic fever | *Unknown* |
| Whitewater Arroyo virus | Western United States | Whitewater Arroyo hemorrhagic fever | *Neotoma albigula* |

*Mus musculus*, the common house mouse, is both the natural host and reservoir for LCMV. The virus is transferred vertically from one generation to the next within the mouse population by intrauterine infection. Hamsters are also competent reservoirs. Although heavily infected with LCMV, rodents that acquire the virus transplacentally often remain asymptomatic because the virus is not cytolytic and because congenital infection in rodents provides them with immunologic tolerance for the virus. Throughout their lives, mice and hamsters infected with LCMV shed the virus in large quantities in nasal secretions, saliva, milk, semen, urine, and feces [2,3].

Postnatal humans acquire LCMV by inhalation of aerosolized virus, by direct contact with fomites contaminated with infectious virus, or by receiving transplanted tissues from an infected donor. Human-to-human horizontal infection has not been documented (except when infected tissues are transplanted), but human-to-human vertical transmission does occur and is the basis for congenital LCMV infection. When a woman acquires LCMV during pregnancy, LCMV can be passed to the fetus transplacentally, presumably during maternal viremia [9]. The virus may also be acquired by the fetus during the intrapartum period [6].

## *Epidemiology*

LCMV is endemic in wild mice throughout temperate regions [10,11]. and probably exists as an infectious pathogen wherever the genus *Mus* has been introduced (every continent but Antarctica). An epidemiologic study has demonstrated that 9% of the house mice in urban Baltimore are infected with LCMV, and that substantial clustering occurs where the prevalence is higher [12]. Serologic studies have demonstrated that 5.1% of healthy black women in Birmingham, Alabama and 4.7% of adults in Baltimore, Maryland possess antibodies to LCMV, indicating previous exposure and infection [12,13]. Similar serologic findings have recently been reported for an inner city of Argentina [14].

Acquired LCMV infections can occur year-round. However, most LCMV infections in humans occur during the late autumn and winter months, reflecting seasonal variations in the cohabitation of humans with mice. The cold months of autumn and winter drive wild mice indoors. The mice carry LCMV with them, thus increasing the likelihood of a human infection.

The incidence and prevalence of congenital LCMV infection are unknown. Although the published case reports of LCMV infection during pregnancy demonstrate that LCMV can be a severe neuroteratogen, it is not known whether the profoundly affected infants described in the case reports represent the typical outcome of gestational LCMV infection, or whether they represent only the most severely affected cases. No prospective clinical or epidemiologic studies of congenital LCMV infection have been conducted. Information regarding the incidence and spectrum of LCMV-induced teratogenicity is further limited by the fact that LCMV is not one of the infectious agents for which infants with a suspected congenital infection are routinely checked. Therefore, congenital LCMV infection, similar to many other congenital infections, might produce a spectrum of pathologic effects ranging from minimal to profound. The high prevalences of infected mice and of seropositive postnatal humans suggest that congenital LCMV infection is an underdiagnosed disease, and that the virus is responsible for more cases of congenital neurological and vision dysfunction than has previously been recognized [15–17].

## *Pathogenesis*

### Acquired LCMV Infection

Both acquired and congenital LCMV disease are caused by the combination of infection with the virus and the host immune response to the infection. In cases of acquired LCMV infection, the virus typically enters the human via aerosol and is deposited in the lung, where initial viral replication occurs [18]. The hilar lymph nodes and lung parenchyma are important sites of viral growth. Interstitial lung infiltrates and lung edema may reflect this parenchymal lung infection with LCMV. The virus then travels via the blood stream to other organs, where further infection and replication occur. Eventually, the virus reaches the choroid plexus, leptomeninges, and ventricular ependymal linings, where the virus often replicates to high titers and where the inflammatory response produces the characteristic pathology and symptoms of meningitis that give the virus its name.

The immune response in acquired LCMV infection is both protective and deleterious. On the one hand, the immune response is critically important to clearance of the virus and to protection against repeat infection. On the other hand, the cellular immune response underlies the symptoms of disease [3].

## Congenital LCMV Infection

Transplacental infection of the fetus is the basis for most cases of congenital LCMV infection. In some cases, the fetus may acquire the virus during the intrapartum period, presumably by exposure to maternal blood or vaginal secretions during maternal viremia.

Within the human fetus, the brain is the principal target of LCMV infection and is the organ most commonly pathologically affected (Fig. 8.1) [1]. Neuronal populations undergoing mitosis are particularly vulnerable to LCMV infection and are an important site of LCMV replication [9,20]. Microencephaly, periventricular calcifications, cerebellar hypoplasia, focal cerebral destruction, and gyral dysplasia are common pathologic effects of congenital LCMV infection

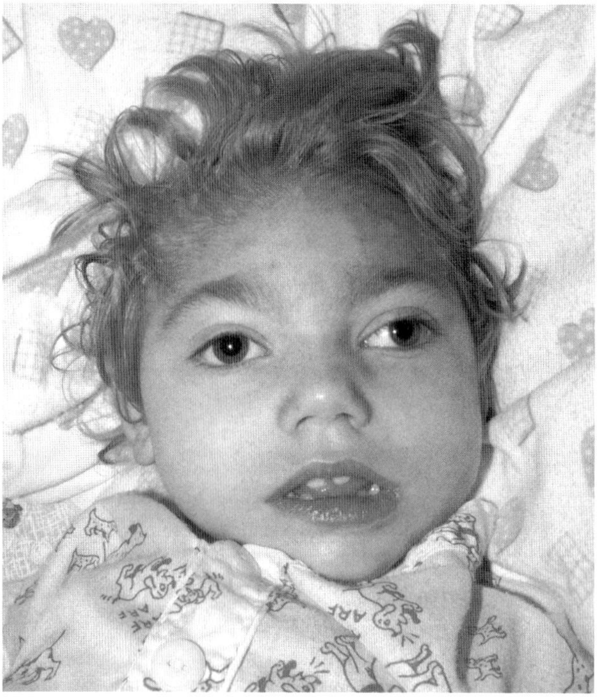

**Fig. 8.1** A 3-year-old child with congenital LCMV infection. The child is microcephalic, blind, mentally retarded, and has spastic cerebral palsy and epilepsy. All of these features are typical of congenital infection with LCMV.

(Figs. 8.2 and 8.3).These pathologic changes reflect both the tropism of the virus for replicating neuroblasts and disrupted brain development induced by dysfunction or loss of immature or replicating neurons [9,19,20].

The mechanism by which LCMV damages the fetal human brain is unknown. However, it is likely that the hydrocephalus commonly observed in children with congenital LCMV is caused by ependymal inflammation within the ventricular system, particularly at the cerebral aqueduct, with a secondary blockage of CSF egress. The sites of focal cerebral destruction probably reflect focal inflammatory lesions, and the periventricular calcifications are probably caused by the infection and death of mitotically active neuronal precursors of the subependymal periventricular region (Fig. 8.2). The cortical dysgenesis (Fig. 8.3) evident in many children with congenital LCMV infection probably reflects virus-induced disruption of neuronal migration [20].

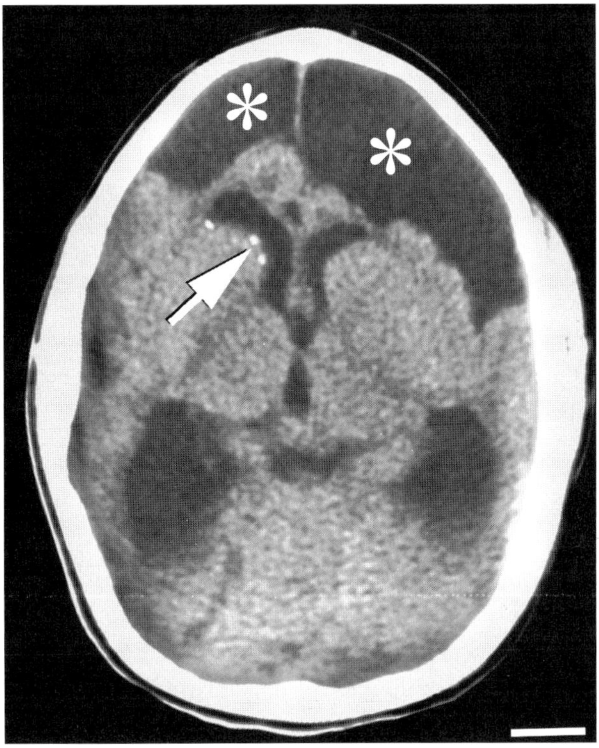

**Fig. 8.2** LCMV infection induces focal destructive lesions and periventricular calcifications within the developing brain. This head computed tomographic scan from a 4-month-old child with congenital LCMV infection reveals bilateral asymmetric regions of encephalomalacia (*asterisks*), strongly suggestive of focal destructive processes. The periventricular calcifications (*arrow*) reflect the specific vulnerability of neuronal precursors to LCMV infection and virus-induced cellular death. The microencephaly in this patient is likely caused by the combination of encephalomalacia and loss of neuronal progenitor cells. Magnification bar, 1 cm.

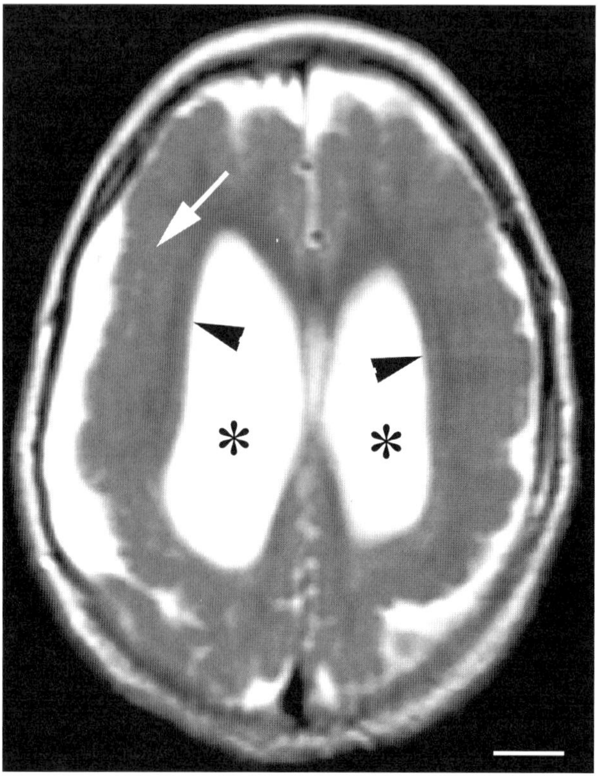

**Fig. 8.3** LCMV infection disrupts neuronal migration in the developing brain. This magnetic resonance imaging scan of a 3-year-old child with congenital LCMV infection demonstrates microencephaly and a deficit of white matter (*arrowheads*) with a compensatory enlargement of the lateral ventricles (*asterisks*). There is also a diminished number of cortical sulci and an abnormally smooth cortical surface (*white arrow*). This abnormal cortical architecture is strongly suggestive of pachygyria, a developmental defect caused by abnormal neuronal migration. Magnification bar, 1 cm.

## *Clinical Manifestations*

The clinical manifestations of LCMV infection depend strongly on the developmental stage of the patient at the time of infection [2,9,21]. In particular, clinical signs and symptoms depend on whether the infection occurs during the prenatal period or during postnatal life.

### Acquired (Postnatal) LCMV Infection

LCMV infection during postnatal life (childhood or adulthood) typically consists of a brief febrile illness from which the patient fully recovers. Classic LCMV infection is a biphasic disease in which the initial symptoms include myalgia, fever, malaise, headache, anorexia, nausea, and vomiting. Defervescence and temporary improvement in constitutional symptoms ensues, often followed by a second phase, consisting of central nervous system (CNS) disease. The symptoms of this CNS phase of the disease are usually those of aseptic meningitis, including headache, nuchal rigidity, fever, vomiting, and photophobia. The entire course of acquired LCMV disease is usually only 1 to 3 weeks [15].

Laboratory abnormalities frequently observed during the initial febrile phase include thrombocytopenia, leukopenia, and mild elevations of liver enzymes. Infiltrates may appear on chest radiographs. The hallmark laboratory abnormality during the second CNS phase of the illness is a CSF pleocytosis. The CSF may contain hundreds to thousands of white blood cells, most of which are lymphocytes. CSF eosinophilia has also been reported [22]. Hypoglycorrhachia and mild elevations of CSF protein can also occur.

The clinical spectrum of acquired LCMV infection is broad. In as many as one third of postnatal infections, the disease is asymptomatic. Other patients develop extraneural disease that extends beyond the usual symptoms and may include orchitis, pneumonitis, myocarditis, parotitis, dermatitis, and pharyngitis [23]. In some patients, the CNS disease may be considerably more severe than just the aseptic meningitis and may include encephalitis and hydrocephalus. Other neurological manifestations include transverse myelitis and Guillain-Barré syndrome. Although recovery is usually complete, fatalities from acquired LCMV infection do occur [5].

Although in the vast majority of postnatal cases the patient acquires LCMV from an infected rodent, the virus can also be acquired through transplantation of infected tissue. In December 2003 and April 2005, two groups of solid organ transplant recipients developed signs and symptoms of infection days to weeks after transplantation [24]. Each cluster of patients had received tissue from a common donor. The transplant recipients developed severe disease, including encephalopathy, abdominal pain, coagulopathy, thrombocytopenia, graft dysfunction, fever, and leukocytosis. In some of the recipients, diarrhea, renal failure, rash, and seizures also developed. LCMV was identified as the infective agent in all patients of both clusters. Seven of the eight organ recipients died. One recipient survived, after receiving ribavirin and reduced levels of immunosuppressive therapy. Neither donor had clinical or laboratory signs of infection. No source of LCMV infection was found in the 2003 cluster. However, in the 2005 cluster, the donor had had contact with a pet hamster infected with LCMV [24].

The severe illness induced by LCMV in the transplant recipients probably stemmed from the substantial immunosuppression—especially T-cell depletion—that accompanied their transplantations. Little is known regarding LCMV infection in immunocompromised patients. However, in a clinical trial investigating the possible antitumor effect of LCMV, patients with advanced lymphomas were inoculated with the virus, and all died with disseminated infection within several weeks of inoculation [25].

## Congenital LCMV Infection

Human fetal infection with LCMV can induce spontaneous abortion and death of the fetus [26]. Among the surviving fetuses, the two cardinal signs of congenital LCMV infection are vision impairment and brain dysfunction [9,27].

The vision impairment is principally caused by chorioretinitis and the formation of bilateral chorioretinal scars. The most common location of the chorioretinal scarring is in the periphery of the fundus, although the macula may also be involved [16]. Other ocular abnormalities reported in congenital LCMV infection include optic atrophy, nystagmus, vitreitis, strabismus, microphthalmos, and cataracts [17]. The cerebral hemispheres often have sites of focal injury and neuronal migrational defects in congenital LCMV infection. Thus, in addition to the retinal injuries, cortical dysfunction also probably underlies some of the vision deficits in this disorder.

Although the vision impairment induced by congenital LCMV infection is often severe, the effect of LCMV on overall cerebral function causes the greatest disability. Prenatal infection with LCMV often leads to either macrocephaly or microencephaly. The macrocephaly observed in infants with congenital LCMV is almost invariably caused by a noncommunicating hydrocephalus, presumably reflecting inflammation and blockade of the cerebral aqueduct. The microencephaly accompanying congenital LCMV infection is caused by a virus-induced failure of brain growth (Fig. 8.1). In addition to hydrocephalus and microencephaly, other abnormalities of brain structure commonly observed in congenital LCMV infection include periventricular calcifications, cortical dysplasia, focal cerebral destruction, and cerebellar hypoplasia (Figs. 8.2 and 8.3) [19]. The reason for differences in forms of neuropathology among children with congenital LCMV infection is unknown, but may be caused by differences in gestational age at the time of infection. Indeed, recent work in an animal model has demonstrated that the nature and severity of LCMV-induced neuropathology within the developing brain depends strongly on the developmental stage of the animal at the time of infection [28].

Brain function in children with congenital LCMV infection is often severely and permanently impaired. Mental retardation, cerebral palsy, ataxia, epilepsy, and decreased visual acuity are common neurological sequelae [29].

Unlike many other congenital infections, LCMV does not typically induce systemic manifestations. Birth weight is typically appropriate for gestational age. Skin rashes and thrombocytopenia, which are common in several other prominent congenital infections, are unusual in congenital LCMV infection. Hepatosplenomegaly is only rarely observed, and serum liver enzyme levels are usually normal. Auditory deficits are unusual.

The principal differential diagnoses of congenital LCMV infection are the other infectious pathogens that can cross the placenta and damage the developing fetus [9]. These infectious agents are linked conceptually by the acronym "TORCHS" and include *Toxoplasma gondii*, rubella virus, cytomegalovirus, herpes simplex virus, and syphilis. Cytomegalovirus and toxoplasmosis may be particularly difficult to differentiate from LCMV, because infection with any of these three infectious agents can produce microencephaly, intracerebral mineralization, and chorioretinitis [30].

Although clinical clues may aid in distinguishing one congenital infection from another, definitive identification of the causative infectious agent usually requires laboratory data, including cultures and serologic studies.

Of all of the congenital infections, toxoplasmosis most closely mimics congenital LCMV infection. Microencephaly, hydrocephalus, chorioretinitis, and intracranial calcifications are hallmarks of congenital infection with either pathogen. Approximately 10% of newborns infected with *Toxoplasma gondii* will exhibit hepatosplenomegaly, jaundice, and rash [31]. These systemic signs are usually absent in congenital LCMV infection. The two infections also tend to differ neuroradiographically. In cases of congenital toxoplasmosis, the intracranial mineralization tends to be diffuse within the brain parenchyma. In contrast, in congenital LCMV infection, the mineralizations are typically periventricular. However, congenital infection with toxoplasmosis and LCMV are so clinically similar that differentiating among them requires laboratory testing. The diagnosis of congenital toxoplasmosis can be established by serologic studies and confirmed by detecting the infectious organisms in tissues, blood, or CSF.

The prognosis for children with congenital LCMV infection is generally poor. A meta-analysis of all reported cases of congenital LCMV infection revealed a mortality rate of 35% by 21 months of age [19]. Of those who survive, most have severe neurodevelopmental disorders, including microencephaly, poor somatic growth, profound vision impairment, severe epilepsy, spastic weakness, and profound mental retardation [29]. However, some of these children have only moderate neurological and mental handicaps, and some congenitally infected children have had a normal outcome. Developmental regression is virtually absent.

## *Diagnosis*

Acute acquired human LCMV infections can be diagnosed by isolation of the virus from CSF, blood, urine or nasopharyngeal secretions. More commonly, the infection is diagnosed presumptively by the characteristic cellular and chemical changes in the CSF and serologically by elevated anti-LCMV antibody titers.

It is possible that some infants born with congenital LCMV infection still harbor the virus, in which case, the infection can be diagnosed by isolating the virus from CSF [32]. However, by the time of birth, many babies prenatally infected with LCMV no longer harbor the virus. Thus, congenital LCMV infection is usually diagnosed by means of serologic testing. The immunofluorescent antibody test detects both IgM and IgG and has greater sensitivity than the more widely available complement fixation method [33]. The immunofluorescent antibody test is commercially available, and its specificity and sensitivity make it an acceptable diagnostic tool. An even more sensitive test for the detection of congenital LCMV infection is the enzyme-linked immunosorbent assay (ELISA), which measures titers of LCMV IgG and IgM and is performed at the Centers for Disease Control and Prevention (CDC). Polymerase chain reaction has recently been used as a means of detecting LCMV RNA in an infected infant [34]. The use of polymerase chain reaction offers exciting possibilities for both prenatal and postnatal detection of LCMV infection. However, LCMV is not known to induce persistent infections in humans, and the time course of viral clearance from an infected human fetus is unknown. A fetus may sustain substantial brain damage from LCMV but effectively clear the virus, and may have no LCMV RNA to be detected by polymerase chain reaction in the postnatal period.

## *Treatment*

Effective antiviral therapy for acquired or congenital LCMV infection is not yet available, although some evidence suggests that ribavirin may be helpful [24]. Ribavirin exerts activity against LCMV in vitro [35], and seems to have helped one patient who acquired the infection via transplant [24]. At best, however, its effectiveness in vivo is unproven. Thus, treatment for LCMV infection is principally supportive and directed toward treatment of complications.

Children with hydrocephalus caused by congenital LCMV infection often require placement of a ventriculoperitoneal shunt during infancy. Seizures in congenital LCMV infection are often difficult to control and require administration of multiple antiepileptic medications. The mental retardation induced by congenital LCMV infection is often profound. In most cases, affected children should be referred for educational intervention during early life. The spasticity accompanying congenital LCMV infection is often severe. Although physical therapy can help to maintain range of motion and minimize painful spasms and contractures, spasticity mediations and/or implantation of a baclofen pump is often necessary and helpful.

## *Prognosis*

Complications in children with congenital LCMV infection are nonspecific and consist of the medical problems that commonly arise in children with ventriculoperitoneal shunts, severe epilepsy, and static encephalopathy. These complications include shunt failure or infection, drooling, aspiration pneumonia, injuries from falls, and joint contractures.

## *Prevention*

No vaccine exists to prevent infection with LCMV. However, measures can be taken to reduce the risk of LCMV infection. In particular, infection can be controlled by eliminating access of rodents to human living spaces and by limiting rodent infestation in animal and food storage areas.

Congenital LCMV infection will not occur unless a woman contracts a primary infection with LCMV during pregnancy. Because rodents, especially house mice, are the principal reservoir of LCMV, women can reduce their risk of contracting LCMV by minimizing their exposure to the secretions and excretions of mice. This can be accomplished most effectively by eliminating cohabitation with mice. Pregnant women should also avoid contact with pet rodents, especially mice and hamsters. Laboratory personnel who work with rodents have an increased risk of infection with LCMV. Pregnant women who work in animal care facilities or laboratories at research institutions should wear gloves, gowns, and face masks to avoid potential aerosolized or secreted LCMV. All animal colonies should be tested periodically for LCMV [36].

## *Other Arenavirus Infections of Humans*

In addition to LCMV, several other arenaviruses are pathogenic in humans. These pathogens are linked not only by their common virionic structure and by their ecology involving rodent hosts, but also by their propensity to produce acute hemorrhagic fevers in humans. The diseases induced by each of these viruses range from mild infections to severe life-threatening acute febrile illnesses in which shock is a frequent feature. Headache, lethargy, fever, myalgia, abdominal pain, and conjunctivitis are early common signs in all of these infections. Encephalopathic signs with tremor, seizures, and altered consciousness may occur in the South American hemorrhagic fevers and severe Lassa fever.

In the wake of the September 11, 2001 terrorist attacks on the United States, greater emphasis has been placed on the potential of bioterrorism. As pathogens that can produce acute hemorrhagic fevers, the arenaviruses are listed by the CDC and by the National Institute of Allergy and Infectious Diseases (NIAID) as Category A Priority Pathogens. These viruses rank as high-priority agents and as a risk to United States national security because they are easily disseminated, have the potential for major public health impact, and could induce public panic and social disruption [37,38].

### Lassa Fever

Lassa fever is caused by infection with the Lassa fever virus. This arenavirus is endemic in western Africa and is named after the town in Nigeria where the first cases were identified [39]. Lassa fever virus causes no, or only mild symptoms, in 80% of infected people. In the remaining 20%, however, it may cause severe multisystem disease [40]. In western Africa, Lassa fever virus induces several hundred thousand infections per year, of which, approximately 5000 are fatal. In some hospitals of western Africa, more than 10% of all hospitalized patients have Lassa fever, underscoring the major public health impact of this disease [41].

The natural reservoirs of Lassa fever virus are rodents of the genus *Mastomys*. These rat-like rodents are numerous in western Africa, breed frequently, produce large numbers of offspring, and readily invade human dwellings. For these reasons, the virus is efficiently spread from infected rodents to humans.

In addition to the fever, chest pain, headache, gastrointestinal symptoms, and conjunctivitis that accompany infection with the other arenaviruses, Lassa fever virus commonly produces an exudative pharyngitis. Neurological dysfunction is common and includes hearing loss, tremor, and encephalitis [42,43]. Death rates are high for pregnant women and particularly for their fetuses, approximately 95% of whom die in utero when the mother is infected.

Unlike the other arenaviruses, Lassa fever can be treated effectively with intravenous ribavirin. This therapy is most effective when administered during the first week of illness. Development of an effective vaccine against Lassa fever virus is a research goal [44,45].

## Argentine Hemorrhagic Fever

Argentine hemorrhagic fever (AHF) is caused by infection with the Junin virus, which is carried by the corn mouse (*Calomys musculinis*). The disease is endemic in the central pampas region of Argentina, where several hundred cases occur annually, principally in agricultural workers.

The clinical picture of infection with this virus is classic viral hemorrhagic fever, similar to Lassa fever, except that thrombocytopenia and florid bleeding are more common in AHF than in Lassa fever [46]. The case fatality rate for AHF is as high as 33%. This mortality rate can be greatly reduced by treatment of patients within the first 8 days of illness with plasma from convalescent patients. A live attenuated Junin vaccine has been developed that protects against AHF [47].

## Bolivian Hemorrhagic Fever

Bolivian hemorrhagic fever is caused by infection with the Machupo virus. The disease is endemic in the El Beni region of Bolivia, where it is carried by the rodent *Calomys callosus*. The clinical signs and course in Bolivian hemorrhagic fever are very similar to those of AHF. Mortality is 25 to 35%. The most recent outbreak of Bolivian hemorrhagic fever was reported in 1994. Infection occurred in seven members of a single family, six of whom died of the disease [48].

## Venezuelan Hemorrhagic Fever

Venezuelan hemorrhagic fever (VHF) is caused by infection with the Guanarito virus [49]. VHF was first reported as an outbreak (15 cases with 9 fatalities) in the Portuguesa state of Venezuela in 1989. To date, VHF has been limited to Venezuela, where it continues to induce outbreaks in isolated hamlets. *Sigmidon alstoni*, the cotton rat, is the principal reservoir for Guanarito virus in nature and is the source of infection for humans [50]. Recent land use changes in Venezuela, especially the conversion of deciduous forests to agricultural lands, have created both larger and more favorable habitats for *Sigmidon alstoni*, and more opportunities for rodent–human contact [51].

VHF has a clinical presentation and course similar to AHF [52]. Thrombocytopenia, bleeding, and neurological dysfunction are prominent signs. The reported case fatality rate is 34%. However, it is likely that some, and perhaps many, milder cases are undetected.

## Sabia Virus Infection

Sabia virus was first isolated in São Paulo, Brazil, in 1990 from an agricultural engineer who presented with a hemorrhagic fever syndrome. The patient ultimately died, and necrosis of the liver was found at autopsy [53]. The infecting agent was identified as an arenavirus. Molecular studies have shown that it is distinct from all other members of the Arenaviridae and shares a progenitor with Junin, Machupo, Tacaribe, and Guanarito viruses [54]. Sabia virus infected a virologist in 1994, once again resulting in a hemorrhagic fever syndrome. This patient was promptly treated with intravenous ribavirin with an apparent virologic response and clinical improvement. The reservoir for Sabia virus in nature remains unknown, but is assumed to be a rodent in the community of Sabia, Brazil, where the only known natural infection has occurred. Although information is sparse, it is assumed that Sabia virus is acquired as an aerosol and has a high morbidity and mortality [55].

## Whitewater Arroyo Virus Infection

Whitewater Arroyo virus (WAV) was identified in 1996 as a viral zoonosis that produces persistent infection in white-throated woodrats (*Neotoma albigula*) in New Mexico [56]. Since then, the known geographic range of the virus has expanded to include all of the southwestern United States [57]. In addition, in the year 2000, WAV was identified as a human pathogen after it produced two fatal cases of acute hemorrhagic fever [58]. The geographic range of woodrats reaches from Canada to Central America and includes most of the contiguous United States. Thus, the geographic range of WAV may extend far beyond the southwestern United States. Because infection with this virus can be fatal, the public health impact of WAV is potentially substantial.

**Acknowledgments** This work was supported by Public Health Service grant K08 NS02007-01A2 from the National Institute of Neurological Disorders and Stroke, by research grant 1-01-217 from the March of Dimes Birth Defects Foundation, by the John Martin Fund for Neuroanatomic Research, by a Carver Medical Research Initiative Grant, by research grants from the Children's Miracle Network, and by a Young Investigator Award from the Child Neurology Society to DJB.

## References

1. Rowe WP, Murphy FA, Bergold GH, et al. Arenaviruses: proposed name for a newly defined virus group. *J Virol* 1970; 5:651–652.
2. Buchmeier MJ, Zajac AJ. Lymphocytic choriomeningitis virus. In: Ahmed R, Chen I (eds.), *Persistent viral infections*, New York: Wiley, 1999; 575–605.
3. Buchmeier MJ, Bowen MD, Peters CJ. Arenaviridae: the viruses and their replication. In: *Field's Virology*, 2001, DM Knipe and PM Howley (eds.), Edition 4, Lippicott Williiams & Wilkins, Philadelphia, pp. 1635–1668.
4. Armstrong C, Lillie RD. Experimental lymphocytic choriomeningitis of monkeys and mice produced by a virus encountered in studies of the 1933 St. Louis encephalitis epidemic. *Public Health Rep* 1934; 49:1019–1022.
5. Meyer HM Jr, Johnson RT, Crawford IP, Dascomb HE, Rogers NG. Central nervous system syndromes of "viral" etiology: a study of 713 cases. *Am J Med* 1960; 29:334–347.
6. Komrower GM, Williams BL, Stones PB. Lymphocytic choriomeningitis in the newborn. Probable transplacental infection. *Lancet* 1955; 1:697–698.
7. Barton LL, Budd SC, Morfitt WS, et al. Congenital lymphocytic choriomeningitis virus infection in twins. *Pediatr Infect Dis J* 1993; 12:942–946.
8. Larsen PD, Chartrand SA, Tomashek KM, Hauser LG, Ksiazek TG. Hydrocephalus complicating lymphocytic choriomeningitis virus infection. *Ped Infect Dis J* 1993; 12:528–531.
9. Bonthius NE, Karacay B, Bonthius DJ. Congenital lymphocytic choriomeningitis virus infection. In: *MedLink-Neurobase*, 2003, S Gilman (ed.), Edition 4, Arbor Publishing Corporation, San Diego.
10. Lehmann-Grube F. Portraits of viruses: arenaviruses. *Intervirology* 1984; 22:121–145.
11. Ambrosio AM, Feuillade MR, Gamboa GS, Maiztegui JI. Prevalence of lymphocytic choriomeningitis virus infection in a human population of Argentina. *Amer J Trop Med* 1994; 50:381–386.
12. Childs JE, Glass GE, Korch GW, Ksiazek TG, Leduc JW. Lymphocytic choriomeningitis virus infection and house mouse (*mus musculus*) distribution in urban Baltimore. *Amer J Trop Med Hyg* 1992; 47:27–34.
13. Stephensen CB, Blount SR, Lanford RE, et al. Prevalence of serum antibodies against lymphocytic choriomeningitis virus in selected populations from two U.S. cities. *J Med Virol* 1992; 38:27–31.
14. Riera L., Castillo E, Del Carmen Saavedra M, et al. Serological study of the lymphocytic choriomeningitis virus (LCMV) in an inner city of Argentina. *J Med Virol* 2005; 76:285–289.
15. Jahrling PB, Peters CJ. Lymphocytic choriomeningitis virus: a neglected pathogen of man. *Arch Pathol Lab Med* 1992; 116:486–488.
16. Mets MB, Barton LL, Khan AS, Ksiazek TG. Lymphocytic choriomeningitis virus: an underdiagnosed cause of congenital chorioretinitis. *Am J Ophthalmol* 2000; 130:209–215.
17. Barton LL, Mets MB. Congenital lymphocytic choriomeningitis virus infection: decade of rediscovery. *Clin Infect Dis* 2001; 33:370–374.
18. Danes L, Benda R, Fuchsova M. Experimental inhalation with the lymphocytic choriomeningitis virus (WE strain) of the monkeys of the *Macacus cynomolgus* and *Macacus rhesus* species. *Bratisl Lek Listy* 1963; 43:21–34.
19. Wright R, Johnson D, Neumann M, Ksiazek TG, Rollin P, Keech RV, Bonthius DJ, Hitchon P, Grose CF, Bell WE, Bale JF. Congenital lymphocytic choriomeningitis virus syndrome: A disease that mimics congenital toxoplasmosis or cytomegalovirus infection. *Pediatrics* 1997;100:1–6. URL: http://www.pediatrics.org/cgi/content/full/100/1/e9.
20. Bonthius DJ, Mahoney JC, Buchmeier MJ, Taggard DA. Critical role for glial cells in the propagation and spread of lymphocytic choriomeningitis virus in the developing rat brain. *J Virol* 2002; 76(13):6618–6635.
21. Bonthius DJ, Karacay B. Meningitis and encephalitis in children: an update. *Neurol Clinics North Amer* 2002; 20:1013–1038.

22. Chesney PJ, Katcher ML, Nelson DB, Horowitz SD. CSF eosinophilia and chronic lymphocytic choriomeningitis virus meningitis. *J Pediatr* 1979; 94:750–752.
23. Lewis JM, Utz JP. Orchitis, parotitis and meningoencephalitis due to lymphocytic choriomeningitis virus. *N Engl J Med* 1961; 265:776–780.
24. Fischer SA, Graham MB, Kuehnert MJ, et al. Transmission of lymphocytic choriomeningitis virus by organ transplantation. *New Engl J Med* 2006; 354:2235–2249.
25. Horton J, Hotchin JE, Olson KB, Davies JNP. The effects of MP virus infection in lymphoma. *Cancer Res* 1971;31:1066–1068.
26. Biggar R, Woodall J, Walter P, Haughie G. Lymphocytic choriomeningitis outbreak associated with pet hamsters: fifty seven cases from New York state. *JAMA* 1975; 232:494.
27. Barton LL, Peters CJ, Ksiazek TG. Lymphocytic choriomeningitis virus: an unrecognized teratogenic pathogen. *Emerg Inf Dis* 1995; 1:152–153.
28. Bonthius DJ, Karacay B, Mahoney J, Bonthius NE. Gestational age determines the outcome of congenital LCM virus infection in humans: confirmation in an animal model. *J Neurovirol* 2006; 12:8.
29. Larsen PD, Wright R. Early clinical manifestations and long-term outcome in children with symptomatic congenital lymphocytic choriomeningitis virus infection. *Neurology* 2001; 56: A39–40.
30. Bale JF, Murph JR. Congenital infections and the nervous system. *Pediatr Clin North Amer* 1992;39:669–690.
31. Koppe JG, Loewer-Sieger DH, De Roever-Bonnet H. Results of 20-year follow-up of congenital toxoplasmosis. *Lancet* 1986; 1:254.
32. Schulte DJ, Comer JA, Erickson BR, et al. Congenital lymphocytic choriomeningitis virus: an underdiagnosed cause of neonatal hydrocephalus. *Ped Inf Dis J* 2006; 25:560–562.
33. Lehmann-Grube F, Kallay M, Ibscher B, Schwartz R. Serologic diagnosis of human infections with lymphocytic choriomeningitis virus: comparative evaluation of seven methods. *J Med Virol* 1979; 4:125–136.
34. Enders G, Varho-Gobel M, Lohler J, Terletskain-Ladwig E, Eggers, M. Congenital lymphocytic choriomeningitis virus infection: an underdiagnosed disease. *Ped Infect Dis J* 1999; 18:652–655.
35. McCormick JB, King IJ, Webb PA, et al. Lassa fever: effective therapy with ribavirin. *New Engl J Med* 1986;314:20–26.
36. Dykewicz CA, Dato VM, Fisher-Hoch SP. Lymphocytic choriomeningitis outbreak associated with nude mice in a research institute. *JAMA* 1992; 267:1349–1353.
37. Centers for Disease Control and Prevention (CDC) 2002. URL: http://www.bt.cdc.gov/agent/agentlist.asp.
38. National Institute of Allergy and Infectious Diseases (NIAID) 2002. URL: http://www.niaid.nih.gov/dmid/bioterrorism/bandc_priority.htm.
39. Frame JD, Baldwin JM Jr, Gocke DJ, Troup JM. Lassa fever, a new virus disease of man from west Africa. I. Clinical description and pathological findings. *Am J Trop Med Hyg* 1970; 19:670–676.
40. Bausch DG, Rollin PE, Demby AH, Coulibaly M, Kanu J, Conteh AS, et al. Diagnosis and clinical virology of Lassa fever as evaluated by enzyme-linked immunosorbent assay, indirect fluorescent-antibody test, and virus isolation. *J Clin Microbiol* 2000; 38:2670–2677.
41. Birmingham K, Kenyon G. Lassa fever is unheralded problem in West Africa. *Nature Med* 2001; 7:878.
42. Cummins D, McCormick JB, Bennett D, et al. Acute sensorineural deafness in Lassa fever. *JAMA* 1990; 264:2093–2096.
43. Cummins D, Bennett D, Fisher-Hoch SP, et al. Lassa fever encephalopathy: clinical and laboratory findings. *J Trop Med Hyg* 1992; 95:197–201.
44. Fisher-Hoch SP. McCormick JB. Towards a human Lassa fever vaccine. *Rev Med Virol* 2001; 11:331–341.
45. Geisbert TW, Jones S, Fritz EA, et al. Development of a new vaccine for the prevention of Lassa fever. *PLoS Med* 2005; 2(6):e183.

46. Harrison LH, Halsey NA, McKee KT Jr, Peters CJ, Barrera Oro JG, Briggiler AM, Feuillade MR, Maiztegui JI. Clinical case definitions for Argentine hemorrhagic fever. *Clin Infect Dis* 1999; 28:1091–1094.
47. Maiztegui JI, McKee KT Jr, Barrera Oro JG, Harrison LH, Gibbs PH, Feuillade MR, Enria DA, Briggiler AM, Levis SC, Ambrosio AM, Halsey NA, Peters CJ. Protective efficacy of a live attenuated vaccine against Argentine hemorrhagic fever. AHF Study Group. *J Infect Dis* 1998; 177:277–283.
48. Centers for Disease Control and Prevention (CDC). International notes: Bolivian hemorrhagic fever: El Beni Department, Bolivia 1994. *MMWR* 43(50); 943–946.
49. Weaver SC, Salas RA, de Manzione N, Fulhorst CF, Duno G, Utrera A, Mills JN, Ksiazek TG, Tovar D, Tesh RB. Guanarito virus (Arenaviridae) isolates from endemic and outlying localities in Venezuela: sequence comparisons among and within strains isolated from Venezuelan hemorrhagic fever patients and rodents. *Virology* 2000; 266:189–195.
50. Tesh RB, Wilson ML, Salas R, De Manzione NM, Tovar D, Ksiazek TG, Peters CJ. Field studies on the epidemiology of Venezuelan hemorrhagic fever: implication of the cotton rat Sigmodon alstoni as the probable rodent reservoir. *Am J Trop Med Hyg*. 1993; 49:227–235.
51. Pan American Health Organization. Venezuelan hemorrhagic fever (VHF). *Epidemiological Bulletin* 1995; 16 (3). URL: http://165.158.1.110/english/sha/be953vhf.htm.
52. de Manzione N, Salas RA, Paredes H, et al. Venezuelan hemorrhagic fever: clinical and epidemiological studies of 165 cases. *Clin Infect Dis* 1998; 26:308–313.
53. Lisieux T, Coimbra M, Nassar ES, et al. New arenavirus isolated in Brazil. *Lancet* 1994; 343:391–392.
54. Gonzalez JP, Bowen MD, Nichol ST, Rico-Hesse R. Genetic characterization and phylogeny of Sabia virus, an emergent pathogen in Brazil. *Virology* 1996; 221:318–324.
55. Armstrong LR, Dembry LM, Rainey PM, Russi MB, Khan AS, Fischer SH, Edberg SC, Ksiazek TG, Rollin PE, Peters CJ. Management of a Sabia virus-infected patient in a US hospital. *Infect Control Hosp Epidemiol* 1999; 20:176–182.
56. Fulhorst CF, Bowen MD, Ksiazek TG, et al. Isolation and characterization of Whitewater Arroyo virus, a novel North American arenavirus. *Virology* 1996; 224:114–120.
57. Fulhorst CF, Charrel RN, Weaver SC,Ksiazek TG, Bradley RD, Milazzo ML, Tesh RB, Bowen MD. Geographic Distribution and Genetic Diversity of Whitewater Arroyo Virus in the Southwestern United States. *Emerg Infect Dis* 2001; 7:403–407.
58. Byrd RG, Cone LA, Commess BC, et al. Fatal illness associated with a New World arenavirus—California, 1999-2000. *MMWR* 2000; 49:709–711.

# Chapter 9
# Orthopoxviruses

José R. Romero, M.D., F.A.A.P.

## Smallpox

### Introduction

Smallpox (variola) is an ancient disease. Physical evidence for its existence dates to the second millennium B.C. in Egypt [1,2]. The eradication of smallpox stands as a medical and public health triumph as the sole disease that has been successfully eliminated from the world.

The last natural case of smallpox occurred in the Merca District of Somalia in 1977 and the last known human case of smallpox occurred in Birmingham, England in 1978 [3,4]. In May 1980, the World Health Organization (WHO) certified the world free of smallpox. Because cessation of vaccination against smallpox occurred in 1982, today, most of the world's population is susceptible to infection. Recent concerns that variola virus could be released accidentally or deliberately has prompted renewed interest in this disease and its complications.

### Epidemiology

Variola is a member of the *Poxviridae* family of viruses within the genus orthopoxvirus [5]. Other members of the genus include vaccinia (smallpox vaccine), monkeypox, cow-pox, and additional animal poxviruses. Variola is a lipid-enveloped, brick-shaped virus that possesses a massive (~200 kbp) single-stranded linear DNA genome. Recent phylogenetic analysis has inferred the existence of three variola clades that correspond to geographic origin and case–fatality rates [6].

Humans are the only reservoir of variola. Before its eradication, smallpox was found worldwide. Although seasonal restriction of transmission does not occur, the cool, dry winter and spring months favor the transmission of variola virus. The principle mode of transmission is via inhalation of infected aerosols and droplets. However, the virus may be spread through direct contact with the lesions and eschars as well

L.L. Barton and N.R. Friedman (eds.), *The Neurological Manifestations of Pediatric Infectious Diseases and Immunodeficiency Syndromes.*

as via fomites such as bedding and clothing. Attack rates among unimmunized individuals range from 37 to 88% [7,8].

## *Pathogenesis*

The pathogenesis of smallpox in humans is based on data from animal poxviruses as well as studies in humans [8,9]. After inhalation of infected respiratory secretions, viral replication in the mucous membranes of the upper respiratory tract ensues with spread to the regional lymph nodes, and is followed by a short-lived period of viremia. The viremia seeds the liver, spleen, and distant sites of the reticuloendothelial system. A period of latency lasting 4 to 14 days then follows, during which, viral replication occurs in the seeded organs. A second period of viremia then ensues, during which, viral infection of the capillary epithelium of the dermal layer of the skin occurs. During the subsequent prodromal phase, the mucous membranes of the mouth and pharynx are infected. Infection of the skin results in the dermatologic manifestations of smallpox.

Large quantities of variola virus are detectable in the skin lesions and oropharyngeal secretions. Additionally, high titers of virus are found in the liver, spleen, bone marrow, kidneys, and lymph nodes. The host immune response limits viral spread through production of cytotoxic T cells and B cells. Neutralizing antibodies appear during the first week of illness.

Two principle forms of smallpox exist: variola major and minor. Variola major accounted for the majority of disease worldwide and carried a fatality rate of 30%. Variola minor, also known as alastrim or amaas, is a much milder form of smallpox that is seen in the Americas and parts of Africa. Less than 1% of persons with variola minor died [10]. The WHO has further classified variola major into five types: ordinary, modified, flat, hemorrhagic, and variola sin eruptione [7].

## *Clinical Manifestations [7,8]*

The mean incubation period for smallpox is 10 to 12 days (range, 7–17 days). The onset of the illness is heralded by the abrupt appearance of a 2- to 3-day prodrome consisting of severe headache, high fever, and backache. The prodrome renders the patient rapidly prostrate. The exanthem is preceded by 1 day by an enanthem that involves the hard palate, pillars of the fauces, and tongue.

The exanthem of smallpox first appears on the face and extremities and exhibits a centrifugal pattern in density. It begins as small erythematous macules that evolve to 2- to 3-mm papules and, subsequently, vesicles measuring 2 to 5 mm. The progression from one phase to the next takes 1 to 2 days and occurs in unison, so that, by the seventh day, all lesions are in a pustular state. The pustules gradually enlarge to 4 to 6 mm in diameter and become umbilicated. The pustules then crust and separate, leaving a hypopigmented area. Lesions on the palms and soles persist the longest.

Non-neurological complications of smallpox included arthritis, which generally involved the elbows. This complication occurred in approximately 2% of cases and affected mostly children. Panophthalmitis, keratitis, and secondary blindness were seen in approximately 1% of patients. Orchitis was a rare complication.

## *Neurological Manifestations*

Knowledge of the occurrence of the central nervous system (CNS) complications of smallpox dates to the early 1700s [11,12]. However, it was not until the first half of the 20th century that clear, detailed clinical and histopathologic descriptions of smallpox-associated encephalomyelitis appeared [11–13].

The reported incidence of encephalitis among smallpox patients varies between variola major and minor. Rao noted an incidence of 1 in 500 cases of variola minor whereas Marsden reported an occurrence of 1 in 2,000 cases of variola major [10,14]. The incidence of encephalitis in association with variola major or minor far exceeds the 1 in 100,000 cases seen in association with smallpox vaccination (i.e., postvaccinal encephalitis). Given the significant occurrence of encephalomyelitis as a complication of smallpox, it is surprising that so few reports exist detailing its clinical characteristics [11–13].

Almost all of what is known regarding smallpox encephalomyelitis is based on case reports by Hurst and Marsden [11–13], and, in particular, their compilation of 11 cases and review of the medical literature published in 1932 [12]. Nine of the 11 cases occurred in children or adolescents. Four deaths were reported among the 11 cases.

Their report described two clinical presentations, "encephalic" and "spinal," depending on the predominance of symptoms of the encephalitic or myelitic component of CNS disease. However, it should be borne in mind that nearly all of the reported cases had components of both.

In smallpox encephalomyelitis, the onset of CNS symptoms occurs from 5 to 13 days after the appearance of the smallpox rash and is never insidious. Fever may also be present early in the course, but then subsides. Depending on the degree and extent of involvement of the brain, brainstem, and spinal cord, various combinations of neurological signs and symptoms may occur. Early CNS symptoms consist of somnolence, and speech or gait disturbances. The somnolence may progress to stupor and, ultimately, coma. The latter may last for several weeks. Somnolence may be a minor component of myelitic cases in which paralysis dominates the clinical presentation. Headache in association with back and extremity pain is common. Nuchal rigidity and Kernig sign may be present.

Superficial and deep tendon reflex abnormalities are common. Abdominal reflexes become absent early and may be followed by loss of deep tendon reflexes. Plantar reflexes may be absent or extensor. Paraplegia, pareses, and paralysis may occur. Paralysis tends to be flaccid in nature and associated with the loss of deep tendon reflexes. Even in cases in which encephalitis is the major clinical component, disturbances of motor function may be present. Sensory loss may accompany motor disturbances and represents the transverse nature of the myelitis.

Loss of voluntary sphincter control presenting as urinary retention or urinary and fecal incontinence is common. The patient may experience periods of emotional lability, in particular, during the recovery phase of the illness. Trismus, dysphagia, and excessive salivation may occur. The absence of reports of seizures is notable.

Evaluation of the cerebrospinal fluid (CSF) demonstrates a pleocytosis of generally no more than 500 cells/mm$^3$ [12]. If the CSF is sampled early in the course of the illness, a high percentage of polymorphonuclear cells may be present. Later, the pleocytosis is comprised of lymphocytes and monocytes. The CSF protein concentration is mildly to moderately increased (50–180 mg/dl), and the glucose level is normal.

## *Pathogenesis and Neuropathology*

Smallpox encephalomyelitis is thought to be caused by an abnormal host response to poxvirus antigens or antigen–antibody complexes that localize to neural tissue [9]. The predominant histologic feature is that of acute perivascular demyelination [12]. The perivascular space shows a lymphocytic infiltration. The areas of demyelination contain lymphocytes and pleomorphic microglia. Rarely, necrosis of the anterior horn cells may be seen. However, this is a decidedly unusual occurrence.

## *Diagnosis*

Because the reported cases of smallpox predate the advent of cell culture, no reports document an attempt to the isolate variola virus from the CSF. Additionally, no reports provide information regarding the electroencephalographic findings in this condition. Thus, the diagnosis of smallpox encephalitis is primarily a clinical one based on the timing of the onset and the constellation of neurological symptoms. Reports of pyogenic meningitis exist in association with smallpox and must be excluded by examination and culture of the CSF.

## *Treatment*

Treatment is supportive in nature. In their series, Marsden and Hurst report the use of human convalescent smallpox serum administered intrathecally to three patients, two of whom survived [12]. Without a large controlled clinical trial, it is not possible to state whether this therapy is beneficial for patients with smallpox encephalitis.

## References


1. Ruffer MA, Ferguson AR. Note on an eruption resembling that of variola in the skin of a mummy of the twentieth dynasty (1200–1100 BC). *J Pathology Bacteriol* 1911; 15:1–3.
2. Fenner F, Isao A, Henderson DA, Jezek Z, Ladnyi ID. The History of Smallpox and its Spread Around the World. *Smallpox and its Eradication.* 1988. Fenner F, Isao A, Henderson DA, Jezek Z, Ladnyi ID (eds). World Health Organization, Geneva, pp 209–244.
3. Fenner F, Isao A, Henderson DA, Jezek Z, Ladnyi ID. *Somalia and Djiboui.* 1988. Fenner F, Isao A, Henderson DA, Jezek Z, Ladnyi ID (eds). World Health Organization, Geneva, pp 1037–1067.
4. Fenner F, Isao A, Henderson DA, Jezek Z, Ladnyi ID. Smallpox in Non-Endemic Countries. *Smallpox and its Eradication.* 1988. Fenner F, Isao A, Henderson DA, Jezek Z, Ladnyi ID (eds). World Health Organization, Geneva, pp 1069–1101.
5. Moss B. Poxviridae: The viruses and their replication. *Fields Virology.* 2001. Knipe DM, Howley PM, Griffin DE, Lamb RA, Martin MA, Roizman B, Straus SE (eds). 4th ed. Lippincott Williams & Wilkins, Philadelphia, pp 2849–2884.
6. Esposito JJ, Sammons SA, Frace AM, Osborne JD, Olsen-Rasmussen M, Zhang M, Govil D, Damon IK, Kline R, Laker M, Li Y, Smith GL, Meyer H, Leduc JW, Wohlhueter RM. Genome sequence diversity and clues to the evolution of variola (smallpox) virus. *Science.* 2006; 313:807–812.
7. Fenner F, Isao A, Henderson DA, Jezek Z, Ladnyi ID. The Clinical Features of Smallpox. *Smallpox and its Eradication.* 1988. Fenner F, Isao A, Henderson DA, Jezek Z, Ladnyi ID (eds). World Health Organization, Geneva, pp 2–68.
8. Breman JG, Henderson DA. Diagnosis and management of smallpox. *N Engl J Med* 2002; 346:1300–1308.
9. Fenner F, Isao A, Henderson DA, Jezek Z, Ladnyi ID. The Pathogenesis, Pathology and Immunology of Smallpox and Vaccinia. *Smallpox and its Eradication.* 1988. Fenner F, Isao A, Henderson DA, Jezek Z, Ladnyi ID (eds). World Health Organization, Geneva, Switzerland, pp 121–168.
10. Marsden JP. Variola minor: a personal analysis of 13,686 cases. *Bull Hyg* 1948; 23:735–746.
11. Troup AG, Hurst EW. Disseminated encephalomyelitis. *Lancet* 1930; 2:566–569.
12. Marsden JP, Hurst EW. Acute perivascular myelinoclassis ("acute disseminated encephalomyelitis") in smallpox. *Brain* 1932; 55:181–225.
13. Marsden JP. Acute perivascular myelinoclasis "acute disseminated encephalomyelitis." *Lancet* 1934; 2:871–872.
14. Rao AR. *Smallpox.* 1972. The Kothari Book Depot, Bombay.

# Chapter 10
# Retroviruses

**Lemuel Aigbivbalu, M.D., Ayesha Mirza, M.D., and Mobeen H. Rathore, M.D., C.P.E., F.A.A.P.**

## Neurological Manifestations of HIV and HIV-Associated Infections

### *Introduction*

Since the first recognition of acquired immunodeficiency syndrome (AIDS) in the early 1980s, much progress has been made in understanding the pathogenesis, treatment, and opportunistic infections associated with human immunodeficiency virus (HIV) infection. Pediatric AIDS was described in 1983 and, within a very short time, neurological involvement was reported in children.

Significant advances have been made since then, both in laboratory and clinical research related to individual opportunistic infections. In addition, the use of highly active antiretroviral therapy (HAART) has dramatically increased, changing the epidemiology and presentation of opportunistic infections among children and adults. As with HIV-infected adults, substantial decreases in mortality and morbidity, including opportunistic infections, have been observed among children receiving HAART. However, even though the number of opportunistic infections has decreased, the relative prevalence of AIDS-defining infections remains similar to that observed in the pre-HAART era [1].

HIV-associated infections causing neurological disorders can occur during any stage of HIV disease. However, some infections occur with greater frequency in advanced HIV disease. Many opportunistic infections seen in adults with HIV infection are a result of reactivation of previous (latent) infections. This is not often the case in children who are perinatally infected. Adolescents who acquire HIV infection postnatally are, in contrast, likely to have opportunistic infections with similar pathogenetic mechanisms as in adults. Neurological disorders may be caused by HIV itself, complications of immunosuppression, or metabolic complications of antiretroviral therapy [2]. The focus of this chapter will primarily be those disorders resulting from complications of immunosuppression, in particular, opportunistic infections.

L.L. Barton and N.R. Friedman (eds.), *The Neurological Manifestations of Pediatric Infectious Diseases and Immunodeficiency Syndromes.*

## *Clinical Manifestations*

HIV replication within $CD4^+$ lymphocytes results in $CD4^+$ cell destruction and immunosuppression. In adult patients, an absolute $CD4^+$ cell count below 200 cells/$mm^3$ is associated with an increased risk of opportunistic infection, with severe or even fatal consequences. In children, the absolute $CD4^+$ cell count below which the risk of the opportunistic infections is highest and immunocompromise considered severe, is age dependent (Table 10.1). Although the incidence of opportunistic infections has significantly declined with the use of HAART, lesser degrees of immunosuppression still predispose to disease with potentially devastating neurological consequences (e.g., tuberculosis [TB] or syphilis).

All of these infections may be classified according to the area of the nervous system affected (i.e., central or peripheral). The central nervous system (CNS) disorders may be further categorized into those that affect the meninges, parenchymal lesions (focal or diffuse), or spinal cord (Table 10.2).

### Central Nervous System

CNS infections in patients with HIV infection overlap those that infect non-HIV immunocompetent patients. These are listed in Table 10.2 and discussed in other sections of this book. This section is restricted to a discussion of diseases unique to HIV-infected patients.

#### Cryptococcal Meningitis

*Cryptococcus neoformans* is a fungus with a worldwide distribution. Although exposure is common, natural resistance is high and disease infrequent [3–5].

**Table 10.1** Age-specific CD4+ T-lymphocyte count and percentage of total lymphocytes

| Immunologic definitions | <12 mo | | 1–5 y | | 6–12 y | |
|---|---|---|---|---|---|---|
| | uL | % | uL | % | uL | % |
| 1: No evidence of suppression | ≥1500 | ≥25 | ≥1000 | ≥25 | ≥500 | ≥25 |
| 2: Evidence of moderate suppression | 750–1499 | 15–24 | 500–999 | 15–24 | 200–499 | 15–24 |
| 3: Severe suppression | <750 | <15 | <500 | <15 | <200 | <15 |

Modified from Centers for Disease Control and Prevention. 1994 revised classification system for human immunodeficiency virus infection in children less than 13 years of age. Official authorized addenda: human immunodeficiency virus infection codes and official guidelines for coding and reporting ICD-9CM. *MMWR*. 1994; 43 (RR-12):1–19

**Table 10.2** Summary of neurological disorders of HIV-associated infections

| Etiologic agent | Area of nervous system affected | Disease/syndrome | Clinical manifestations | *Range of absolute CD4 count (per $mm^3$) | Diagnostic studies | Treatment |
|---|---|---|---|---|---|---|
| ***Cryptococcus neoformans*** | Diffuse lesions in brain, esp. basal ganglia & cortical gray matter | Meningoencephalitis or cryptococcoma | Headache, dizziness, somnolence, behavioral changes, cranial nerve palsies | < 200 | CT/MRI: edema, cryptococcoma;<br>CSF: opening pressure; cryptococcal antigen & fungal cultures | Amphotericin B plus flucytosine initially, followed by oral/iv fluconazole therapy; lifelong suppressive therapy may be needed |
| ***Treponema pallidum*** | Parenchyma (cerebral cortex) or meningovascular | Neurosyphilis | Hemiplegia, hemiparesis, meningitis, general paresis, tabes dorsalis | Any CD4 count | CSF: reactive VDRL; elevated protein, leukocytosis | Penicillin G IV x<br>10-14 days; repeat lumbar puncture every six months until CSF normal |
| ***Mycobacterium tuberculosis*** | Parenchyma (esp. base of brain) and meninges of brain & spinal cord | Tuberculoma, meningitis | Headache, meningismus, seizures, or symptoms of cord compression | Any CD4 count | CT/MRI: tuberculomas/ granulomas;<br>CSF: *M. tuberculosis* PCR, low glucose, lymphocytic predominance | INH, Rifampin, PZA and ethambutol or an aminoglycoside, (streptomycin, or amikacin); PZA and ethambutol can be discontinued after 2 months; minimum Rx is 12 months |
| ***Toxoplasma gondii*** | Diffuse brain lesions, occasional spinal cord masses | Toxoplasmic encephalitis | Wide range including, altered mental status, seizures, hemiparesis | <200 | CT/ MRI: multiple ring-enhancing lesions<br>Toxoplasma IgG serology helpful | Pyrimethamine + folinic acid + sulfadiazine for ≥ 6 weeks with lifelong suppressive therapy |
| **JC virus** | Cerebral white matter, cerebellum & brainstem | Progressive multifocal leukoencephalopathy | Hemiparesis, cognitive disturbance & visual field defects | ?? | CT/MRI: non-enhancing lesions primarily in cerebral white matter;<br>Stereotactic brain biopsy | Highly active anti-retroviral treatment (HAART) |
| ***Nocardia spp.*** | Parenchyma | Brain abscess | Depends on location | ?? | CT/MRI: space-occupying lesion;<br>Stereotactic brain biopsy | Trimethoprim-sulfamethoxazole + ceftriaxone and an aminoglycoside for the first 4-12 weeks duration Rx 6-12 months |

(continued)

**Table 10.2** Summary of neurological disorders of HIV-associated infections (continued)

| Etiologic agent | Area of nervous system affected | Disease/syndrome | Clinical manifestations | *Range of absolute CD4 count (per $mm^3$) | Diagnostic studies | Treatment |
|---|---|---|---|---|---|---|
| ***Salmonella spp.*** | Parenchyma | Brain abscess | Depends on location | ?? | CT/MRI: space-occupying lesion;<br>Stereotactic brain biopsy | Third-generation cephalosporin × 1-2 weeks followed by oral fluoroquinolone or cephalosporin |
| **Herpes simplex virus** | Medial temporal & inferior frontal lobes, spinal cord | Meningoencephalitis, acute myelopathies | Headache, seizures, fever, | Any CD4 | CT/MRI: edema, contrast enhancement or hemorrhage in medial temporal or inferior frontal lobes<br>EEG abnormalities<br>CSF: HSV DNA PCR & abnormal parameters | Acyclovir |
| **Herpes zoster virus** | Meninges, cerebral blood vessels, spinal cord | Meningoencephalitis, ependymitis, cranial nerve palsies, cerebral angiitis, acute myelopathies | Altered mental status, focal cranial nerve deficits, strokes or TIAs | Any CD4 | CT/MRI: hemorrhagic or ischemic changes<br>CSF: HZV DNA PCR | Acyclovir |
| **Cytomegalovirus** | Meninges, spinal cord, peripheral nerves | Meningoencephalitis, necrotizing ependymitis, progressive lumbosacral radiculopathy, mononeuropathy multiplex | Altered mental status, bilateral leg weakness progressing to paraplegia, urinary retention, constipation; cranial or peripheral neuropathies | <50 | CT/MRI: periventricular white matter disease<br>CSF: CMV PCR | Ganciclovir and/or foscarnet |

* Based on adult patients. For children use age appropriate cutoff for severe immunesuppression;

+ See chapter on tubeculosis for treatment in areas with high level of resistance; INH = isoniazid; PZA= pyrazinamide; TIAs= transient ischemic attack

However, there was a dramatic increase in new cases of cryptococcal meningitis after the appearance of AIDS. Infection occurs more commonly in infected adults as opposed to children. Infected children usually have severe immune suppression (CD4 <200) [1]. Currently, 80 to 90% of cases of cryptococcosis occur in AIDS patients.

CNS cryptococcosis may have an acute or insidious onset. The acute onset of the disease is seen more commonly in AIDS patients. Complaints may be mild (e.g., headache, dizziness, irritability, or somnolence) or more severe, with behavioral changes, clumsiness, confusion, obtundation, or seizures. Diplopia, decrease in visual acuity, facial numbness, or weakness may also occur. HIV-positive patients may also be asymptomatic initially.

Among HIV-infected children with CNS disease, cerebrospinal fluid (CSF) cell count, glucose and protein levels may be virtually normal, but opening pressure is usually elevated. Indicators of high risk are abnormal mental status, CSF cryptococcal antigen titer greater than 1:1,024, and CSF white blood cell count less than 20 cells/mm$^3$ [6].

Cryptococcal meningitis is fatal if not treated. There are no controlled treatment trials in the pediatric population. Current recommendations are based on data obtained from adults. Amphotericin B in combination with flucytosine is recommended for the first 2 weeks of treatment. Once the patient is stable, these may be discontinued, and either intravenous or oral fluconazole started for at least another 8 weeks or until CSF cultures become sterile. Because treatment of cryptococcosis in patients with AIDS is seldom curative, maintenance therapy with fluconazole should be continued until the patient's CD4 count rises above the age appropriate cutoff of normal (Table 10.1) and is maintained at that level for at least 6 months [7]. The safety of discontinuation of secondary prophylaxis after immune reconstitution with HAART among children has not been extensively studied.

## Neurosyphilis

Between 1986 and 1994, there was a rapid increase in the incidence of syphilis in the heterosexual population, primarily women and children [8]. However, between 1991 and 2004, there was a 19.8% average yearly decrease in the rate of primary and secondary syphilis reported among women; after this, an average yearly 17% decrease in the rate of congenital syphilis [9]. Concomitant infection with HIV is common, and the two diseases may enhance the acquisition and transmission of each other [10]. Syphilis tends to have a more aggressive course in HIV-infected patients, with a greater tendency for development of neurological disease, especially uveitis. Other neurological manifestations include meningitis, cerebritis, and deafness [11,12].

In an HIV-infected adolescent with a positive test for syphilis, a lumbar puncture is indicated to determine whether neurosyphilis is present. A repeat lumbar puncture is indicated every 6 months if the initial CSF specimen showed pleocytosis. The patient should be retreated at 6 months if the cell count has not decreased or at 2 years if the CSF is still abnormal [13]. There have been several reports of treatment failures in co-infected persons [12]. The management of HIV-infected infants and children who have syphilis is not different from non-HIV-infected infants and children.

## Tuberculosis

Although the number of cases of extrapulmonary TB increased dramatically in the mid-1980s, largely because of co-infection with HIV, there has been a 46% decrease in the overall number of cases of TB reported to the Centers for Disease Control and Prevention (CDC) since 1992. The number of cases of multidrug-resistant TB also decreased from 2.5% in 1993 to 1% in 2004 [1].

The clinical presentation of tuberculous disease among children with HIV infection is similar to that among children without HIV infection. Younger children are, however, more likely to progress more rapidly from infection to active disease than older children and adults, and may not be recognized as having tuberculous disease because they may have negative skin tests and fewer symptoms of disease. CNS TB manifests as meningitis or tuberculomas. If branches of the middle cerebral artery are involved, hemiparesis may ensue. Tuberculomas and space-occupying lesions in the brain, occur more frequently in HIV-infected patients [14,15].

## Toxoplasmosis

In most immunocompetent persons, there are no symptoms of infection with *Toxoplasma gondii*. However, asymptomatic latent or chronic infection ensues with persistence of cysts in tissues. In adolescents with AIDS, toxoplasmosis is usually the result of reactivation of latent infection. Reactivation is thought to be a result of cyst rupture with release of organisms that subsequently proliferate and destroy tissue in the immunodeficient individual. Perinatal transmission of *Toxoplasma gondii* from women without HIV infection who have chronic *Toxoplasma* infection acquired before pregnancy is uncommon. However, in the setting of HIV co-infection, perinatal transmission of *Toxoplasma* has been observed among women with chronic *Toxoplasma* infection (transmission rate $<4\%$), presumably because of reactivation and replication of the organism and among women with severe immune suppression [1].

AIDS-defining infection of the CNS with *Toxoplasma gondii* is uncommon among HIV-infected children. It was reported as an AIDS-indicator condition in less than 1% of pediatric AIDS cases, even before the advent of HAART [1].

In AIDS patients, toxoplasmic encephalitis (TE) is the most common manifestation of toxoplasmosis and is a frequent cause of focal CNS lesions [16]. In most cases of TE among HIV-infected children, infection is considered to have occurred in utero. More rarely, it has also been reported among older HIV-infected pediatric patients, presumably with primary acquired toxoplasmosis. TE can present with a wide range of clinical signs, such as altered mental status, seizures, cerebellar signs, cranial nerve abnormalities, sensory abnormalities, meningismus, movement disorders, and neuropsychiatric disturbances. The onset is usually subacute with focal neurological signs, but in up to 25% of patients it can present abruptly with seizures or cerebral hemorrhage. Common initial manifestations are hemiparesis and/or speech abnormalities. Diffuse TE also occurs in AIDS patients and is acute in onset and rapidly fatal. There are no focal neurological deficits, with global cerebral dysfunction. Chorioretinitis may be seen in association with CNS disease.

Head computed tomographic (CT) scans in diffuse disease can show cerebral atrophy or the results may be normal [17]. In approximately 80% of AIDS patients with TE, CT scans of the brain show multiple ring-enhancing lesions [18]. Solitary lesions have also been reported. The presence of IgG antibodies to *Toxoplasma* in serum and multiple ring-enhancing lesions on contrast CT or magnetic resonance imaging (MRI) scanning has a predictive value of 80% for TE [19]. MRI scanning with gadolinium contrast has a greater sensitivity for detection of lesions than CT. The differential diagnosis of CNS lesions in AIDS patients should also include lymphoma, which is more likely when there is a solitary lesion. Positron emission tomography (PET) scans can be helpful in distinguishing *Toxoplasma* abscesses from primary CNS lymphoma, but the accuracy is not high and this test is not widely available [1].

The indications for brain biopsy are: a single lesion on CT or MRI scan, a negative *Toxoplasma* IgG antibody test, inadequate clinical response to appropriate anti-*Toxoplasma* treatment, or suspected toxoplasmosis in patients considered compliant with prophylactic trimethoprim-sulfamethoxazole (TMP-SMX) therapy.

Antimicrobial therapy of *T. gondii* is the same as in HIV-uninfected children. Empiric treatment for *T. gondii* should be initiated in patients with multiple ring-enhancing lesions on MRI scan, positive *Toxoplasma* IgG, and absolute CD4 counts less than the appropriate cutoff for age. A clinical response generally is noted in 1 week and improvement on CT or MRI scan in 2 weeks. Lifelong suppressive therapy is maintained, because there is a high rate of relapse. Primary prophylaxis with TMP-SMX or dapsone, if allergic to sulfonamides, is recommended for patients with CD4 counts below 200 or age appropriate cutoff (Table 10.1) and positive *Toxoplasma* IgG titers [20]. Patients on HAART, who have CD4 counts above the appropriate cutoff for age that are maintained for at least 6 months, may discontinue primary prophylaxis [21]. The safety of discontinuation of secondary prophylaxis after immune reconstitution with HAART among children has not been extensively studied.

### Progressive Multifocal Leukoencephalopathy

Progressive multifocal leukoencephalopathy (PML), caused by the Jakob-Creutzfeldt (JC) virus, occurs in approximately 4 to 7% of immunodeficient patients, including those with AIDS [22]. Approximately 60 to 80% of the U.S. and European populations demonstrate serologic evidence of previous exposure to this virus. Usually the virus is acquired in childhood and patients are asymptomatic. It is unclear whether PML is the result of reactivation or a primary infection in the immunocompromised host.

In the pre-HAART era, the prognosis was extremely poor in HIV-infected patients, with death usually occurring within 6 months of diagnosis. Aggressive antiretroviral therapy has resulted in marked clinical and radiographic improvement [23].

## Bacterial Brain Abscess

Bacterial brain abscesses have been associated with HIV infection. The most prevalent microorganisms reported in AIDS patients are *Nocardia* spp. and *Salmonella* spp. All patients with pulmonary nocardiosis should be evaluated to exclude CNS disease [24]. There is a 20- to 100-fold increased risk of salmonellosis in HIV-infected patients in comparison with the general population [25]. There is an even greater risk of severe invasive disease in persons with AIDS when compared with immunocompetent persons, resulting in fulminant diarrhea, recurrent bacteremia, and CNS invasion [26].

The classic triad of fever, headache, and focal neurological deficit may occur in less than 50% of patients with brain abscess. In addition, the diminished inflammatory response in immunocompromised patients may further mask symptoms [24].

Salmonellosis should be treated with intravenous antibiotics (e.g., third-generation cephalosporins) for 1 to 2 weeks, followed by 4 weeks with an oral antibiotic (depending on the susceptibility) to decrease the risk of recurrence [27].

## Viral Encephalitis

### *Herpes Simplex Virus*

Herpes simplex virus (HSV) infections have been rarely reported in AIDS patients. In these patients, the onset is more insidious with a more chronic course than observed in immunocompetent persons. However, prompt empiric therapy with acyclovir is recommended for patients presenting with fever, headache, and seizures for which there is no apparent etiology. Herpetic skin or mucosal lesions may be present. Among children with suspected HSV encephalitis, detection of HSV by polymerase chain reaction (PCR) in the CSF is the diagnostic test of choice.

### *Varicella-Zoster Virus*

Varicella-zoster virus (VZV) infection occurs in approximately 8 to 11% of HIV-infected patients [28]. CNS involvement may be manifested by meningoencephalitis or encephalitis, cranial nerve palsies, and ependymitis. In adult patients, the rare complication, granulomatous cerebral angiitis, results in strokes or transient ischemic attacks (TIAs). The presence of these manifestations should prompt suspicion of VZV encephalitis in children with AIDS [27]. VZV cultures as well as PCR for VZV from the CSF should be obtained, and the patient started on high-dose acyclovir (40–60 mg/kg/d) [1]. Other reported complications include retinitis and acute retinal necrosis [28]. Rash may precede or follow the neurological signs and symptoms, or may be absent.

### *Cytomegalovirus*

Infection with human cytomegalovirus (CMV) is common and usually inapparent; acquisition of CMV can occur during infancy, early childhood, or adolescence. HIV-infected children seem to be at greater risk for acquisition of CMV infection during early childhood than children without HIV infection. CMV causes 8 to 10% of pediatric AIDS-defining illness. HIV-infected children with CMV co-infection seem to have accelerated progression of HIV disease compared with those without CMV.

CNS manifestations of CMV include subacute encephalopathy, myelitis, and polyradiculitis (primarily seen in adults, but rarely reported in children). CSF findings are nonspecific, and up to 20% of children have completely normal CSF findings. CMV infection versus disease may be difficult to diagnose in HIV-infected children. Virus may be isolated in cell culture from body fluids or peripheral blood leukocytes. In addition to this, detection of CMV antigen or detection by PCR are more specific methods. Quantitative CMV PCR may also be used to monitor response to therapy. Ganciclovir is the treatment of choice for disseminated disease. The dose is 5 mg/kg/dose twice daily for 14 to 21 days, followed by lifelong maintenance therapy. Foscarnet is a therapeutic alternative for ganciclovir-resistant CMV [1].

## Fungal Encephalitis

Fungal encephalitis in AIDS patients may be caused by *Candida albicans*, *Aspergillus spp.*, and mucormycosis (especially among adolescents who are injection drug users). In endemic areas, coccidioidomycosis and histoplasmosis have also been associated with meningoencephalitis in AIDS patients. A brain biopsy is necessary for definitive diagnosis and appropriate antifungal therapy.

## HIV Encephalopathy

Encephalopathy, as a direct result of HIV, has been well documented in HIV-infected children [29]. The prevalence of HIV encephalopathy in a cohort of children with perinatally acquired HIV infection in the period before the availability of HAART was 21%, and the survival time of these children was significantly reduced [30]. In this cohort, encephalopathy was frequently the first (67%) or the only (27%) AIDS-defining condition. Encephalopathic children were more likely to be worse clinically, to be more immunosuppressed, and were likely to have higher viral loads compared with children without encephalopathy. The majority of cases of HIV encephalopathy were diagnosed in the first 2 years of life [30,31]. Early antiretroviral therapy with HAART has decreased the prevalence of encephalopathy, in both children and adults [32,33]. There are few data regarding the prevalence of encephalopathy in children with perinatal HIV infection since the routine use of HAART, and almost no data for adolescents who did not acquire HIV infection perinatally.

Several forms of encephalopathy are described in the literature, each with specific signs and patterns of progression. They may manifest as progressive, static, or indolent processes and vary according to the age and treatment of the infected child. Infants with a developing neurological system who have aggressive HIV disease and progressive encephalopathy have the highest morbidity and mortality rate.

The first sign of progressive encephalopathy is often a behavioral change, such as deterioration of play, and progressive apathy. In all cases, there is impairment in three areas: cognitive, behavioral, and motor skills. Depending on the age of the child and the severity of the disease, the initial signs and progression will vary.

Motor impairment manifests itself as developmental delays or loss of developmental milestones. In school-aged children, clumsiness or a spastic gait may be the first motor impairment exhibited. Some children are noted to have psychomotor slowing. With advancing disease, bilateral pyramidal tract signs, such as spastic diparesis and spastic quadriparesis, occur [34]. Extrapyramidal and cerebellar signs, such as rigidity, ataxia, and abnormal posturing, may also be seen.

Cognitive impairment can be seen with decreased vocalization, loss of previous language skills, and apathy in the infant and toddler. In school-aged children, progressive encephalopathy may present with loss of interest in school performance, decreased attention, decreased cognitive abilities and verbal expression, and apathy.

Behavioral impairment becomes the most obvious in the older toddler or school-aged child who is affected. Emotional lability, attention deficits, attention deficit/hyperactivity disorder and conduct disorders, lack of interest, and apathy are often noted by parents and teachers.

Neurological function was assessed in children with perinatally acquired HIV infection enrolled in an antiretroviral treatment trial (not using HAART by current standards) [35]. Neurological examinations and age-appropriate neuropsychologic/neurocognitive testing were performed. The prevalence of abnormalities associated with encephalopathy was defined. The most frequent motor abnormalities were increased tone, decreased strength, gait disturbances, psychomotor retardation, and poor head control. Approximately 50% of the children in the youngest age group exhibited motor dysfunction; 21% of the entire cohort had cognitive deficiencies. Children with the lowest IQ scores at follow-up and those with motor dysfunction were at the highest risk of progression [35].

Some children will follow a more static or indolent course. During plateau periods, the child may gain further cognitive, language, and socially adaptive skills, but the rate of acquisition of these skills may be at a rate different from the norm. During the plateau period, motor impairment may be static but hyperreflexia, clumsiness, or even a mild spastic gait may be present. Unfortunately, these children will continue to have periods of progression and deterioration. Longer survivals are associated with a static course, but overall, the mortality rate in HIV-infected patients is higher in those with encephalopathy. The time of onset of progressive encephalopathy to death averaged 8 months in one study. A large majority of these patients will have concurrent opportunistic infections that contribute to the higher mortality rate.

*Neuropathology of HIV-Related Encephalopathy*

HIV-1 belongs to the Lentiviridae subfamily of retroviruses; it invades the CNS shortly after primary infection. The virus does not infect neurons, but infects the microglia, macrophages, and astrocytes within the CNS. HIV infection originates from the migration of infected microcytes into the CNS via the blood–brain barrier. Several products of these activated microcytes are neurotoxins, such as tumor necrosis factor and interleukin-1bNF-a, and they damage oligodendria and myelin. Apoptosis in neurons occurs because of cytokines, eicosanoids, phospholipid mediators, HIV gene products, and actual viral proteins that are secreted by infected macrophages. The proinflammatory cytokines secreted impair glial and neuronal function and interfere with neurotransmitters.

Gross brain studies reveal cerebral atrophy with ventricular enlargement and sulci widening. Microscopic studies show reactive microglia, macrophages, and multinucleated giant cells, along with calcific vasculopathy, predominantly in the basal ganglia and frontal white matter. Leukoencephalopathy is demonstrated by myelin pallor and loss and diffuse astrocytosis in the white matter.

*Diagnosis of HIV-Associated Encephalopathy*

Neuroimaging studies are important to exclude other diagnostic possibilities, such as *Toxoplasma* encephalitis, PML, or primary CNS lymphoma. The most common findings in HIV-associated encephalopathy include cerebral atrophy and white matter changes. Calcifications of the basal ganglia and frontal matter are commonly seen on CT scan, and abnormal high signals in white and deep gray matter are seen on MRI. Enlargement of the subarachnoid spaces and ventricles has also been noted.

Cortical atrophy has been seen on CT and MRI scan, more pronounced in children younger than 30 months of age. Of this group, 50.8% of the children had head circumferences below the fifth percentile compared with only 31.5% of those without cortical atrophy [35].

CSF evaluations are necessary to exclude other infectious causes, but the findings are nonspecific in HIV encephalopathy. Typically, the CSF may be normal or demonstrate slightly elevated protein and a pleocytosis. No specific finding is diagnostic of encephalopathy. In adult patients, elevations of neopterin and B2-microglobulin have been correlated with increasing dementia. Although high viral loads can be present, they do not always correlate with presence or degree of encephalopathy. Some studies have shown that the CSF of children with progressive encephalopathy demonstrates elevations in interleukin-6 and interleukin-1b, which are not detected in asymptomatic children.

Increasing evidence suggests that aggressive HAART therapy may halt or even reverse signs of encephalopathy and that AIDS dementia symptoms may be partially reversible in adult patients on HAART. There are several reports of impressive improvement in neurological function in children with recent-onset encephalopathy started on HAART [36].

## Spinal Cord

### Acute Myelopathies

Acute myelopathies may be caused by spinal cord compression or acute viral infections. Spinal cord compression is a neurological emergency, presents as acute back pain, leg weakness or numbness, and bladder or bowel dysfunction. The causes in HIV-infected patients include TB, bacterial spinal abscesses, and metastases caused by lymphoma [27]. Acute infections by VZV, HSV, and CMV have also been reported as causes of acute myelopathies [37–39].

## Peripheral Nervous System

### Peripheral Neuropathy

Peripheral neuropathy is the most common neurological complication of HIV infection in adults, but infrequently described in pediatric cases. Early in the epidemic, many children died before acquiring adequate language skills to describe symptoms or developed encephalopathy that prevented recognition of signs and symptoms of peripheral neuropathy [40]. With improved treatments and prolonged survival, more affected children are being recognized.

Peripheral neuropathy may present as an inflammatory demyelinating polyneuropathy, mononeuropathy, mononeuritis multiplex, polyradiculopathy, or distal sensory polyneuropathy (DSP). In individuals on HAART, it may be difficult to distinguish neuropathy caused by HIV versus drug-induced neuropathy, because the symptoms are similar. One study looked at the prevalence and characteristics of peripheral neuropathy in a cohort of children. The most common neurological findings included distal paresthesias and/or pain plus diminished ankle jerks and/or diminished vibration sense. Nerve conduction studies (NCS) revealed axonal changes. Approximately one-third of the children had features consistent with peripheral neuropathy [40].

The symptoms, clinical findings, diagnosis, and treatment have been well established in adults, but are less clear in pediatrics. Generally, the symptoms first occur distally, with dysesthesias first appearing on the soles with subsequent proximal progression. As the symptoms ascend and reach mid-leg level, involvement of the upper extremities becomes apparent, initially on the fingertips. Pain and paresthesias are the primary complaints in children, as in adults, but do not seem to be as severe. Pain is often described as a burning sensation in the feet or fingertips. Motor involvement may be minimal and only noticed by the clinician with diminished or absent ankle reflexes [41].

Neurological examination may show diminished distal vibratory sensation, diminished or absent deep tendon reflexes, hypotonia, distal muscle weakness, and diminished tactile sensation. NCS may show either low amplitudes or small alterations in conduction velocities or latencies in the sural nerve or the absence of the F response in the peroneal nerve. A normal NCS does not exclude early neuropathy. Small fiber involvement may be associated with a normal NCS result, but a reduction in nerve fiber density may be demonstrated on skin biopsy, affirming the presence of neuropathy and correlating with severity.

There are no current recommendations for treatment of DSP in children. Moreover, it may be very difficult to distinguish between HIV- and antiretroviral-related peripheral neuropathy. Approximately one-third of HIV-infected children will develop HIV-associated peripheral neuropathy. Because these children experience less pain than adults, damage to peripheral nerves may be more advanced when brought to the clinician's attention. Therefore, meticulous neurological examinations need to be routinely performed to detect early signs of this process. Intervention with treatment for the underlying HIV disease is presently the only treatment that may prevent further nerve damage. Because of the high risk of encephalopathy and opportunistic infections in this advanced group, peripheral neuropathy can often be overlooked or misdiagnosed, but should be an important consideration in the care of HIV-infected pediatric patients.

### Progressive Lumbosacral Polyradiculopathy

Progressive lumbosacral polyradiculopathy caused by CMV is rare in children. It is treatable and important to recognize, because it may be debilitating or lethal if untreated. It usually occurs in patients with advanced disease and a very low CD4 count (<50 cells/mm$^3$ in adults). The characteristic presentation is of bilateral leg weakness with progression to difficulty walking. The speed of disease progression is rapid, and flaccid paraplegia may develop in 1 to 2 weeks. If the lower sacral roots are involved, patients may experience urinary retention, constipation, or obstipation. On physical examination, deep tendon reflexes in the lower extremities may be decreased or absent. Although sensory deficits are rare, sensory loss may be apparent over the perineal or perianal areas. Dysthesias or back pain may also be present.

CSF pleocytosis supports the diagnosis of progressive lumbosacral polyradiculopathy. Approximately 50% of patients have a CSF white blood cell count greater than 500 cells/mm$^3$, with 40 to 50% polymorphonuclear cells. The CSF protein level may be elevated and the glucose level decreased. Viral cultures of the CSF yield CMV in 50 to 75% of patients with these findings. The diagnostic test of choice, however, is CMV PCR of the CSF. Recommended therapy includes ganciclovir and/or foscarnet [27].

### Mononeuropathy Multiplex

Mononeuropathy multiplex (MM) is a rare occurrence in AIDS patients. It is associated with the most severe immunosuppression and very low CD4$^+$ counts. It is thought to be caused by CMV infection of nerves or their blood supply [27]. There may be a similar self-limited syndrome in early HIV infection that may be caused by an autoimmune phenomenon.

The presentation of MM may be subacute, with asymmetric sensory and motor deficits in the distribution of peripheral nerves or spinal roots. Cranial neuropathies may be apparent as well. CMV-associated MM may affect several limbs or cranial nerves or may affect the recurrent laryngeal nerve, resulting in hoarseness and vocal cord weakness [27]. Untreated CMV-related MM is progressive and generally overlaps a more diffuse neuropathic process, such as DSP or progressive polyradiculopathy [41].

## References

1. Mofenson LM, Oleske J, Serchuck L, Van Dyke R, Wilfert C. Treating opportunistic infections among HIV-exposed and infected children: recommendations from CDC, the National Institutes of Health, and the Infectious Diseases Society of America. *Clin Infect Dis*. 2005; 40:S1–84.
2. Belman AL. HIV-1 infection and AIDS. *Neurol Clin*. 2002; 20:983–1011.
3. Mitchell TG, Perfect JR. Cryptococcosis in the era of AIDS-100 years after the discovery of *Cryptococcus neoformans*. *Clin Microbiol Rev*. 1995; 8:515–548.
4. Levitz SM. The ecology of *Cryptococcus neoformans* and the epidemiology of cryptococcosis. *Rev Infect Dis*. 1991; 13:1163–1169.
5. Atkinson AJ Jr, Bennett JE. Experience with a new skin test antigen prepared from *Cryptococcus neoformans*. *Am Rev Respir Dis*. 1968; 97:637–643.
6. Saag M, Powderly WG, Cloud GA, et al. Comparison of amphotericin B with fluconazole in the treatment of acute AIDS-associated cryptococcal meningitis. The NIAID Mycoses Study Group and the AIDS Clinical Trials Group. *N Engl J Med*. 1992; 326:83–89.
7. Bartlett JG. *The 2002 Abbreviated Guide to Medical Management of HIV Infection*. 1st ed. Johns Hopkins University, Division of Infectious Diseases.
8. Ansell DA, Hu T, Straus M, Cohen M, Sherer R. HIV and syphilis seroprevalence among clients with sexually transmitted diseases attending a walk-in clinic at Cook County Hospital. *Sex Transm Dis*. 1993; 21:93–97.
9. Centers for Disease Control and Prevention. *Sexually Transmitted Disease Surveillance 2004 Supplement, Syphilis Surveillance Report*. Atlanta, GA: US Department of Health and Human Services, Centers for Disease Control and Prevention, December 2005.
10. Theus SA, Harrich DA, Gaynor R, Radolf JD, Norgard MV. *Treponema pallidum*, lipoproteins, and synthetic lipoprotein analogues induce human immunodeficiency virus type 1 gene expression in monocytes via NF-kappaB activation. *J Infect Dis*. 1998; 177:941–950.
11. Johns DR, Tierney M, Felsenstein D. Alteration in the natural history of neurosyphilis by concurrent infection with human immunodeficiency virus. *N Engl J Med*. 1987; 316:1569–1572.
12. Berry CD, Hooton TM, Collier AC, Lukehart SA. Neurologic relapse after benzathine penicillin therapy for secondary syphilis in a patient with HIV infection. *N Engl J Med*. 1987; 316:1587–1589.
13. Bartlett JG. *Pocket Book of Infectious Disease Therapy: Sexually Transmitted Diseases*. Williams & Wilkins; Rev 2005.
14. Fitzgerald D, Haas DW. *Mycobacterium tuberculosis*. In: Mandell GL, Bennett JE, Dolin R, eds. *Mandell, Douglas, and Bennett's Principles and Practice of Infectious Diseases*. 6th ed. Philadelphia, PA: Elsevier Churchill Livingstone; 2005; 2576–2664.
15. Dube MP, Holtom PD, Larsen RA. Tuberculous meningitis in patients with and without human immunodeficiency virus infection. *Am J Med*. 1992; 93:520–524.

16. Luft BJ, Remington JS. Toxoplasmic encephalitis in AIDS. *Clin Infect Dis*. 1992; 15:211–222.
17. Gray F, Gherardi R, Wingate E, et al. Diffuse "encephalitic" cerebral toxoplasmosis in AIDS. Report of four cases. *J Neurol*. 1989; 236:273–277.
18. Liesenfeld O, Wong SY, Remington JS. Toxoplasmosis in the setting of AIDS. In: Bartlett JG, Merigan TC, Bolognesi D, eds. *Textbook of AIDS Medicine*. 2nd edition. Baltimore: Williams & Wilkins; 1999; 225–259.
19. Haverkos HW. Assessment of therapy for toxoplasma encephalitis. The TE Study Group. *Am J Med*. 1987; 82:907–914.
20. Bartlett JG. *Pocket Book of Infectious Disease Therapy: Management of Complications of HIV*. Williams & Wilkins; Rev 2005.
21. Trikalinos TA, Ioannidis JPA. Discontinuation of *Pneumocystis carinii* prophylaxis in patients infected with human immunodeficiency virus: a meta-analysis and decision analysis. *Clin Infect Dis*. 2001; 33:1901–1909.
22. Said G, Saimot AG, Tardieu M, Lacroix C ed. Opportunistic Infections of the Central Nervous System. In: *Neurological complications of HIV and AIDS*, Chapter 4; W.B Saunders: 1997; pp. 47–116.
23. Baqi M, Kucharcyzk W, Walmsley SL. Regression of progressive multifocal encephalopathy with highly active antiretroviral therapy. *AIDS*. 1997; 11:1526–1527.
24. Tunkel AR. Brain Abscess. In: Mandell GL, Bennett JE, Dolin R, eds. *Mandell, Douglas, and Bennett's Principles and Practice of Infectious Diseases*. 6th ed. Philadelphia, PA: Elsevier Churchill Livingstone: 2005; pp. 1016–1025.
25. Celum CL, Chaisson RE, Rutherford GW, Barnhart JL, Echenberg DF. Incidence of salmonellosis in patients with AIDS. *J Infect Dis*. 1987; 156:998–1002.
26. Miller SI, Pegues DA, Ohl ME. Salmonella species, including *Salmonella typhi*. In: Mandell GL, Bennett JE, Dolin R, eds. *Mandell, Douglas, and Bennett's Principles and Practice of Infectious Diseases*. 6th ed. Philadelphia, PA: Elsevier Churchill Livingstone: 2005; pp. 2344–2356.
27. McGuire D. Neurologic Manifestations of HIV (Section: Clinical Manifestations of HIV). Ed. Peiperl and Volberding, HIV InSite Knowledge Base, in *HIV* online textbook, June 2003. {www.hivinsite.ucsf.edu}.
28. Whitley RJ. Varicella Zoster Virus. In: Mandell GL, Bennett JE, Dolin R, eds. *Mandell, Douglas, and Bennett's Principles and Practice of Infectious Diseases*. 6th ed. Philadelphia, PA: Elsevier Churchill Livingstone: 2005; pp. 1580–1585.
29. Janssen RS, Nwanyanwu OC, Selik RM, Stehr-Green JK. Epidemiology of human immunodeficiency virus encephalopathy in the United States. *Neurology*. 1992; 42:1472–1476.
30. Cooper ER, Hanson C, Diaz C, et al. Encephalopathy and progression of human immunodeficiency virus disease in a cohort of children with perinatally acquired human immunodeficiency virus infection. Women and Infants Transmission Study Group. *J Pediatr*. 1998; 132:808–812.
31. Lobato MN, Caldwell MB, Ng P, Oxtoby MJ. Encephalopathy in children with perinatally acquired immunodeficiency virus infection. Pediatric spectrum of disease clinical consortium. *J Pediatr*. 1995; 126:710–715.
32. Sanchez-Ramon S, Resino S, Bellon Cano JM, Ramos JT, Gurbindo D, Munoz-Fernandez A. Neuroprotective effects of early antiretrovirals in vertical HIV infection. *Pediatr Neurol*. 2003; 29:218–221.
33. Price RW, Yiannoutsos CT, Clifford DB, et al. Neurological outcomes in late HIV infection: adverse impact of neurological impairment on survival and protective effect of antiviral therapy. AIDS Clinical Trials Group and Neurological AIDS Research Consortium Study team. *AIDS*. 1999; 13:1677–1685.
34. Belman AL, Diamond G, Dickson D, et al. Pediatric acquired immunodeficiency syndrome. Neurologic syndromes. *Am J Dis Child*. 1988; 142:29–35.
35. Pearson DA, McGrath NM, Nozyce M, et al. Predicting HIV disease progression in children using measures of neuropsychological and neurological functioning. Pediatric AIDS clinical trials 152 study team. *Pediatrics*. 2000; 106:E76.

36. Mitchell W. Neurological and developmental effects of HIV and AIDS in children and adolescents. *Ment Retard Dev Disabil Res Rev*. 2001; 7:211–216.
37. Dix RD, Bredesen DE, Erlich KS, Mills J. Recovery of herpes viruses from cerebrospinal fluid of immunodeficient homosexual men. *Ann Neurol*. 1985; 18:611–614.
38. Britton CB, Mesa-Tejada R, Fenoglio CM, Hays AP, Garvey GG, Miller JR. A new complication of AIDS: thoracic myelitis caused by herpes simplex virus. *Neurology*. 1985; 35:1071–1074.
39. Tucker T, Dix RD, Katzen C, Davis RL, Schmidley JW. Cytomegalovirus and herpes simplex virus ascending myelitis in a patient with acquired immunodeficiency syndrome. *Ann Neurol*. 1985; 18:74–79.
40. Araujo AP, Nascimento OJ, Garcia OS. Distal sensory polyneuropathy in a cohort of HIV-infected children over five years of age. *Pediatrics*. 2000; 106:E35.
41. Verma A. Epidemiology and clinical features of HIV-1 associated neuropathies. *J Peripher Nerv Syst*. 2001; 6:8–13.
42. Centers for Disease Control and Prevention. 1994 revised classification system for human immunodeficiency virus infection in children less than 13 years of age. Official authorized addenda: human immunodeficiency virus infection codes and official guidelines for coding and reporting ICD-9CM. *MMWR* 1994; 43 (RR-12):1–19.

# Chapter 11
# Neurological Consequences of Antiretroviral Treatment

**Kimberley C. Brown, Pharm.D., Lisa D. Inge, Pharm.D., and Mobeen H. Rathore, M.D., C.P.E., F.A.A.P.**

## Antiretroviral Treatment

### *Introduction*

The human immunodeficiency virus (HIV) is a lentivirus that quickly compromises the immune system of its host [1]. In the early 1980s, acquired immunodeficiency syndrome (AIDS) was described in the United States as a deadly syndrome that mainly affected homosexual men. Twenty-five years later, HIV infection has become a worldwide epidemic; more than 25 million people have died and more than 40 million people are infected [2].

Many of those affected by HIV have varying degrees of disease progression and immune system dysfunction. Both viral and host factors, and likely, their interaction, may predict the risk of HIV disease progression. Approximately 50% of those who remain untreated with antiretroviral (ARV) therapy will progress to AIDS, which is defined as having an AIDS-defining illness or a $CD4^{+}$ cell count of less than 200 cells/μL. As the severity of the disease worsens, pathologic abnormalities of the brain may manifest. This may be a direct result of HIV infection or indirectly, a result of opportunistic infections or psychological/psychiatric disease. Furthermore, complications may also result from adverse effects related to ARV therapy.

### *Central and Peripheral Nervous System Abnormalities*

Neurological and psychiatric disorders have been described and include peripheral neuropathies, myelopathy, focal cerebral mass lesions, opportunistic infections, vascular abnormalities, seizures, encephalopathies, developmental delays, mania, and depression (for details, see Chapter 10) [3,4].

Eggers and colleagues described HIV encephalopathy (HIVE) as a "direct manifestation of HIV infection of the central nervous system" [5]. Two types of encephalopathy have been described in HIV-infected children: progressive and

L.L. Barton and N.R. Friedman (eds.), *The Neurological Manifestations of Pediatric Infectious Diseases and Immunodeficiency Syndromes.*

static. Ultimately, the only way to reverse or halt symptoms of encephalopathy is to initiate highly active antiretroviral therapy (HAART) and establish intervention programs [6]. Early investigations of HIV-positive children with encephalopathy who were treated with continuous infusion zidovudine (AZT/ZDV) for several months demonstrated improved IQ scores that remained improved after several months of testing [7]. A more recent study confirmed the association between the decline of HIVE and the advent of HAART [8].

Mitochondrial toxicity, caused by usage of the nucleoside/nucleotide reverse transcriptase inhibitors (NRTIs), manifests as neuropathy, myopathy, or cardiomyopathy. This toxicity is thought to be a result of the varying affinity of these medications for the eukaryotic mitochondrial DNA polymerase gamma [9]. Mitochondrial DNA polymerase gamma is inhibited by the NRTIs because they act as alternative substrates for the enzyme. Thus, NRTIs cause the reduction or mutation of mitochondria and may lead to increased lactate production, fat accumulation, hepatic steatosis, pancreatitis, lipodystrophy, and pancytopenias. Recently published data also suggest that mitochondrial toxicity reduces neuronal integrity via the loss of N-acetylaspartate (NAA), resulting in lower measured levels of NAA and decreased cognitive function [10].

A 1999 study from France involving 4,392 uninfected or HIV-indeterminate children born to HIV-positive women who received zidovudine or zidovudine/lamivudine identified 12 children who developed mitochondrial dysfunction during the first months of life; 2 of these children developed severe neurological disease and died [11]. A subsequent review was performed that included more than 20,000 infants born to HIV-infected mothers who had participated in perinatal prevention trials in the United States. There were 353 deaths in this group of infants. A review of this group of infants did not confirm the findings of the French study [12]. Poirier compared infants born to HIV-infected and uninfected women and documented a correlation between mitochondrial DNA in cord blood and peripheral blood leukocytes at ages 1 and 2 years in both groups. Infants in this study who were born to HIV-infected mothers with in utero zidovudine (ZDV, AZT) exposure had less mitochondrial DNA compared with those infants without ZDV exposure, whether born to HIV-infected or uninfected women [13]. However, the European Collaborative Study evaluated 1,008 HIV affected children who were exposed to ARV drugs in utero and did not find any clinical manifestations suggestive of mitochondrial abnormalities [14]. Furthermore, only a few maternal toxicities were observed in the Women and Infants Transmission Study; there was one patient who was diagnosed with lactic acidosis who received AZT and lamivudine during early study visits and the combination of stavudine, didanosine, and saquinavir during later study visits [15]. Current perinatal guidelines, as well as both stavudine and didanosine package inserts, warn of the increased risk of fatal lactic acidosis/hepatic steatosis occurring in pregnant women taking the stavudine plus didanosine combination [9,16,17].

Peripheral neuropathy can be caused by viral pathogens, autoimmune processes, and vitamin and mineral deficiencies, but is most often caused by adverse effects of ARVs [18]. Mitochondrial toxicity associated with nucleoside analogs may lead to peripheral neuropathy. The dideoxynucleosides (stavudine, didanosine, and zalcitabine) have been associated with a 15 to 30% incidence of sensory neuropathy in

HIV-infected individuals, but all of the NRTIs may contribute to symptoms. Previous studies related peripheral neuropathy to a deficit in acetylcarnitine levels, but further investigation is needed [19,20]. Five cases of Guillain-Barré syndrome reported to the adverse event reporting service of the U.S. Food and Drug Administration (FDA) were related to lactic acidosis and treatment with ddI and d4T [21].

## *Highly Active Antiretroviral Therapy (HAART)*

HAART has provided substantial clinical benefit to individuals infected with HIV. Since the advent of HAART, there has been a significant reduction in morbidity and mortality of AIDS-related illnesses. However, despite the progress, ARVs have severe long-term adverse effects that overlap the symptoms of HIV.

Currently, there are 27 ARV medications in five classes approved for use in adolescents and adults (Table 11.1). Many of the current ARV formulations are neither approved nor appropriate for children. These classes include the NRTIs, non-NRTIs (NNRTIs), protease inhibitors, and a fusion inhibitor. Exposure to ARV therapy for prophylaxis or treatment of HIV infection in infants, children, and adolescents occurs during two distinct periods; first, when a developing fetus is in utero, and then during treatment of confirmed infection. Current consensus guidelines do not provide any specific recommendations regarding the management of HIV-related neurological impairment. Of note, many of the agents have been associated with central nervous system (CNS) toxicity.

**Table 11.1** Antiretroviral agents

| Nucleoside/nucleotide reverse transcriptase inhibitor (NRTI) | Non-nucleoside reverse transcriptase inhibitor (NNRTI) | Protease inhibitor (PI) | Entry inhibitor | CCR5 entry inhibitor | Integrase inhibitor |
|---|---|---|---|---|---|
| Zidovudine (AZT, Retrovir)<br>Abacavir (Ziagen)<br>Didanosine (Videx)<br>Emtricitabine (Emtriva)<br>Lamivudine (Epivir)<br>Stavudine (Zerit)<br>Zalcitabine (Hivid)<br>Tenofovir (Viread) | Delavirdine (Rescriptor)<br>Efavirenz (Sustiva)<br>Nevirapine (Viramune) | Amprenavir (Agenerase)<br>Indinavir (Crixivan)<br>Nelfinavir (Viracept)<br>Ritonavir (Norvir)<br>Saquinavir (Invirase, Fortavase)<br>Lopinavir/Ritonavir (Kaletra)<br>Atazanavir (Reyataz)<br>Fosamprenavir (Lexiva)<br>Tipranavir (Aptivus)<br>Darunavir (Prezista) | Enfuvirtide (Fuzeon) | Maraviroc (Selzentry) | Isentress (Raltegravir) |

## In Utero Exposure to ARVs

Mother-to-infant transmission accounts for 90% or more of childhood HIV-1 infections [16]. Zidovudine (ZDV, AZT, Retrovir) monotherapy administered after the first trimester of pregnancy has been shown to decrease the risk of HIV vertical transmission by 66%. HAART, consisting of at least a three-drug regimen during pregnancy, has resulted in an even greater reduction in the rate of transmission, to approximately 1% [22,23]. Zidovudine monotherapy is the only ARV that had proven efficacy in preventing mother-to-child transmission (MTCT). Zidovudine should be used during pregnancy, labor, and delivery, and is recommended as monotherapy in HIV-exposed neonates for the first 6 weeks of life (with rare exceptions) [24]. Because of the dramatic reduction of MTCT, the benefits of using ZDV during pregnancy outweighs the risks. However, one study detected birth defects in 8 of 104 ZDV-exposed infants. These defects ranged from minor abnormalities to conditions such as asymptomatic atrial septal defect and pectus excavatum [25].

The NNRTIs efavirenz and delavirdine are not recommended during pregnancy. Efavirenz has a 15% incidence of anencephaly, anophthalmia, cleft palate, or microphthalmia in primates and there are reports of myelomeningocele in humans [26–28]. The documented neurological toxicity of ARV medications in the developing fetus or mother during pregnancy is limited.

## Pediatric and Adolescent ARV Exposure

ARV therapy is the cornerstone of management of HIV infection in children and adolescents. If infection is documented, current pediatric guidelines recommend initiation of combination therapy (HAART) based on age, $CD4^+$ cell percentage, and the number of plasma HIV RNA copies per milliliter. These ARV medications have been proven to markedly decrease HIV-associated morbidity and mortality. HIV infection has, thus, become a chronic rather than an invariably fatal disease [29]. Although current pediatric treatment guidelines provide information and recommendations for the use of a limited number of ARV medications, resistance and clinical conditions often require the clinician to go beyond these recommendations to provide optimal care.

## Pharmacokinetics of HAART and the CNS

One of the initial sites of entry of HIV is the CNS. Unfortunately, most currently available ARVs have poor CNS penetration because of the blood–brain barrier. Once the integrity of the blood–brain barrier is compromised, it is more vulnerable to the vagaries of HIV infection. Furthermore, infected macrophages can persist in the CNS for extended periods, making the CNS a reservoir for HIV infection. This can cause prolonged damage to the CNS given the long half-life of the macrophage. In addition, data support the existence of a separate viral reservoir of HIV and the independent evolution of HIV within the CNS. In this case, plasma viral load may not reflect the cerebrospinal fluid (CSF) viral load. Initiating a regimen that will control HIV in the CSF and plasma may produce the best treatment outcomes.

The penetration of ARVs across the blood–brain barrier varies, mainly because each drug has a different degree of protein binding in plasma, and only free and unbound drug are able to cross the blood–brain barrier (Table 11.2). Emerging data suggest that ARV therapy with better CNS penetration may be preferable for patients with neurological disease, to maximize the likelihood of suppressing CSF HIV viral replication [30,31]. Agents shown to have the best CSF penetration include ZDV, stavudine, abacavir, nevirapine, and indinavir. The chemical profile of many ARVs currently in development suggests that their CNS penetration will be negligible. In addition to the absolute drug concentration in the CSF, one must consider how effectively the drug inhibits viral replication. Cunningham observed that resistance patterns in the CSF and the plasma differed; thus, therapeutic options should be chosen accordingly [32]. Data regarding the importance of CNS penetration and resistance profiles will become increasingly important as new agents are introduced into the armamentarium.

## *Nucleoside/Nucleotide Analog Reverse Transcriptase Inhibitors*

NRTIs and the nucleotide, Tenofovir, inhibit HIV reverse transcriptase, which is responsible for the transcription of RNA to DNA. These drugs are phosphorylated and converted to active drug. The NRTIs also bind to and inhibit eukaryotic DNA polymerase gamma, the enzyme responsible for mitochondrial DNA synthesis, causing some degree of mitochondrial dysfunction. As stated previously, this

**Table 11.2** Protein binding of antiretroviral agents

| Protease inhibitor | Protein binding |
|---|---|
| Amprenavir | 90% |
| Atazanavir | 86% |
| Indinavir | 60–65% |
| Nelfinavir | >98% |
| Ritonavir | 98–99% |
| Saquinavir | 98% |
| Lopinavir/Ritonavir | 98–99% |
| Tipranavir | >99% |
| Darunavir | 95% |

inhibition may be responsible for organ dysfunction, including peripheral neuropathy, myopathies, cardiomyopathy, pancreatic dysfunction, rare ototoxicity, lactic acidosis, and fatty liver [33–36]. All patients treated with nucleoside analogs who have any unexplained neurological deterioration should be evaluated for lactic acidosis to provide for earlier intervention and potential reversal of this process [37].

Zidovudine (ZDV, AZT, Retrovir) has been shown to be effective in the treatment of CNS HIV infection [22,29,38], because of its ability to penetrate the CNS. HIV-related encephalopathy is often seen as the AIDS-defining illness in perinatally infected children [22]. Treatment with zidovudine monotherapy has been shown to improve cognitive functioning and may halt or reverse encephalopathy in some patients. HAART may also improve neurological function in children as well as dementia in adult patients [39–43]. Zidovudine penetration into the CNS may result in confusion, agitation, mania, and insomnia in fewer than 5% of patients during the first year. Other side effects include severe headaches, malaise, and fatigue. A rare association with seizures, especially in cases of overdose, has also been reported [44,45]. Zidovudine, although not directly associated with peripheral neuropathy, has also been associated with myalgias and myopathy with long-term therapy. Cardiomyopathy has also been reported in children receiving ZDV. In the pre-HAART era, zidovudine was used as monotherapy and at higher doses (up to 2,000 mg/d). Mania and depression were observed in individuals with no previous psychiatric history [45].

Within the group of nucleosides exists a select group identified as the dideoxynucleosides (ddN) reverse transcriptase inhibitors, which include didanosine (Videx), stavudine (Zerit), and zalcitabine (Hivid was infrequently used in the HAART area and production ceased in 2006). These medications have been associated with the development of peripheral neuropathy, in particular, distal sensory polyneuropathy, in children [34,46,47]. These sensory neuropathies are more likely to occur with higher doses, lower $CD4^+$ cell counts, higher viral loads, and increasing age [46–50]. Sensory neuropathies also occur in up to 34% of HIV-infected children and are of lesser severity than those observed in adults [34,51]. Improvement in the neuropathy is often preceded by an initial period of worsening of symptoms or "coasting," which may last several weeks. In most adult patients, improvement in symptoms may be seen within 2 weeks of removal of the drug, if the neuropathy is drug related [52,53].

Didanosine (ddI, Videx) less commonly causes sensory neuropathies, most often in patients with low $CD4^+$ counts [34,51,53].Although its CNS penetration has been shown to improve neuropsychometric test scores, didanosine has been associated with nervousness in approximately 27% of children. Optic neuritis and a reversible asymptomatic peripheral retinal depigmentation have also been observed in less than 5% of children receiving high-dose didanosine [16,41,54].

Stavudine (d4T, Zerit) has also been used to halt psychomotor deterioration. It has been shown to produce peripheral sensory neuropathies in up to 12 to 15% of patients. Symptoms tend to improve soon after the drug is discontinued. There is a synergistic neurotoxicity when didanosine and stavudine are used together or in combination with hydroxyurea. Neurotoxicity presents as early as 4 months after initiation of therapy in adults [34,41,46,53,55].

Lamivudine (3TC, Epivir) exerts little or no mitochondrial toxicity *in vitro* and has only been associated with peripheral neuropathy. In general, this medication is very well tolerated, other than complaints of headaches in some patients [36,52,56].

Abacavir (ABC, Ziagen) has limited mitochondrial toxicity as well, but may produce headaches in 16% of children. Adverse neuropsychiatric reactions have been reported in two adult women co-infected with hepatitis B or C. A second case report described an HIV-infected individual who presented with "persecutory delusion, mutism, posturing and catatonia". All symptoms resolved with discontinuation. On rechallenge of the regimen, minus abacavir, no evidence of psychosis was noted [57]. To date, no such events have been observed in children [52,58,59].

Tenofovir (TNF, Viread), although not currently approved for use in children, has limited mitochondrial and CNS penetration. When used in combination with didanosine, levels of didanosine are increased between 40 and 60%. Dose adjustment must, therefore, be made to decrease the risk of ddI-induced peripheral neuropathy, pancreatitis, and potential lactic acidosis [16,60,61].

Emtricitabine (FTC, Emtriva) was approved for pediatric use in 2005. Emtricitabine has very little mitochondrial toxicity or neurological effect. There is no information regarding CNS penetration; however, in clinical studies, emtricitabine had a higher rate of headache than lamivudine [62].

## *New Non-Nucleoside Reverse Transcriptase Inhibitors*

Two NNRTIs are currently available for treatment of HIV-1 infection: efavirenz and nevirapine. These medications noncompetitively bind to HIV reverse transcriptase [63]. Because of inconvenient dosing of delavirdine and the lack of availability of a liquid formulation, this medication was rarely used, and production has been discontinued. Both efavirenz and nevirapine penetrate the CSF. High CSF concentrations are achieved because of their lipophilicity and long elimination half-life [64,65]. Efavirenz has been associated with a 45% incidence of CNS side effects in children, including dizziness, headache, confusion, stupor, impaired concentration, agitation, amnesia, hallucinations, and abnormal or vivid dreams. Although most patients experience sedation, insomnia has also been observed. These side effects are usually transient, with a 2- to 4-week duration, during which time, drug levels in the CNS level off as a consequence of autoinduction of drug metabolism.

Spanish researchers determined that 10 (58.8%) of 17 patients had CNS-related adverse events that ranged from insomnia and vivid dreams to severe depression and suicidal ideation. Investigators also found that mean efavirenz levels were higher for patients experiencing neuropsychiatric symptoms, however, only 4 patients (23.5%) required discontinuation of the drug [66]. Nontransient side effects include psychiatric effects of anxiety, depression, and suicidal ideation, especially in psychiatrically vulnerable patients [26,45,53] Teglas et al. observed adverse CNS reactions in 36% of children. Increased appetite occurred in three children and necessitated drug discontinuation because of excessive weight gain [67]. Nevirapine-related attempted suicide has been reported in adults, however, this is not frequently seen [63,68].

## Protease Inhibitors

Protease inhibitors bind to and inhibit viral protease, with little effect on the host cell proteases. Penetration of these medications into the CNS and across the placenta is hindered by a number of factors. Extensive protein binding of all protease inhibitors except indinavir limits drug transport, as does the presence of an efflux transporter pump P-glycoprotein, which is present in the brain and placenta [69,70]. Indinavir and saquinavir are the only protease inhibitors that have adequate concentrations in the CNS. These protease inhibitors do not seem to have the neurological side effects observed with NRTIs or NNRTIs, and they have been shown to halt viral replication in the CNS. One study in AIDS found that despite the high levels of protein binding of lopinavir/ritonavir, the concentrations of the medications were adequate to inhibit HIV replication [71]. The addition of a protease inhibitor to two nucleoside analogs has been shown to improve HIV-associated motor slowing and HIVE [42,53,64,72]. However, the entire class has the ability to interact with the cytochrome P-450 enzyme system, increasing the risk of potential drug–drug interactions with multiple other medications.

Postmarketing studies have revealed that tipranavir (Aptivus) has been associated with fatal and nonfatal intracranial hemorrhage (ICH). Of 6,840 patients evaluated in clinical trials, 14 developed ICH; 8 were fatal. Many of these patients had other medical conditions or were receiving concomitant medications that may have caused or contributed to these events. No pattern of abnormal coagulation parameters has been observed in patients in general, or preceding the development of ICH. Therefore, routine measurement of coagulation parameters is not currently indicated in the management of patients taking tipranavir [73].

Darunavir (Prezista) was approved by the FDA in July of 2006. Similar to other protease inhibitors, it is highly protein bound (95%). The drug's safety and efficacy has not been established in the pediatric population [74].

## Fusion Inhibitors

Enfuvirtide (T-20, Fuzeon) is a fusion inhibitor in a new class of ARV drugs called "Entry Inhibitors." This drug prevents the attachment of the transmembrane glycoprotein 41 of HIV-1 to the chemokine co-receptor located on the $CD4^+$ cell. This prevents the insertion of the viral material into the $CD4^+$ cell, and inhibits advanced viral replication. Enfuvirtide does not affect intracellular biochemical pathways and, therefore, is unlikely to cause metabolic complications. Nor is it metabolized by the cytochrome P-450 enzyme system, thus, the risk of drug interactions is low. Enfuvirtide is approximately 92% protein bound, a probable limitation to penetration of the blood–brain barrier [75,76]. However, the drug may control HIV replication in the CSF through its effects on systemic infection [77]. Piliero and colleagues have reported a fatal case of T-20-associated Guillain-Barré syndrome [78].

## *Summary*

The use of ARV medications has not only provided a significant reduction in perinatal transmission, but has also improved the neurological prognosis of pediatric as well as adult patients infected with HIV. The physiologic challenges of the placenta and the blood–brain barrier may limit the effects of some of these medications because of poor penetration or altered pharmacokinetics [69]. Zidovudine, stavudine, abacavir, efavirenz, nevirapine, and indinavir offer better penetration and, thus, treatment of neurological manifestations. However, all components of HAART contribute to the treatment of neurological manifestations of HIV infection by reduction of viral load and elevation of the $CD4^+$ counts. Nevertheless, adverse neurological events may arise from the use of these same medications. Future ARV therapy must take into account the potential for poor penetration into the sanctuary sites, including the CNS, or inadequate peripheral viral suppression as well as the potential for the development of drug resistance. CNS penetration, although desirable, remains a two-edged sword.

## References

1. Gabuzda DH, Hirsch MS. Neurologic manifestations of infection with human immunodeficiency virus. Clinical features and pathogenesis. *Ann Intern Med.* 1987; 107:383–391.
2. Global Report on the AIDS epidemic. *UNAIDS.* May 2006.
3. Spudich SS, Huang W, Nilsson AC, Petropoulos CJ. HIV-1 chemokine coreceptor utilization in paired cerebrospinal fluid and plasma samples: a survey of subjects with viremia. *J Inf Dis.* 2005; 191:890–898.
4. Rabkin JG, Ferrando S. A 'second life' agenda. Psychiatric research issues raised by protease inhibitor treatments for people with human immunodeficiency virus or the acquired immunodeficiency syndrome. *Arch Gen Psych.* 1997; 54:1049–1053.
5. Eggers C, Hertogs K, Sturenberg HJ. Delayed central nervous system virus suppression during highly active antiretroviral therapy is associated with HIV encephalopathy, but not with viral drug resistance or poor central nervous system drug penetration *AIDS.* 2003; 17:1897–1906.
6. Tamula MA, Wolters PL, Walsek C. Cognitive decline with immunologic and virologic stability in four children with human immunodeficiency virus disease. *Pediatrics.* 2003; 112:679–684.
7. Brouwers P, Moss H, Wolters P. Effects of continuous infusion Zidovudine therapy on neuropsychologic functioning in children with symptomatic human immunodeficiency virus. *J Pediatr.* 1990; 117:980–985.

8. Chiriboga CA, Fleishman S, Champion S, Gaye-Robinson L, Abrams EJ. Incidence and prevalence of HIV encephalopathy in children with HIV infection receiving highly active anti-retroviral therapy (HAART). *J Pediatr*. 2005; 146:402–407.
9. Alimenti A, Burdge DR, Ogolvie GS, et al. Lactic acidemia in human immunodeficiency virus-uninfected infected infants exposed to perinatal antiretroviral therapy. *Pediatr Infect Dis J*. 2003; 22:782–788.
10. Schweinberg BC, Taylor MJ, Alhassoon OM. Brain mitochondrial injury in human immunodeficiency virus—seropositive (HIV+) individuals taking nucleoside reverse transcriptase inhibitors. *J Neurovirol*. 2005; 11:356–364.
11. Blanche S, Tardieu M, Rustin P, et al. Persistent mitochondrial dysfunction and perinatal exposure to antiretroviral nucleoside analogues. *Lancet*. 1999; 354;1084–1089.
12. The Perinatal Safety Review Working Group. Nucleoside exposure in the children of HIV-infected women receiving antiretroviral drugs: absence of clear evidence for mitochondrial disease in children who died before 5 years of age in five United States cohorts. *J Acquir Immune Defic Syndr*. 2000; 25:261–268.
13. Poirier MC, Divi RL, Al-Harthi L, et al. Long-term mitochondrial toxicity in HIV-uninfected infants born to HIV-infected mothers. *J Acquir Immune Defic Syndr*. 2003; 33:175–183.
14. European Collaborative Study. Exposure to antiretroviral therapy in utero or early life: the health of uninfected children born to HIV-infected women. *J Acquir Immune Defic Syndr*. 2003; 32:380–387.
15. Tuomala RE, Watts DH, Li D, et al. Improved obstetric outcomes and few maternal toxicities are associated with antiretroviral therapy, including highly active antiretroviral therapy during pregnancy. *J Acquir Immune Defic Syndr*. 2005; 38:449–473.
16. Didanosine, Videx. Bristol Myers Squibb, Product Information. 2006.
17. Stavudine, Zerit. Bristol Myers Squibb, Product Information. 2006.
18. Brew B. The peripheral nerve complications of human immunodeficiency virus (HIV) infection. *Mus Ner*. 2003; 28:542–552.
19. Osio M, Muscia F, Zampini L, et al. Acetyl-l-carnitine in the treatment of painful antiretroviral neuropathy in human immunodeficiency virus patients: an open label study. *J Periph Nerv Sys*. 2006; 11:72–76.
20. Famularo G, Moretti S, Marcellini S, et al. Acetylcarnitine deficiency in AIDS patients with neurotoxicity on treatment with antiretroviral nucleoside analogues. *AIDS*. 1997; 11:185–190.
21. Marcus K, Truffa M, Boxwell D. Recently identified adverse events secondary to NRTI therapy in HIV-infected individuals: cases from the FDA's reporting system (abstract LB14). In: *Programs and Abstracts of the 9th Conference on Retroviruses and Opportunistic Infections* (Seattle) 2002.
22. Mitchell W. Neurological and developmental effects of HIV and AIDS in children and adolescents. *Ment Retard Dev Disabil Res Rev*. 2001; 7:211–216.
23. Sullivan JL, Luzuriaga K. The changing face of pediatric HIV-1 infection. *N Engl J Med*. 2001; 345:1568–1569.
24. Connor EM, Sperling RS, Gelber R, et al. Reduction of maternal-infant transmission of human immunodeficiency virus type infant transmission of human immunodeficiency virus type 1 with zidovudine treatment. Pediatric AIDS Clinical Trials Group Protocol 076 Study Group. *N Engl J Med*. 1994; 331:1173.
25. Kumar RM, Hughes PF, Khurranna A. Zidovudine use in pregnancy: a report on 104 cases and the occurrence of birth defects. *J Acq Imm Def Synd*. 1994; 7:1034.
26. Efavirenz, Sustiva. Bristol Myers Squibb, Product Information. 2006.
27. Minkoff H. Human immunodeficiency virus infection in pregnancy. *Obstet Gynec*. 2003; 101:797–810.
28. Watts DH. Management of human immunodeficiency virus in pregnancy. *N Engl J Med*. 2002; 346:1879–1891.
29. Gisslen M, Hagberg L. Antiretroviral treatment of central nervous system HIV-1 infection: a review. *HIV Med*. 2001; 2(2):97–104.

30. Tamula MA, Wolters PL, Walsek C. Cognitive decline with immunologic and virologic stability in four children with human immunodeficiency virus disease. *Pediatrics*. 2003; 112:679–684.
31. DeLuca A, Ciancio B, Larussa D, et al. Correlates of independent HIV-1 replication in the CNS and of its control by antiretrovirals. *Neurol*. 2002; 59:342–347.
32. Cunningham P, Smith D, Satchell C, Cooper D, Brew B. Evidence for independent development of reverse transcriptase inhibitor resistance patterns in the cerebrospinal fluid. *AIDS*. 2000; 14:1949–1954.
33. Belman AL. HIV-1 infection and AIDS. *Neurol Clin*. 2002; 20:983–1011.
34. Cherry CL, McArthur JC, Hoy JF. Nucleoside analogues and neuropathy in the era of HAART. *J Clin Virol*. 2003; 26:195–207.
35. Brinkman K, ter Hofstede HG, Hadewych JM. Adverse effects of reverse transcriptase inhibitors: mitochondrial toxicity as common pathway. *AIDS*. 1998; 12:1735–1744.
36. Kakuda TN. Pharmacology of nucleoside and nucleotide reverse transcriptase inhibitor-induced mitochondrial toxicity. *Clin Therap*. 2000; 22:685–708.
37. Church JA, Mitchell WG, Gonzalez-Gomez I. Mitochondrial DNA depletion, near-fatal metabolic acidosis, and liver failure in an HIV-infected child treated with combination antiretroviral therapy. *J Pediatr*. 2001; 138:748–751.
38. Husstedt I, Frohne L, Bockenholt S. Impact of highly active antiretroviral therapy on cognitive processing in HIV infection: cross-sectional and longitudinal studies of event-related potentials. *AIDS Res Hum Retro*. 2002; 18:485–490.
39. Antinouri A, Giancola ML, Grisetti S. Factors influencing virological response to antiretroviral drugs in cerebrospinal fluid of advanced HIV-1 infected patients. *AIDS*. 2002; 16:1867–1876.
40. Arendt G, Giesen HV, Hefter H. Therapeutic effects of nucleoside analogues on psychomotor slowing in HIV infection. *AIDS*. 2001; 15:493–500.
41. Raskino CR, Pearson DA, Baker CJ. Neurologic, neurocognitive and brain growth outcomes in human immunodeficiency virus-infected children receiving different nucleoside antiretroviral regimens. *Pediatrics*. 1999; 104:1–10.
42. Price RW, Yiannoutsos CT, Clifford DB. Neurological outcomes in late HIV infection: adverse impact of neurological impairment on survival and protective effect of antiviral therapy. *AIDS*. 1999; 13:1677–1685.
43. Rauch DM, Stover ES. Neuroscience research in AIDS. *Prog Neuropsychopharmacol Biol Psychiatry*. 2001; 25:231–257.
44. Calamandrei G, Valanzano A, Puopolo M. Developmental exposure to the antiretroviral drug zidovudine increases brain levels of brain-derived neurotropic factor in mice. *Neuroscience Letters*. 2002; 333:111–114.
45. Treisman GJ, Kaplina AI. Neurologic and psychiatric complications of antiretroviral agents. *AIDS*. 2002; 16:1201–1215.
46. Simpson DM, Haidich A, Schitto G, et al. Severity of HIV-associated neuropathy is associated with plasma HIV-1 RNA levels. *AIDS*. 2002; 16:407–412.
47. Keswania SC, Pardoa CA, Cherry CL, et al. HIV-1 associated sensory neuropathies. *AIDS*. 16:2105–2117.
48. Geraci AP, Simpson DM. Neurological manifestations of HIV-1 infection in the HAART era. *Comp Ther*. 2001; 27:232–241.
49. Geraci AP, Di Rocco AD, Simpson DM. Neurologic complications of AIDS. *Neurologist*. 2001; 7:82–97.
50. Wulff EA, Simpson DM. Neuromuscular complications of the human immunodeficiency virus type 1 infection. *Semin Neurol*. 1999:19:157–164.
51. Araujo A, Nascimneto OJ, Garcia OS. Distal sensory polyneuropathy in a cohort of HIV-infected children over five years of age. *Pediatrics*. 2000; 106:E35.
52. Moyle G. Clinical manifestations and management of antiretroviral nucleoside analog-related mitochondrial toxicity. *Clinical Therapeutics*. 2000; 22:911–936.

53. Dalakas M. Peripheral neuropathy and antiretroviral drugs. *J Periph Nerv Syst.* 2001; 6:14–20.
54. Pediatric Antiretroviral Drug Information, DHHS Pediatric Guidelines. 2006.
55. Reliquet V, Mussini JM, Lafeuillade A. Peripheral neuropathy during stavudine-didanosine antiretroviral therapy. *HIV Med.* 2001; 2:92–96.
56. Lamivudine, Epivir. Glaxo Wellcome, Product Information. 2002.
57. Foster R. Antiretroviral therapy-induced psychosis: case report and brief review of the literature. *HIV Med.* 2003; 4:139–144.
58. Abacavir, Ziagen. Glaxo Wellcome, Product Information. 2002.
59. Colebunders R, Hilbrands R, DeRoo A. Neuropsychiatric reaction induced by abacavir. *Am J Med.* 2002; 113:616.
60. Tenofovir, Viread. Gilead, Product Information. 2006.
61. Pharmacokinetics of Viread. Gilead, 2003.
62. Emtrictabine (FTC, Emtriva). Gilead, Product Information. 2006.
63. Maddocks S, Dwyer D. The role of non-nucleoside reverse transcriptase inhibitors in children with HIV-1 infection. *Pediatric Drugs.* 2001; 3:681–702.
64. Wynn HE, Brundage RC, Fletcher CV. Clinical implications of CNS penetration of antiretroviral drugs. *CNS Drugs.* 2002; 16:595–609.
65. Glynn SL, Yazanian M. In vitro blood-brain barrier permeability of nevirapine compared to other HIV antiretroviral agents. *J Pharma Sci.* 1998; 87:306–310.
66. Gutierrez F, et al. Prediction of neuropsychiatric adverse events associated with long-term efavirenz therapy, using plasma drug level monitoring. *Clin Infect Dis.* 2005; 41:1648–1653.
67. Teglas JP, Quartier P, Treluyer JM, et al. Tolerance of efavirenz in children. *AIDS.* 2001; 15:241–243.
68. Wise ME. Neuropsychiatric complications of nevirapine treatment. *BMJ.* 2002; 324:879.
69. Marzolini C, Christoph R, Decosterd LA Transplacental passage of protease inhibitors at delivery. *AIDS.* 2002; 16:889–893.
70. Mirochnick M. Antiretroviral pharmacology in pregnant women and their newborns. *Ann N Y Acad Sci.* 2000; 918:287–297.
71. Capparelli EV, Holland D, Okamotot C, et al. Lopinavir concentrations in cerebrospinal fluid exceed the 50% inhibitory concentration for HIV. *AIDS.* 2005; 19:949–952.
72. Martin C, Sonnerborg A, Svensson O, et al. Indinavir-based treatment of HIV-1 infected patients; efficacy in the central nervous system. *AIDS.* 1999; 13:1227–1232.
73. Tipranvir (Aptivus). Boehringer Ingelheim, Product Information. 2006.
74. Darunavir (Prezista). Tibotec, Product Information. 2006.
75. Enfuvirtide, Fuzeon. Roche, Product Information. 2003.
76. Church JA, Cunningham C, Hughes M, et al. Safety and antiretroviral activity of chronic subcutaneous administration of T-20 in human immunodeficiency virus 1-infected children. *Pediatr Infect Dis J.* 2002, 21:653–659.
77. Price RW, Palmatier R, Wring S, et al. Enfuvirtide cerebrospinal fluid pharmacokinetics: a potential tool to analyze CSF HIV origin and the therapeutic role of local drug penetration. (abstract 402). In: *Programs and Abstracts of the 12th Conference on Retroviruses and Opportunistic Infections* (Boston) 2005.
78. Piliero P, Fish DG, Preston S, et al. Guillain-Barré syndrome associated with immune reconstitution. *Clin Infect Dis.* 2003; 36:111–114.

# Chapter 12
# Papovaviruses

**Diane C. Halstead, Ph.D. and Mobeen H. Rathore, M.D., C.P.E., F.A.A.P.**

## JC Virus and Progressive Multifocal Leukoencephalopathy

### *Introduction*

Progressive multifocal leukoencephalopathy (PML) is a demyelinating opportunistic disease caused by JC virus (JCV), a member of the subfamily *Polyomavirus* in the family *Papovaviridae*. JCV infects the myelin-producing oligodendrocytes of the brain and produces a multifocal distribution of demyelinated plaques in the white matter, leading to neurological disease characteristic of PML.

### *Epidemiology*

Serology is of limited value in providing a laboratory diagnosis of PML. Serology is, however, helpful in establishing the prevalence of infection with JCV. Based on JCV antibody detection, clinically inapparent primary infections occur early in life and with worldwide distribution. Ten percent of 5-year-old children, 65% of 17-year-old adolescents, and 76 to 92% of adults are seropositive for JCV [1,2]. A significant number (5%) of healthy individuals have JCV DNA in their peripheral blood, supporting the theory that a high percentage of the population is latently infected [3]. Most PML patients have been found to have preexisting JCV antibody and do not show a rise in antibody titer during disease progression. Serum and cerebrospinal fluid (CSF) from these patients lack IgM antibodies and are devoid of a rise in IgG titer during the course of illness [4]. suggesting that reactivation rather than primary infection occurs with JCV [2,5].

PML, a once thought to be rare demyelinating disease of the central nervous system (CNS) in older individuals, has increased significantly in recent years because of the increased use of immunosuppressive agents for transplant patients, an increased prevalence of chronic and neoplastic diseases, and an overwhelming global spread of HIV. In fact, PML is found in 3.8% of AIDS patients with neurological

L.L. Barton and N.R. Friedman (eds.), *The Neurological Manifestations of Pediatric Infectious Diseases and Immunodeficiency Syndromes.*

abnormalities [6]. Deaths related to PML increased fourfold from 1.5/10,000,000 individuals in 1979 to 6.1/10,000,000 individuals in 1987. The increase began in 1984 with the AIDS epidemic [6]. PML is an AIDS-defining disease according to the Centers for Disease Control and Prevention surveillance case definition [7]. It is estimated that 85% of reported PML cases are in patients who have AIDS [8]. Before the AIDS pandemic, the average age of onset was 50 to 70 years, but this has shifted to individuals 20 to 50 years old. Although the incidence of PML in children is unknown, it has been reported in pediatric patients with AIDS and other immunosuppressive diseases [9,10]. More young adults with PML will undoubtedly be seen as the incidence of AIDS increases; therefore, the diagnosis of HIV infection should be considered in patients with PML.

## *Pathogenesis*

Polyomaviruses, including JCV, are ubiquitous, hardy, non-enveloped viruses whose genetic information is divided equally between two DNA strands. There is only one serotype of JCV, i.e., *Polyomavirus hominis* type 2, but many variants based on differences in the regulatory region of the genome. The virus is fastidious and difficult to grow in culture, taking up to 7 weeks in some cases. Humans seem to be the natural host for this virus [11]. How JCV transmission occurs has not been determined, although there is speculation that the virus requires sustained close contact and enters the host via the respiratory or gastrointestinal tract. Up to 50% of renal and bone marrow transplant recipients have been found to excrete JCV in their urine for days to several months after transplantation [12]. Whether viruria is a vehicle for transmission remains to be seen. Recent studies provide evidence for frequent transmission of JCV from parent to child [13]. Whether JCV can be transmitted to the fetus during primary maternal infection is still unresolved.

Another virus in the same family, *Polyomavirus hominis* type 1, BK virus causes a latent infection in the urogenital tract during childhood [14]. At 10 years of age, 50% of individuals have detectable BK antibody and, by adulthood, more than 70% are seropositive. BK virus may reactivate in approximately 5% of healthy individuals with low-level replication and viruria. High-level replication is a hallmark of nephropathy after renal transplantation and hemorrhagic cystitis in bone marrow transplant patients. Polyomavirus-associated nephropathy (PVAN) occurs in approximately 1 to 10% of patients with allograft dysfunction and 50% of cases with allograft loss within the first 2 years of transplantation. Early diagnosis of PVAN based on cytology and histological examination is associated with improved outcome after reduction of immunosuppression. BK viral infection may be identified by examining renal tubular epithelial cells for enlarged nuclei and viral inclusions and confirmed based on immunohistochemical staining of the large tumor antigen (LTag).

## Clinical and Neurological Manifestations

PML has an insidious onset and patients often present with speech and vision impairment, hemiparesis, and mental deterioration. The particular neurological manifestations of the disease depends on the area of brain involved and may be generalized (altered mental status, personality changes, delirium, dementia, or headache) or focal (hemiparesis). Cortical blindness and sensory abnormalities often occur later in the course of illness [15]. Visual field defects, ataxia, aphasia, and cranial nerve deficits have also been described. Focal and generalized seizures are an infrequent complication. Spinal cord involvement is rare. Death usually ensues within 3 to 6 months after onset. Most cases of PML seem to occur after immunosuppression [5], a key factor in reactivation of latent virus in the kidney. Immunosuppression is also a major contributing factor in the development of fatal, demyelinating disease of the CNS because of invasion of the oligodendrocytes in the brain. Viral reactivation in the urinary tract has been reported in patients receiving kidney or bone marrow transplants, immunosuppressive therapy, pregnancy, chronic disease, and primary immunodeficiency diseases, such as HIV or conditions associated with T-cell deficiencies [12,16]. JCV most likely disseminates hematogenously from the kidneys and/or bone marrow to the brain via B cells [17,18].

## Neuropathology

JCV-induced demyelination of subcortical white matter occurs as a result of the destruction of the oligodendrocytes because they are responsible for myelination of the axons that project from the neuronal cell bodies. Multiple discrete foci of demyelination tend to coalesce into large CNS lesions, particularly in the gray–white matter junction of the cerebral hemispheres. Unusual regions, such as the temporal lobes, basal ganglia, brainstem, and cerebellum, may be affected in patients with AIDS. Necrosis may be seen on gross examination, particularly in those who are severely immune compromised [19]. The microscopic appearance of the brain is characteristic (*vide infra*).

Although the oncogenic potential of JCV has been demonstrated *in vitro* and in animal models, to date the role JCV plays in the development of human brain tumors is speculative. JCV has been shown to infect human astrocytes, resulting in neoplastic transformation and multifocal astrocytomas [20]. Rencic et al. have provided evidence for oncogenicity in humans by detecting JCV DNA and tumor antigen in the brain of an immunocompetent patient with oligoastrocytoma [21]. Boldorini, likewise, reported the presence of JCV DNA in the brain of a 9-year-old immunocompetent child with pleomorphic xanthoastrocytoma [22 ]. Medullo blastoma, a malignant invasive tumor of the cerebellum, represents one of the most common CNS neoplasms in children, with 70% occurring in children younger than 16 years old. Krynska et al. have provided evidence to support the role of JCV in developing medulloblastomas by identifying DNA sequences in a significant number of tumor samples [23]. Because infection with JCV occurs in early childhood, it is possible that detection of JCV within human medulloblastomas results from initial primary exposure to the virus. Detection of JCV sequences may not establish a cause and effect relation to this CNS neoplasm, but it does provide a basis for additional studies to establish the role of JCV in the pathogenesis of pediatric medulloblastomas [23]. Laghi has provided evidence that JCV DNA is present in malignant colorectal epithelial tissue [24]. There was 10 times more JCV DNA in cancerous tissue than in normal colonic tissue, again pointing to the role of JCV in the development of human cancer.

## *Diagnosis*

Neuroimaging is particularly useful in diagnosing PML. On computerized tomographic (CT) scans, non-enhancing subcortical hypodense lesions can be detected, especially in the parietooccipital area [15]. Magnetic resonance imaging (MRI) scanning is superior to CT scanning, particularly in detecting early lesions and determining the number of lesions [25]. Electroencephalography may show focal slowing that corresponds to white matter lesions and may be used to corroborate the presence of a lesion(s) seen by neuroimaging, but is generally considered insensitive and nonspecific for use as a diagnostic test for PML.

Lumbar punctures are used primarily to exclude other illnesses because CSF findings are generally nonspecific in PML. A lymphocytic pleocytosis ($\leq$25 white blood cells/ml) and mildly elevated total protein may be observed in a small percentage of patients. The most reliable and accurate method for diagnosis is the use of a brain biopsy to detect the characteristic pathology, including hyperchromatic, enlarged oligodendroglial nuclei and intranuclear inclusion bodies, bizarre astrocytes with enlarged pleomorphic nuclei, and foamy macrophages in the center of demyelinated lesions [15]. Infected oligodendrocytes with eosinophilic, intranuclear inclusions containing JC viral particles, viral DNA and antigen, and hyperchromatic staining are particularly concentrated at the edge of the lesion. Their presence is required for presumptive diagnosis [26].

In addition, JCV DNA in situ hybridization and electron microscopy to detect virions may be used [15]. Polymerase chain reaction (PCR) can also be used to detect JCV DNA in CSF and, in some cases, peripheral lymphocytes [27,28]. Based on reports of high sensitivity and specificity of PCR using CSF, less invasive lumbar punctures rather than brain biopsies may become the standard when establishing a diagnosis of PML. Diagnosis of PML is based on the presentation of the classic triad of symptoms, visual, motor, and cognitive impairments, [12]. along with positive laboratory findings.

## *Treatment*

Although the prognosis of PML patients is grim, the progression of disease seems to be related to the degree of immunosuppression [15]. Whereas patients with AIDS have a very rapid course, leading to death in 2 to 4 months from presentation, patients showing a reversal in immunosuppression may survive for extended periods of time. Remission of PML in non-AIDS patients has been reported to occur spontaneously and after decreased immunosuppressive therapy [29]. In HIV-infected patients, highly active antiretroviral therapy significantly increases survival in patients with AIDS-related PML [30]. There have been rare, if any, randomized double-blind studies of therapeutic regimens for the treatment of PML. Several nucleoside analogs have been used with limited success. There have been conflicting results with the use of cytosine arabinoside administered by the intrathecal or intravenous route, recombinant interferon alpha-2a administered subcutaneously, and cidofovir. Currently, there are no antiviral drugs that have been specifically identified to target JCV. In the meantime, immunomodulating agents may offer some hope in the treatment of PML.

## References


1. Shah KV. Polyomaviruses. In: Fields BN, Knipe DM, Howley PM eds. *Fields Virology*, 3rd ed. New York, NY: Raven Press; 1996; 2027–2043.
2. Walker DL, BL Padgett. The epidemiology of human polyomaviruses. In: Sever J, Madden D, eds. *Polyomaviruses and Human Neurological Disease*, New York, NY: Alan R Liss, Inc; 1983; 99–106.
3. Tornatore C, Berger JR, Houff SA, et al. Detection of JC virus DNA in peripheral lymphocytes from patients with and without progressive multifocal leukoencephalopathy. *Ann Neurol*. 1992; 31:454–462.
4. Walker DL. Progressive multifocal leukoencephalopathy: an opportunistic viral infection of the central nervous system. In: Vinken PJ, Bruyn GW, eds. *Handbook of Clinical Neurology*. New York, NY: Elsevier/North-Holland Publishing Co; 1978; 307–329.
5. Padgett BL, Walker DL. Virologic and serologic studies of progressive multifocal leukoencephalopathy. *Prog Clin Biol Res*. 1983; 105:107–117.
6. Holman RC, Janssen RS, Buehler JW, Zelasky MT, Hooper WC. Epidemiology of progressive multifocal leukoencephalopathy in the United States: analysis of national mortality and AIDS surveillance data. *Neurology*. 1991; 41(11):1733–1736.
7. Centers for Disease Control and Prevention. 1993 Revised classification system for HIV infection and expanded surveillance case definition for AIDS among adolescents and adults. *MMWR*. 1992; 41:1–20.
8. Berger JR, Concha M. Progressive multifocal leukoencephalopathy: the evolution of a disease once considered rare. *J Neurovirol*. 1995; 1:5–18.
9. Berger JR, Scott G, Albrecht J, Belman AL, Tornatore C, Major EO. Progressive multifocal leukoencephalopathy in HIV-1 infected children. *AIDS*. 1992; 6:837–841.
10. Katz DA, Berger JR, Hamilton B, Major EO, Post MJ. Progressive multifocal leukoencephalopathy complicating Wiskott-Aldrich syndrome. Report of a case and review of the literature of progressive multifocal leukoencephalopathy with other inherited immunodeficiency states. *Arch Neurol*. 1994; 51:422–426.
11. Frisque RJ, White PA III. The molecular biology of JCV, causative agent of progressive multifocal leukoencephalopathy. In: Roos RP, ed. *Molecular Neurovirology*. Totowa, NJ: Humana Press; 1992; 25–158.
12. Shah KV. Papovaviruses. In: Specter S, Hodinka RL, Young SA, eds. *Clinical Virology Manual*. Washington, DC: ASM Press; 2000; 374–383.
13. Kunitake T, Kitamura T, Guo J, Taquchi F, Kawabe K, Yogo Y. Parent-to-child transmission is relatively common in the spread of the human polyomavirus JC virus. *J Clin Microbiol*. 1995; 33(6):1448–1451.

14. Hirsch HH. BK virus: Opportunity makes a pathogen. *Clin Infect Dis*. 2005; 41:354–360.
15. Major EO, Amemiya K, Tornatore CS, Houff SA, Berger JR. Pathogenesis and molecular biology of progressive multifocal leukoencephalopathy, the JC virus-induced demyelinating disease of the human brain. *Clin Microbiol Rev*. 1992; 5:49–73.
16. Shah K. Polyomaviruses. In: Fields BN, Knipe DM, Chanock RM, Hirsh MS, Melnick JL, Monath TP, Roizman B, eds. *Virology*. New York, NY: Raven Press; 1990; 1609–1624.
17. Houff SA, Major EO, Katz DA, et al. Involvement of JC virus-infected mononuclear cells from the bone marrow and spleen in the pathogenesis of progressive multifocal leukoencephalopathy. *N Engl J Med*. 1988; 318:301–305.
18. Finkelstein SD. Polyomaviruses and progressive multifocal leukoencephalopathy. In: Connor DH, Chandler FW, Schwartz DA, Manz HJ, Lack EE, eds. *Pathology of Infectious Diseases*. Stamford, CT: Appleton & Lange; 1997; 265–272.
19. Richardson EP, Webster HF. Progressive multifocal leukoencephalopathy; its pathological features. In: Sever JL, Madden DI, eds. *Polyomaviruses and Human Neurological Diseases*. New York, NY: Liss; 1983:191.
20. Sima AA, Finkelstein SD, McLachlan DR. Multiple malignant astrocytomas in a patient with spontaneous progressive multifocal leukoencephalopathy. *Ann Neurol*. 1983; 14:183–188.
21. Rencic A, Gordon J, Otte J, et al. Detection of JC virus DNA sequence and expression of the viral oncoprotein, tumor antigen, in brain of immunocompetent patient with oligoastrocytoma. *Proc Natl Acad Sci USA*. 1996; 93:7352–7357.
22. Boldorini R, Caldarelli-Stefano R, Monga G, et al. PCR detection of JC virus DNA in the brain tissue of a 9-year old child with pleomorphic xanthoastrocytoma. *J Neurovirol*. 1998; 4:242–245.
23. Krynska B, Del Valle L, Croul S, et al. Detection of human neurotropic JC virus DNA sequence and expression of the viral oncogenic protein in pediatric medulloblastomas. *Proc Natl Acad Sci USA*. 1999; 96:11519–11524.
24. Laghi L, Randolph AE, Chauhan DP, et al. JC virus DNA is present in the mucosa of the human colon and in colorectal cancers. *Proc Natl Acad Sci USA*. 1999; 96:7484–7489.
25. Post MJ, Sheldon JJ, Hensley GT, et al. Central nervous system disease in acquired immunodeficiency syndrome: prospective correlation using CT, MR imaging and pathologic studies. *Radiology*. 1986; 158:141–148.
26. Burger PC, Vogel FS. *Surgical Pathology of the Nervous System and Its Coverings*, 1982, 2nd ed., John Wiley & Sons, New York, pp. 195–203.
27. Henson J, Rosenblum M, Furneaux H. A potential diagnostic test for PML: PCR analysis of JC virus DNA. *Neurology* 1991; 41(Suppl 1):338.
28. Telenti A, Aksamit AJ Jr, Proper J, Smith TF. Detection of JC virus DNA by polymerase chain reaction in patients with progressive multifocal leukoencephalopathy. *J Infect Dis*. 1990; 162:858–861.
29. Greenlee JE. Progressive multifocal leukoencephalopathy. In: Aminoff MJ, Goetz CG, eds. *Handbook of Clinical Neurology*. Amsterdam, The Netherlands: Elsevier Science B.V.; 1998; 399–430.
30. Giudici B, Vaz B, Bossolasco S, et al. Highly active antiretroviral therapy and progressive multifocal leukoencephalopathy: effects on cerebrospinal fluid markers of JC virus replication and immune response. *Clin Infect Dis*. 2000; 30:95–99.

# Section II
# Bacteria

# Chapter 13
# Bacterial Meningitis

**Barbara Stechenberg, M.D.**

## Bacterial Meningitis

### *Introduction*

Bacterial meningitis, an inflammation of the meninges caused by a bacterial infection, is a medical emergency. The mortality of untreated disease approaches 100%; even with optimal therapy, there remains significant morbidity and mortality. Case fatality rates in developed countries vary with the etiologic agent, ranging from 0 to 15% [1].

### *Epidemiology*

Etiologic agents causing meningitis vary with the age of the child. For infants younger than 1 month of age, the etiologic agents are group B streptococci followed by *S. pneumoniae*, *Escherichia coli*, and *Listeria monocytogenes*. Presentation in the first week of life, particularly the first few days, suggests vertical transmission. Later onset suggests nosocomial or community acquisition and may include other Gram-negative organisms as well as staphylococcal species.

Before the introduction of *Haemophilus influenzae* type b conjugate vaccines, *H. influenzae* was the most common cause of meningitis in children older than 1 month of age. By 1995, the most frequent cause of bacterial meningitis in the United States in children 1 to 24 months of age was *Streptococcus pneumoniae*, followed by *Neisseria meningitidis*, group B streptococcus, and *H. influenzae* [2]. In children older than 2 years of age, *N. meningitidis* becomes more common than *S. pneumoniae*. However, any organism can produce meningitis in a susceptible individual. Outside of the neonatal period, the child between 6 and 12 months of age is at greatest risk for meningitis; 90% of reported cases are in children 1 month to 5 years of age. However, the epidemiology is again shifting with the widespread use of conjugate pneumococcal, as well as the *H. influenzae* vaccine.

L.L. Barton and N.R. Friedman (eds.), *The Neurological Manifestations of Pediatric Infectious Diseases and Immunodeficiency Syndromes.*

## *Pathogenesis*

Most cases of bacterial meningitis occur through hematogenous spread. There is initial infection or colonization of the upper respiratory tract, with subsequent invasion of the blood and seeding of the meninges with resultant inflammation. Less commonly, meningitis develops from a contiguous focus of infection, such as the sinuses or mastoids. Fractures through the paranasal sinuses from head trauma may precede meningitis, particularly with *S. pneumoniae* as the cause. Direct invasion may occur in children with meningomyelocele or dermoid sinus tracts. Children with mechanical hardware, such as ventriculoperitoneal (or other) shunts for hydrocephalus, are at increased risk for meningitis with skin flora, such as *Staphylococcus epidermidis,* as well as from the more common organisms. Recently, an association between cochlear implants and meningitis, particularly *Streptococcus pneumoniae*, has been reported [3].

Clinical meningitis that occurs when bacteria enter the subarachnoid space is a result of the complex interaction of components of the bacteria and the host inflammatory response. This results in the disruption of the blood–brain barrier and neuronal injury. Various cell wall products of meningeal pathogens induce a cascade of immune activation that includes the release of cytokines, chemokines, proteolytic enzymes, and oxidants that result in cell injury [4].

## *Clinical and Neurological Manifestations*

The signs and symptoms of meningitis are variable and depend on the age of the patient. The younger the child, the more nonspecific the findings. A history suggestive of a preceding upper respiratory illness is elicited in 75% of patients. Nausea, vomiting, fever, and anorexia are commonly seen. Older children may have complaints that are more specific, such as severe headache, photophobia, and neck or back pain. Seizures before diagnosis occur in 20 to 30% of children and are associated with other signs and symptoms of meningitis [5].

On initial examination, the level of consciousness is highly variable. Most children are irritable or lethargic or both. Approximately 10% or less are comatose on admission. A stiff neck is reported in 60 to 80% of children [6]. Kernig and Brudzinski signs are indicative of meningeal irritation and are often present; their absence, however, does not exclude the diagnosis of meningitis. Increased intracranial pressure is universal and undoubtedly accounts for the headache. Young infants may have a tense or bulging fontanelle. Papilledema is uncommon; its presence should provoke a search for subdural empyema, brain abscess, or venous sinus occlusion. Signs of sepsis, such as hypotension, petechiae, or purpura, may be seen, particularly in patients with meningococcal disease. Early mortality in bacterial meningitis is often related to septic shock.

Focal neurological signs may be present on admission. They are related to increased intracranial pressure and decreased cerebral blood flow, causing occlusive vasculitis, thrombosis of cortical veins, or cortical necrosis. Sixth nerve palsies are primarily related to increased intracranial pressure. Other cranial nerves, especially the eighth nerve may be involved.

## *Neuropathology*

The invasion of bacteria into the subarachnoid space produces meningeal exudates of variable thickness. The purulent material may be widely distributed, but often accumulates around veins and venous sinuses, in the depth of the sulci, over the convexity of the brain, and within the basal cisterns. Hydrocephalus is more common in neonates than in older children, but may occur with adhesive thickening of the arachnoid and extensive exudates at the base of the brain. Vascular changes include polymorphonuclear infiltrates extending to the subintimal regions of small vessels, thrombosis of cortical veins, and, rarely, occlusion of major venous sinuses and subarachnoid hemorrhage secondary to necrotizing arteritis. Subdural effusions occur commonly and are usually transient; they rarely develop into subdural empyema. Cerebral edema results from alteration in cerebral blood flow, intracranial blood volume, and permeability of cerebral vasculature caused by the immune response. Brain abscess formation is very rare, except in the case of neonatal meningitis caused by certain organisms, such as *Citrobacter koseri* and *Enterobacter sakazakii*.

## *Diagnosis*

A definitive diagnosis of meningitis requires examination and culture of cerebrospinal fluid (CSF). Early diagnosis and appropriate management is imperative to prevent morbidity and mortality. Delay of lumbar puncture for computed tomographic imaging is unnecessary in most patients unless there are focal neurological findings or coma. If lumbar puncture is contraindicated or cannot be performed, antimicrobial therapy should not be delayed. However, the time period between antibiotic administration and negative CSF cultures may be shorter than previously appreciated [7,8]. In neonates, sepsis is accompanied by meningitis in 20 to 25% of cases, therefore, CSF evaluation is important [9]. Antigen detection studies have been used in pretreated patients to make an etiologic diagnosis, but they are fraught with false positive and false negative findings and, thus, not generally used. Polymerase chain reaction of the CSF is not commercially available.

CSF analysis usually demonstrates cloudy fluid with an increased white blood cell count (predominantly polymorphonuclear leukocytes), a low glucose concentration, a high protein concentration, and a positive Gram stain and culture for the causative organism. In pneumococcal meningitis, the Gram stain is positive in 90% of cases [10]. In rare cases, the CSF will appear normal but will grow an important pathogen. If an unusual organism, such as *Staphylococcus aureus*, or an enteric organism beyond the newborn period is isolated, an underlying anatomic or immunologic abnormality should be sought.

## Treatment

Antimicrobial therapy should be initiated with bactericidal agents [7]. The drugs used for empiric therapy need to achieve concentrations in the CSF that will kill the likely organisms (Table 13.1). Vancomycin is added to a third-generation cephalosporin to cover for *S. pneumoniae* with decreased susceptibility to beta-lactam antibiotics.

The addition of corticosteroids to the early management of meningitis in children is controversial [11]. The administration of dexamethasone has shown no survival advantage, but there has been a reduction in neurological complications, particularly deafness, in a subset of patients. A meta-analysis of five studies showed a decrease risk in the corticosteroid groups [12]. A second meta-analysis that evaluated outcome related to organism isolated showed an advantage in *H. influenzae* meningitis, less for other organisms [13]. There is no consensus; the American Academy of Pediatrics suggests that corticosteroids may be beneficial in *H. influenzae* meningitis but does not make a clear recommendation in pneumococcal disease [14].

Adjunctive care should include meticulous monitoring, and avoidance of hyponatremia, hypoglycemia, and hypoxia. Measures to decrease cerebral hypertension (elevation of head of bed to 30 degrees, maintenance of $pCO_2$ concentration between 32 and 35 mmHg, mannitol) and maintain cerebral blood flow are imperative. Placement of an intracranial pressure monitoring device should be considered. Anticonvulsants may be necessary for the treatment of seizures but should not be used prophylactically. Anticoagulation for septic venous sinus thrombosis is controversial. Hydrocephalus requires CSF diversion through the placement of a shunt.

## Prognosis

Permanent neurological sequelae occur in 10 to 36% of children who survive an episode of bacterial meningitis [1,6]. Prognosis is dependent on many factors including 1) age; 2) time course or progression before administration of effective

**Table 13.1** Initial empiric antibiotic therapy of suspected meningitis in healthy children

| Age | Antibiotics |
|---|---|
| Neonates | Ampicillin and cefotaxime (± gentamicin) |
| 1–3 months | Ampicillin and cefotaxime or ceftriaxone |
| >3 months | Cefotaxime or ceftriaxone and vancomycin |

antibiotics; 3) the specific organism; 4) the number or concentration of orgarnisms [15] 5) the rapidity of sterilization of the CSF [16] and 6) the presence of underlying disorders that compromise the host response to infection. In neonates, predictors of adverse outcome include duration of seizures longer than 72 hours, presence of coma, use of inotropes, and leukopenia [17].

Hearing loss is a common sequela of bacterial meningitis [18]. The mechanisms responsible include spread of infection along the auditory canal and cochlear aqueduct, serous or purulent labyrinthitis, and subsequent replacement of the labyrinth with fibrous tissue. Deafness is noted early and is more common in pneumococcal disease. Ataxia may be associated with deafness because both the vestibular and auditory systems may be involved. All children with bacterial meningitis should be evaluated formally with evoked response audiometry (or pure tone audiometry in older children).

Focal neurological findings, such as hemiparesis, quadriparesis, facial palsy, and visual field deficits, can develop early or late in approximately 10 to 15% of children and may persist long term [6,17,19]. Intellectual impairment is seen in some children. Children who develop meningitis before 1 year of age may be at increased risk of poor neurobehavioral outcome; the overall risk of major intellectual deficit is less than 10% [20].

Early seizures that are easily controlled do not usually portend a persistent seizure disorder. Focal seizures and those that are difficult to control or that persist or arise beyond the fourth hospital day course have a greater likelihood of associated neurological sequelae [6]. Recurrent or new seizures after treatment also predict persisting neurological deficits [21].

Subdural effusions are not generally associated with clinical problems and resolve without specific intervention. Unusual complications include transverse myelitis, brain abscess (particularly with *Citrobacter* species), permanent hydrocephalus, and vascular changes in focal intracranial vessels.

## References


1. Baraff LJ, Lee SI, Schriger DL. Outcomes of bacterial meningitis in children: a meta-analysis. *Pediatr Infect Dis J*. 1993; 12:389–394.
2. Schuchat A, Robinson K, Wenger JD, et al: Bacterial meningitis in the United States in 1995. Active Surveillance Team. *N Engl J Med*. 1997; 337:970–976.
3. Whitney CG. Cochlear implants and meningitis in children. *Pediatr Infect Dis J*. 2004; 23:767–768.
4. Scheld WM, Koedel U, Nathan B, Pfister HW. Pathophysiology of bacterial meningitis: mechanism(s) of neuronal injury. *J Infect Dis*. 2002; 186 Suppl 2:S225–233.
5. Green SM, Rothrock SG, Clem KJ. Zurcher RF, Mellick L. Can seizures be the sole manifestation of meningitis in febrile children? *Pediatrics*. 1993; 92:527–534.
6. Kaplan SL. Clinical presentations, diagnosis and prognostic factors of bacterial meningitis. *Infect Dis Clin North Am*. 1999; 13:579–594.
7. Talan DA, Hoffman JR, Yoshikawa TT, Overturf GD. Role of empiric parenteral antibiotics prior to lumbar puncture in suspected bacterial meningitis: state of the art. *Rev Infect Dis*. 1988; 10:365–376.

8. Kanegaye JT, Soliemanzadeh P, Bradley JS. Lumbar puncture in pediatric bacterial meningitis: defining the time interval for recovery of cerebrospinal fluid pathogens after parenteral antibiotic pretreatment. *Pediatrics*. 2001; 108:1169–1174.
9. Sáez-Llorens X; McCracken GH Jr. Bacterial meningitis in children. *Lancet*. 2003; 361:2139–2148.
10. Arditi M, Mason EO, Bradley JS, et al. Three-year multicenter surveillance of pneumococcal meningitis in children: clinical characteristics, and outcome related to penicillin susceptibility and dexamethasone use. *Pediatrics* 1998; 102:1087–1097.
11. Feigin RD. Use of corticosteroids in bacterial meningitis. *Pediatr Infect Dis J*. 2004; 23:355–357.
12. Geiman BJ, Smith AL: Dexamethasone and bacterial meningitis. A meta-analysis of randomized controlled trials. *West J Med*. 1992; 157:27–31.
13. McIntyre PB, Berkey CS, King SM, et al. Dexamethasone as adjunctive therapy in bacterial meningitis. A meta-analysis of randomized clinical trials since 1988. *JAMA*. 1997; 278:925–931.
14. American Academy of Pediatrics. *Redbook: Report of the Committee on Infectious disease*. 27th Edition, Pickering LK (Ed). American Academy of Pediatrics, Elk Grove Village, IL, 2006. p. 530.
15. Feldman WE, Ginsburg CM, McCracken GH Jr, et al. Relation of concentrations of *Haemophilus influenzae* type B in cerebrospinal fluid to late sequelae of patients with meningitis. *J Pediatr*. 1982; 100:209–212.
16. Lebel MH, McCracken GH Jr. Delayed cerebrospinal fluid sterilization and adverse outcome of bacterial meningitis in infants and children. *Pediatrics*. 1989; 83:161–167.
17. Klinger G, Chin CN, Beyene J, Perlman M. Predicting the outcome of neonatal bacterial meningitis. *Pediatrics*. 2000; 106:477–482.
18. Dodge PR, Davis H, Feigin RD, et al. Prospective evaluation of hearing impairment as a sequela of acute bacterial meningitis. *N Engl J Med*. 1984; 311:869–874.
19. Sell SH. Long term sequelae of bacterial meningitis in children. *Pediatr Infect Dis*. 1983; 2:90–93.
20. Anderson V, Anderson P, Grimwood K, Nolan T. Cognitive and executive function 12 years after childhood bacterial meningitis: effect of acute neurologic complications and age of onset. *J Pediatr Psychol*. 2004; 29:67–81.
21. Pomeroy SL, Holmes SJ, Dodge PR, Feigin RD. Seizures and other neurologic sequelae of bacterial meningitis in children. *N Engl J Med*. 1990; 323:1651–1657.

# Chapter 14
# Focal Bacterial Infections and Parameningeal Infections

**Barbara Stechenberg, M.D.**

## Focal Bacterial Infections/Parameningeal Infections

Abscesses may form in many different areas of the nervous system—in the parenchyma of the brain or in the subdural or epidural space. Brain abscess, subdural empyema, cranial epidural abscess, and spinal epidural abscess may occur as a single entity or in combination with each other. They all alter neurological function by compression caused by mass effect, direct destruction, and infarction after inflammatory occlusion of vessels.

## Brain Abscess

### *Introduction*

Brain abscess is a focal collection of infectious material within the brain parenchyma. These abscesses may arise as a complication of a variety of infections, trauma, or surgery. Presentation may be subtle and requires a high index of suspicion.

### *Epidemiology*

Brain abscess is uncommon in children. In a series spanning 24 years, only 74 cases were identified in a large referral children's hospital [1]. The incidence of brain abscess varies by geographic location and access to health care.

### *Pathogenesis*

Bacteria may invade the brain either by direct spread, accounting for 20 to 60% of cases, or through hematogenous spread [2]. Direct spread usually produces a single

L.L. Barton and N.R. Friedman (eds.), *The Neurological Manifestations of Pediatric Infectious Diseases and Immunodeficiency Syndromes.*

focus. Primary infections that may act as sources include subacute and chronic otitis media and mastoiditis, frontal or ethmoid sinusitis, and dental infections. Brain abscesses from ear infections have decreased, whereas sinuses are a more frequent source. Missile injuries from bullets, pencil tips, sticks, or lawn darts have been associated with brain abscess; occasionally it can result from facial trauma or as a complication of a neurosurgical procedure.

Brain abscesses also may arise from hematogenous spread, often producing multiple lesions. These are most commonly located in the distribution of the middle cerebral artery and often situated at the junction of gray and white matter. Underlying infections leading to hematogenous seeding include chronic pulmonary infections, such as lung abscess and empyema; skin infections; intra-abdominal infections; and bacterial endocarditis (2–4% of cases). Recently, infancy and immunosuppression have become important predisposing factors [3]. No primary site or underlying condition can be identified in 20 to 40% of patients with brain abscess.

The microbiologic etiology depends on the site of primary infection. A wide range of organisms, including most bacteria as well as some fungi and parasites, has been recovered. Polymicrobial growth is not uncommon. Anaerobic and Gram-positive organisms are frequently encountered. Aerobic Gram-negative rods are not usually recovered. An exception is the recovery of Citrobacter or Proteus from brain abscesses in neonates associated with meningitis [4].

## *Clinical and Neurological Manifestations*

The clinical manifestations of brain abscess are extremely variable and may be nonspecific, resulting in a delay in diagnosis. During the initial stages, fever, vomiting, malaise, and focal headache may be present. The onset of headache can be gradual or sudden. Unfortunately, in infants and young children, the presence of headache is hard to elicit; nor is fever a reliable sign [5]. Symptoms are typically either generalized as the result of raised intracranial pressure or focal secondary to local mass effect. In infants, a bulging fontanelle caused by raised intracranial pressure may be seen. The classic triad of fever, focal deficits, and headache is seen in less than 30% and meningeal signs in less than 25% of patients [6]. Local neurological signs depend on the site of the lesion (Table 14.1).

Complications of brain abscess include seizures, ventriculitis or meningitis from rupture of the abscess, and obstructive hydrocephalus.

## *Neuropathology*

The histology depends on the age of the lesion and is characteristic of abscesses elsewhere in the body. Early lesions are poorly demarcated and associated with localized edema. After 2 to 3 weeks, central necrosis and liquefaction occur,

**Table 14.1** Neurological findings in brain abscess by location

| Site | Typical origin | Findings |
|---|---|---|
| Frontal lobe | Facial infection | Often silent |
| | Sinus infection, often with orbital disease | Papilledema |
| | | Disturbed behavior |
| | Dental infection | Forced grasp and suck |
| | | Depressed consciousness |
| Temporal lobe | Otogenic | Aphasia |
| | | Homonymous superior quadranopsia |
| | | Mild contralateral facial muscle or arm weakness |
| Parietal lobe | Hematogenous | Often asymptomatic |
| | | Impaired position sense |
| | | Homonymous hemianopsia |
| | | Focal sensory and motor seizures |
| Cerebellar | Otogenic | Vomiting, papilledema, ataxia |
| | | Ipsilateral tremor |
| | | Nystagmus (coarser on gaze toward lesion) |
| | | Ipsilateral arm and leg incoordination |
| Brainstem | Otogenic | Cranial nerve palsies |
| | Hematogenous | Contralateral hemiparesis |

surrounded by neutrophils. A fibrotic capsule develops that can be several millimeters to centimeters in thickness.

## *Diagnosis*

Routine laboratory evaluation is not helpful; leukocytosis and elevated sedimentation rate may or may not be present. Blood cultures are positive in a small percentage of cases. When brain abscess is a consideration, imaging studies should be performed before performance of a lumbar puncture because of the risk of cerebral herniation.

Magnetic resonance imaging (MRI) scanning is the modality of choice for the diagnosis and localization of brain abscesses (Fig. 14.1). It should be performed with gadolinium diethylenetriamine pentaacetic acid for enhancement. Compared with computed tomographic (CT) scanning, MRI scanning is more sensitive for early cerebritis and for picking up satellite lesions; it more accurately estimates the extent of the lesion, and it allows better visualization of the brainstem. Diffusion-weighted MRI scanning allows for differentiating ring-enhancing lesions (brain abscesses) from tumors [7]. If MRI scanning is unavailable, CT scanning with contrast represents a reasonable alternative.

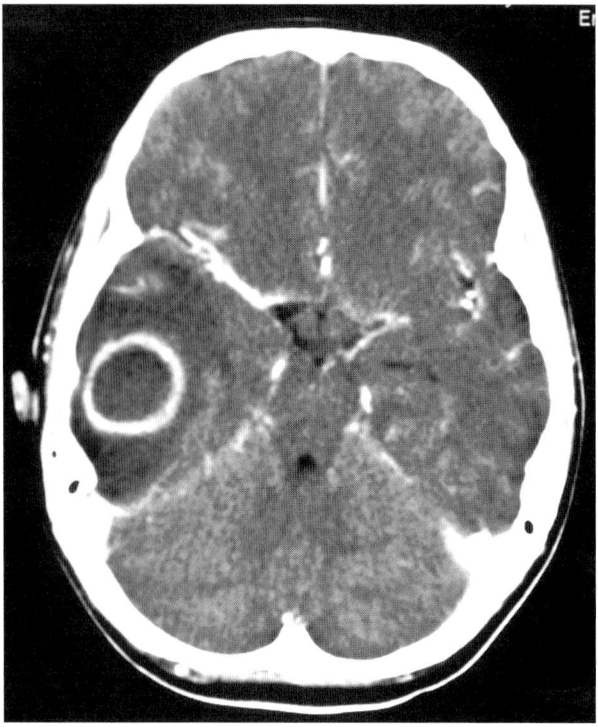

**Fig. 14.1** Right temporal lobe abscess. A contrast-enhanced CT scan shows a thin-walled abscess. The contents of the cavity are of fluid density. Edema surrounds the abscess. The patient was an 8-year-old boy with chronic otitis media and mastoiditis. (Image courtesy of J. Robert Kirkwood, M.D.)

After the diagnosis of brain abscess is established, a careful search for the source of infection is imperative. MRI and CT scanning should include the sinuses and mastoids, depending on the history. Echocardiography also may be helpful.

## *Treatment*

Successful management usually requires a combination of antibiotics and surgical drainage for both diagnostic and therapeutic purposes [8,9]. Initial aspiration of the abscess cavity is important to isolate the organism(s). Isolated medical management is usually limited to very small abscesses, surgically inaccessible abscesses, or those in the early cerebritis stage. Steroids should be considered if there is significant edema or mass effect.

Empiric antibiotic treatment is dictated by the presumed source, but often includes nafcillin or vancomycin, cefotaxime or ceftriaxone, and metronidazole.

Therapy is adjusted when the culture results are available. Treatment trials comparing various regimens are not available in children; however, treatment usually is continued for 4 to 8 weeks. Further surgical drainage is determined by the evolution of lesions by MRI or CT scanning, signs of increased intracranial pressure, and lack of clinical improvement.

Complications such as seizures require anticonvulsant medication, but the prophylactic use of anticonvulsant medication in the absence of seizure or epileptiform discharges on electroencephalogram is controversial. Obstructive hydrocephalus requires CSF relief or diversion through the placement of a shunt (external ventriculostomy shunt). Raised intracranial pressure requires early identification and aggressive management (elevation of head of bed to 30 degrees, maintenance of $pCO_2$ concentration between 32 and 35 mmHg, mannitol).

### *Prognosis*

Mortality from brain abscess currently ranges from 0 to 30%. This improvement from older series is ascribed to earlier diagnosis with CT and/or MRI scanning and the ability to follow patients closely with these modalities [8]. Two thirds of survivors do not develop neurological sequelae [6]. Poor prognostic factors include: rapid progression before hospitalization; severe mental status changes on admission; stupor or coma, and rupture into the ventricle [4]. The latter has a mortality of 80 to 100% and often leaves residual neurological deficits, such as hydrocephalus. Frequently, rupture occurs before diagnosis, presenting suddenly with high fever, shock, meningismus, and altered consciousness. CSF may show 50,000 to 100,000 polymorphonuclear leukocytes/$mm^3$. Neurological sequelae vary with the site and size of the lesion, mass effect, and vascular involvement.

## Subdural Empyema

### *Introduction*

Subdural empyema is a pyogenic infection with similar etiologic agents to brain abscess. Subdural empyema arises in the subdural space between the dura mater and the arachnoid mater. It is relatively rare, occurring as a complication of meningitis in infants, or of paranasal sinusitis and mastoiditis in older children [10]. This spread may be directly from contiguous osteomyelitis or by way of infected veins that penetrate the skull. It is an infrequent complication of intracranial surgery [11]. Because of the anatomy of the subdural space, the infection often extends widely over one or both cerebral hemispheres.

## *Clinical and Neurological Manifestations*

The signs and symptoms of the primary source of infection may vary from absent to prominent. The development of subdural empyema may be heralded by increasingly severe headache, meningismus, high fever, and focal neurological deficits. Focal or generalized seizures and signs of increased intracranial pressure may occur.

## *Diagnosis*

Routine laboratory evaluation is not helpful. The cerebrospinal fluid (CSF) in infants may reflect the association with meningitis, either treated or untreated. In older children, the characteristic CSF findings are increased opening pressure, few to a few hundred polymorphonuclear leukocytes, normal glucose concentration, and elevated protein concentration. The CSF is usually sterile.

Confirmation of the diagnosis of subdural empyema is obtained by contrast enhanced MRI or CT scanning (Fig. 14.2). Because the presentation may be subtle,

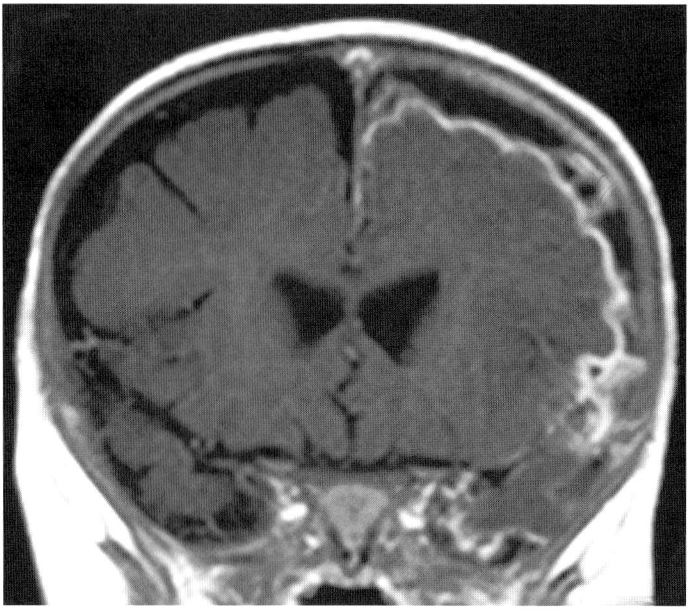

**Fig. 14.2** Left subdural empyema. The coronal gadolinium-enhanced T1-weighted MRI scan shows an extracerebral fluid collection, slightly more intense than CSF. There is contrast enhancement of the meninges and cortical surface, and within the subdural space as well. The patient was an 11-month-old boy with pneumococcal meningitis. (Image courtesy of J. Robert Kirkwood, M.D.)

the early use of these modalities may establish the diagnosis and attenuate the dramatic presentation noted with marked increased intracranial pressure.

### *Treatment*

The empiric antibiotics selected depend on the primary source of infection. For infants, the usual antibiotics, such as vancomycin and ceftriaxone, are appropriate. When sinusitis or mastoiditis is the source, coverage with vancomycin, metronidazole, and ceftriaxone may be started initially [12]. Surgical intervention to make an etiologic diagnosis, to drain the purulent material, and to relieve pressure is imperative. It may be accomplished with multiple burr holes or craniotomy. Adjunctive medical therapy for treating raised intracranial pressure may be required before the surgical drainage (elevation of head of bed to 30 degrees, maintenance of $pCO_2$ concentration between 32 and 35 mmHg, mannitol). Seizures, when present, require anticonvulsant medication.

### *Prognosis*

Mortality and morbidity have been lowered by the use of imaging modalities in early diagnosis [13]. Recent studies cite a mortality rate of 7 to 9%, with 24 to 55% having neurological deficits [11,14].

## Epidural Abscess

Epidural abscesses are rare suppurative infections of the central nervous system. They are less common than subdural abscesses and occur between the dura and the skull or vertebrae of the spine. Because of the rigid bony confines of the skull and spinal column, these lesions can expand to cause compression of the brain or spinal cord, with the development of severe complications or death.

### *Spinal Epidural Abscess*

#### Introduction

Spinal epidural infections may be restricted in extent or, more commonly, extend longitudinally over several segments of the spinal cord because the epidural space offers no resistance to infection. Most abscesses are located posteriorly, especially in children [15,16]. They are rare. In a 27-year review, only 6 of 39 patients were younger than 20 years of age; the youngest was 11 years old [17].

## Pathogenesis

Many spinal epidural abscesses begin as focal pyogenic infections involving the vertebral disc, the junctions between the disc and vertebral body, or the vertebral body itself. In acute cases, the abscesses contain primarily purulent material; granulation tissue is often present in patients presenting after 2 weeks. As the process progresses, the abscess may extend longitudinally in the epidural space, and damage the spinal cord by direct compression or thrombosis and thrombophlebitis of nearby veins.

The leading bacterial pathogen is *Staphylococcus aureus*, which accounts for approximately two thirds of cases [15–20]. Other bacteria include coagulase-negative staphylococci, aerobic Gram-negative bacilli, aerobic streptococci, and, importantly, *Mycobacterium tuberculosis*.

Approximately one third of patients have no identifiable source of the infection. It can occur after hematogenous spread from skin infections, dental abscesses, decubitus ulcers, pharyngitis, and wound infections. It may complicate spinal surgery. Osteomyelitis occurs uncommonly, except in chronic infections. There may be a history of antecedent trauma to the back in as many as one fourth of children [18]. Most children have no predisposing conditions [15,18].

## Clinical and Neurological Manifestations

Fever is almost always present. The abscess itself may cause symptoms in a typical sequence: 1) back pain, often focal and severe; 2) root or radicular pain, often described as "shooting" or "shock-like" in the distribution of the involved nerve root; 3) motor weakness, sensory changes, and bladder or bowel dysfunction; and, finally, 4) paralysis, which can occur rapidly and may become irreversible [21]. However, in young children, this typical presentation may be absent, with root pain seen in only 20% [18].

## Diagnosis

Fever and severe, localized back pain should suggest spinal epidural abscess, especially if there is increased pain on percussion. The diagnosis is established by MRI scan of the spine. If MRI scanning is not available, CT scanning with contrast may reveal the lesion. Once discovered, immediate neurosurgical intervention is necessary to prevent long-term neurological sequelae. Appropriate specimens for stains and cultures are obtained at the time of surgery. Cultures from the abscess content are positive in 90% of patients.

### Treatment

The two principles of therapy are eradication of the organism and reduction and, ultimately, elimination of the inflammatory mass. Early surgical decompression and drainage is critical, although some cases have responded to medical management [22]. Broad coverage with intravenous antibiotics is necessary until the organism is isolated. Initial empiric antibiotics are similar to those for brain abscess, vancomycin, metronidazole, and ceftriaxone or cefotaxime. Duration of treatment should be 4 to 6 weeks, or longer if there is extensive associated osteomyelitis.

### Prognosis

Morbidity is high in adults with at least one third of patients left with permanent neurological sequelae [16,17,19]. However, in children, mortality is low and sequelae are seen in only approximately 20% [15,18].

## *Cranial Epidural Abscess*

### Introduction

Intracranial epidural abscesses are much less common than are those in the spinal region. Because the dura is adherent to the inner aspect of the cranium, these abscesses rarely become large.

### Clinical and Neurological Manifestations

Their presentation is less acute because they are slow growing and well localized. They may spread to the subdural spaces, meninges, or brain. They may also coexist with other lesions, such as osteomyelitis secondary to mastoiditis, or after head injury. Local pain and tenderness associated with fever may be the only signs.

### Treatment

Treatment includes surgical drainage and prolonged antibiotics.

## References

1. Chun CH, Johnson JD, Hofstetter M, and Raff MJ. Brain abscess. A study of 45 consecutive cases. *Medicine* (Baltimore) 1986; 65:415–431.

2. Jadavjii T. Brain abscesses in infants and children. *Pediatr Inf Dis J.* 1985; 4:394–398.
3. Goodkin HP, Harper MB, and Pomeroy SL. Intracerebral abscess in children: historical trends at Children's Hospital Boston. *Pediatrics.* 2004; 113:1765–1770.
4. Foreman SD, Smith EE, Ryan NJ, et al. Neonatal Citrobacter meningitis: pathogenesis of cerebral abscess formation. *Ann Neurol.* 1984; 16:655–659.
5. Seydoux C and Francioli P. Bacterial brain abscesses: factors influencing mortality and sequelae. *Clin Inf Dis.* 1992; 15:394–401.
6. Yogev R and Bar-Meir M. Management of brain abscesses in children. *Pediatr Infect Dis J.* 2004; 23:157–158.
7. Castillo M. Imaging brain abscesses with diffusion-weighted and other sequences. *Am J Neuroradiol.* 1999; 20:1193–1194.
8. Mathisen GE, Johnson JP. Brain abscess. *Clin Infect Dis.* 1997; 25:763–779.
9. Brook I. Brain abscess in children: microbiology and management. *Pediatr Neurol.* 1992; 8:210–214.
10. Farma TW and Wise GR. Subdural empyema in infants, children and adults. *Neurology.* 1973; 23:254–261.
11. Dill SR, Cobb CG, and McDonald CK. Subdural empyema: analysis of 32 cases and review. *Clin Infect Dis.* 1995; 20:372–386.
12. Bockova J and Daniele R. Intracranial empyema (concise reviews of pediatric infectious diseases). *Pediatr Inf Dis J.* 2000; 19:735–737.
13. Zimmerman RD, Leeds NE, Danzinger A. Subdural empyema: CT findings. *Radiology.* 1984; 150:417–422.
14. Bok APL and Peter JC. Subdural empyema: burr holes or craniotomy? *J Neurosurg.* 1993; 78:574–578.
15. Auletta JJ, John CC. Spinal epidural abscess in children: a 15-year experience and review of the literature. *Clin Infect Dis.* 2001; 32:9–16.
16. Danner RL, Harmen BJ. Update on spinal epidural abscess: 35 cases and review of the literature. *Rev Infect Dis.* 1987; 9:265–274.
17. Baker AS, Ojemann RG, Swartz MN, Richardson EP. Spinal epidural abscess. *N Engl J Med.* 1975; 293:463–468.
18. Rubin G, Michowiz SD, Ashkenasi A, et al. Spinal epidural abscess in the pediatric are group: case report and review of the literature. *Pediatr Inf Dis J.* 1993; 12:1007–1011.
19. Nussbaum ES, Rigamonti D, Staudiford H, et al. Spinal epidural abscess: a report of 40 cases and review. *Surg Neurol.* 1992; 38:225–231.
20. Darouiche RO. Spinal epidural abscess. *N Engl J Med.* 2006; 355:2012–2020.
21. Heusner AP. Nontuberculous spinal epidural abscess. *N Engl J Med.* 1948; 239:845–854.
22. Wheeler D, Keiser P, Rigamonti D, et al. Medical management of spinal epidural abscesses: case report and review. *Clin Infect Dis.* 1992; 15:22–27.

# Chapter 15
# *Streptococcus pyogenes*

**Barbara Stechenberg, M.D.**

## Group A Streptococcus

### *Introduction*

Infections caused by group A streptococcus (*Streptococcus pyogenes)* may be followed by major nonsuppurative complications, acute rheumatic fever (ARF) and acute glomerulonephritis (AGN). Both of these illnesses follow the streptococcal infection by an interval during which immunologic mechanisms are triggered. One manifestation of ARF is Sydenham chorea (SC) also known as St. Vitus dance, or rheumatic chorea. Another possible relationship to group A streptococcal infection is postulated for a subgroup of children with neuropsychiatric disorders, pediatric autoimmune neuropsychiatric disorders associated with *Streptococcus pyogenes* (PANDAS).

## Acute Rheumatic Fever

### *Epidemiology*

The incidence of ARF and SC has declined dramatically in the Western world. However, an apparent resurgence of ARF has been seen in some areas of the United States since the mid 1980s [1]. In developing countries, SC is still a common manifestation of ARF. It is seen in approximately 10 to 15% of cases.

SC typically occurs in children 5 to 15 years of age, although it may be seen in younger children. Females are affected more frequently, at a ratio of 2:1. There seems to be a familial predisposition.

L.L. Barton and N.R. Friedman (eds.), *The Neurological Manifestations of Pediatric Infectious Diseases and Immunodeficiency Syndromes.*

## Pathogenesis

Although there is general agreement that ARF results from an interaction between the group A streptococcus and a genetically susceptible host, the pathophysiology is not completely understood. Certain strains are more likely to trigger ARF after untreated pharyngitis. Skin infection with the organism is not associated with ARF. Molecular mimicry, in which antibodies directed against group A streptococcus cross-react with host antigens in genetically susceptible subjects, is thought to be the basis of the immune-mediated pathogenesis [2].

## Clinical and Neurological Manifestations

In 1944, T. Duckett Jones proposed guidelines for the clinical diagnosis of ARF because there are no pathognomonic clinical or laboratory findings. These were revised in 1992 [3] for the diagnosis of an initial attack (Table 15.1). Chorea is the one major criterion that may be seen alone without fever or acute-phase reactants.

The onset of chorea usually occurs 1 to 8 months after the initial streptococcal infection, compared with arthritis or carditis, which occur within 2 to 4 weeks [4]. The onset can be insidious, with several months of symptoms later noted in retrospect. Emotional changes, such as easy crying, inappropriate laughter, or emotional liability, may precede the development of chorea. Regression in school performance may be the initial concern. Additional characteristic findings are uncontrollable movements and facial grimacing. The chorea typically begins with distal movement of the hands, but generalized jerking of the face and feet emerge as the chorea progresses. The movements are irregular and not stereotypical. The movements are continuous while awake, disappear with sleep, and are exacerbated by stress.

The clinical findings can be elicited on examination by several maneuvers: 1) milkmaid's grip, by asking the patient to grip the examiner's finger, demonstrates

**Table 15.1** Modified Duckett Jones criteria for acute rheumatic fever

| Major criteria | Minor criteria |
|---|---|
| Carditis | Clinical |
| Arthritis | Previous rheumatic fever |
| Chorea | Fever |
| Erythema marginatum | Arthralgia |
| Subcutaneous nodules | Laboratory |
| | Prolonged PR interval |
| | Elevated acute phase reactants |

*Requirements:* Evidence of antecedent Group A streptococcal infection.

Two major criteria or one major and at least two minor criteria.

irregular contractions of the muscles of the hand; 2) spooning and pronation of the hands when the arms are extended; 3) wormian movements of the tongue when protruded; and 4) examination of handwriting. The involvement of the tongue can interfere with speech.

Psychiatric symptoms include irritability and distractibility, as well as age-regressed behavior [5]. There seems to be a frequent association with obsessive–compulsive symptomatology. These symptoms typically occur during the first 2 months of ARF, although the obsessive–compulsive symptoms may precede, or occur concomitant with or after the onset of chorea.

Other neurological complications are rare. Isolated cases of seizures, papilledema, pseudotumor cerebri, and blindness from central retinal occlusion have been described. Sensory or cranial nerve involvement is absent. Most patients with SC recover without neurological sequelae.

## *Neuropathology*

Because SC is not a fatal disease, the neuropathology remains incompletely described. However, brain MRI scan findings include increased volume of the caudate, putamen, and globus pallidus compared with controls, [6] increased signal, particularly in the caudate and putamen, and angiographic changes consistent with inflammatory vasculitis [7].

## *Diagnosis*

SC may be the only overt manifestation of ARF. However, echocardiographic studies have confirmed that subclinical carditis is not uncommon [8]. Because the diagnosis of SC is clinical and signs of acute inflammation may be absent, the presence of carditis confirms the diagnosis. Therefore, a careful cardiac examination with echocardiography is warranted.

In SC, evidence by throat culture of streptococcal infections may not be present because of the long latent period. Supportive serologic evidence of previous streptococcal infection should be sought. Antideoxyribonuclease (anti-DNAse) B antibody is more sensitive and tends to remain elevated longer than anti-streptolysin O titers and should be sought when the results of the latter titer are normal. In the absence of carditis or evidence of infection, numerous other diagnoses, such as systemic lupus erythematosus, Wilson's disease, glutaric aciduria type 2, Huntington's disease, Tourette's syndrome, familial benign chorea, thyrotoxicosis, and attention deficit disorder with choreiform movements, should be considered.

## *Treatment*

As for other forms of ARF, antibiotic treatment with penicillin for acute infections should be prescribed for 10 days whether or not pharyngitis is present. Antibiotic prophylaxis to prevent recurrent ARF should then be initiated according to current guidelines: intramuscular benzathine penicillin G every 4 weeks, oral penicillin V twice a day, or sulfadiazine or sulfamethisoxazole once a day [9].

The chorea typically improves gradually, with a mean duration of 12 to 15 weeks, but may persist for 2 years or more. Full recovery ultimately occurs in almost all patients.

Treatment of SC depends on the degree of clinical impairment of motor function and the possibility of self-injury. Several treatments have been reported to be effective, including valproic acid, phenobarbital, haloperidol, pimozide, diazepam, chlorpromazine, and carbamazine. Corticosteroids administered as a brief course may shorten the course of the chorea.

## Pediatric Autoimmune Neuropsychiatric Disorder Associated with *Streptococcus pyogenes* (PANDAS)

The term PANDAS has been used to refer to a group of neuropsychiatric or behavioral disorders, particularly obsessive–compulsive disorder (OCD), Tourette's syndrome, and tic disorder, with a possible relationship to group A streptococcal infections. Swedo and colleagues have proposed an autoimmune pathogenesis for these disorders [10]. Suggested diagnostic criteria include the presence of OCD or a tic disorder; onset between 3 years of age and the onset of puberty; abrupt onset of symptoms or a course characterized by dramatic exacerbations of symptoms; onset or exacerbation of symptoms coincident with group A streptococcal infection; and abnormal results of neurological examination (hyperactivity, choreiform movements, or tics) during an exacerbation. This association has led to intensive investigation into its epidemiology, diagnosis, and potential treatment [11–13].

## References

1. Kaplan EL, Johnson DR, Cleary PP. Group A streptococcal serotypes isolated from patients and sibling contacts during the resurgence of rheumatic fever in the US in the mid-1980's. *J Inf Dis*. 1989; 159:101–103.
2. Kirvan CA, Swedo SE, Heuser JC, Cunningham MW. Mimicry and autoantibody-mediated neuronal cell signaling in Sydenham chorea. *Nat Med*. 2003; 9:914–920.
3. Special writing group of the committee on Rheumatic fever, Endocarditis and Kawasaki Disease. Guidelines for the diagnosis of acute rheumatic fever. *JAMA*. 1992; 268:2069–2073.
4. Nausieda PA, Grossman BJ, Koller WC, et al. Sydenham chorea: an update. *Neurology*. 1980; 30:331–334.

5. Swedo SE, Leonard HL, Schapiro MB, et al. Sydenham's chorea: physical and psychological symptoms of St. Vitus dance. *Pediatrics*. 1993; 91:706–713.
6. Giedd JN, Rapoport JL, Kruesi MJP, Parker C, et al. Sydenham's chorea: magnetic resonance imaging of the basal ganglia. *Neurol*. 1995; 45:2199–2202.
7. Robertson WC, Smith CD. Sydenham's chorea in the age of MRI: a case report and review. *Pediatr Neurol*. 2002; 27:65–67.
8. Elevli M, Celebi A, Tombul T, Gokalp AS. Cardiac involvement in Sydenham's chorea: clinical and Doppler echocardiographic findings. *Acta Paediatr*. 1999; 88:1074–1077.
9. Dajani A, Taubert K, Ferrieri P, Peter, G, et al. Treatment of acute streptococcal pharyngitis and prevention of rheumatic fever: statement for health professionals: Committee on Rheumatic Fever, Endocarditis, and Kawasaki Disease of the Council on Cardiovascular Disease in the Young, the American Heart Association. *Pediatrics*. 1995; 96:758–764.
10. Swedo SE, Leonard HL, Garvey M, Mittleman B, et al. Pediatric autoimmune neuropsychiatric disorders associated with streptococcal infections: clinical description of the first 50 cases. *Am J Psychiatry*. 1998; 155:264–271.
11. Kurlan R, Kaplan EL. The pediatric autoimmune neuropsychiatric disorders associated with streptococcal infections (PANDAS) etiology for tics and obsessive-compulsive symptoms: hypothesis or entity? Practical considerations for the clinician. *Pediatrics*. 2004; 113:883–886.
12. Swedo SE, Leonard HL, Rapoport JL. The pediatric autoimmune neuropsychiatric disorders associated with streptococcal infection (PANDAS) subgroup: separating fact from fiction. *Pediatrics*. 2004; 113:907–911.
13. Mell LK, Davis RL, Owens D. Association between Streptococcal infection and obsessive-compulsive disorder, Tourette's syndrome and tic disorder. *Pediatrics*. 2005; 116:56–60.

# Chapter 16
# *Bordetella pertussis*

**Barbara Stechenberg, M.D.**

## Pertussis

### *Introduction*

Pertussis, or whooping cough, is an acute infectious disease of the respiratory tract caused by *Bordetella pertussis*, or, rarely, by *Bordetella parapertussis*. It occurs worldwide and affects susceptible persons of all ages, although it is most serious in young infants.

### *Epidemiology*

The epidemiology of reported cases of pertussis is strongly affected by the degree of vaccine use. In unvaccinated populations, approximately 10% of reported cases occur in infants younger than 1 year of age, 40% in children 1 to 4 years of age, 45% in children 5 to 9 years old, with few cases in children older than 9 years old. In a highly vaccinated population, such as the United States, 30% of cases are reported in the first year of life, less than 25% in children 1 to 9 years of age, and the remaining cases are reported in older children, adolescents, and adults [1].

### *Pathogenesis*

*B. pertussis* is a small, aerobic Gram-negative rod. It is fastidious and requires special media for transport and isolation. Pertussis is highly contagious. Humans are the only hosts; transmission occurs via aerosolized droplets by close contact.

*B. pertussis* produces multiple antigenic and biologically active products, including pertussis toxin, filamentous hemagglutinin, agglutinogens, adenylate cyclase, pertactin, and tracheal cytotoxin. These products are responsible for the

L.L. Barton and N.R. Friedman (eds.), *The Neurological Manifestations of Pediatric Infectious Diseases and Immunodeficiency Syndromes.*

clinical manifestations of the disease because pertussis is primarily a toxin-mediated disease. The bacteria attach to the respiratory cilia, and produce toxins that paralyze the cilia and cause inflammation and local tissue damage to the respiratory epithelium. This interferes with the clearance of respiratory secretions. The pertussis antigens allow the organism to evade the host defenses; lymphocytosis is promoted but chemotaxis is impaired.

## *Clinical and Neurological Manifestations*

The incubation period is usually 7 to 10 days (range, 4–21 days). Classic pertussis is a lengthy illness with three stages: catarrhal, paroxysmal, and convalescent. Onset is insidious, with symptoms in the catarrhal phase resembling a mild upper respiratory infection with nonspecific cough. Fever may be mild during this period, but usually is minimal throughout the illness. The cough becomes more persistent and frequent during the next 1 to 2 weeks, until the paroxysmal phase, which is characterized by forceful coughing in the form of paroxysms. Classically, these spasms of cough are followed by a single massive inspiration (whoop). This stage may last 1 to 6 weeks. In the convalescent phase, recovery is gradual over weeks to months, with decrease in the number and severity of the paroxysms.

Older persons (adolescents and adults) and those partially protected by vaccine tend to have milder disease that is often misdiagnosed as bronchitis or upper respiratory infection [2]. The inspiratory whoop is often absent. Infants also may have an atypical presentation without a whoop or with apnea as a prominent finding.

## *Neurological Manifestations*

Central nervous system complications are primarily seen in young infants. They occur in the paroxysmal phase. Data from the Centers for Disease Control and Prevention indicate that in 2% of reported patients experience seizures, and less than 0.5% of patients suffer encephalopathy [3]. Severe disease is associated with convulsions, coma, and death. Persistent neurological sequelae may occur, including mental retardation, blindness, seizure disorders, personality or behavioral changes, hemiplegia, paraplegia, and ataxia. These findings are likely related to cerebral hypoxia related to asphyxia. Rarely, subarachnoid and intraventricular hemorrhage may occur [4]. Tetanic seizures associated with severe alkalosis caused by severe posttussive vomiting may also occur. Other rare neurological findings reported include subdural hematoma, spinal epidural hematoma, meningoencephalitis, and apnea [5–7].

## Neuropathology

Pathologic changes in the brain include microscopic and gross cerebral hemorrhage, as well as cortical atrophy. The exact mechanism for the encephalopathy is not known, although hypoxia during coughing spasms is most likely.

## Diagnosis

The diagnosis is usually based on a characteristic history and physical examination, particularly with possible exposure to an older child or adult with persistent cough. The standard laboratory test is the isolation of the organism by culture from a nasopharyngeal specimen. However, the organism has fastidious growth requirements. Successful isolation of the organism is unlikely after the first 2 weeks of illness. Polymerase chain reaction (PCR) offers a rapid, highly sensitive, and specific method for diagnosing pertussis [8]. However, reliable PCR testing is only available in selected laboratories. Serologic testing may be helpful, particularly in patients who have had prolonged illness before diagnosis; however, the efficacy of this testing varies greatly. Direct fluorescent antibody (DFA) testing has been available and is a rapid test. However, performance requires an experienced technologist; therefore, DFA is not generally recommended.

## Treatment

*B. pertussis* is susceptible to erythromycin and other macrolides. If administered during the incubation period or the catarrhal phase, these antibiotics can prevent or modify clinical disease. Treatment initiated after the paroxysmal stage is established does not affect the course of the clinical illness, but will reduce the spread of the organism to contacts. Because of the reported association of infantile hypertrophic pyloric stenosis and orally administered erythromycin, azithromycin should be considered for treatment or prophylaxis of infants younger than 6 months of age. For older infants children and adults, erythromycin, clarithromycin, and azithromycin are appropriate first-line drugs either for prophylaxis of close contacts or for treatment [9,10]. Both clarithromycin and azithromycin have better tissue penetration and longer half-life than erythromycin, requiring fewer doses per day and shorter duration of treatment.

Infants younger than 6 months of age with pertussis often require hospitalization for supportive care, to manage potential apnea, hypoxia, feeding difficulties, and other complications.

## *Prevention*

Universal immunization with pertussis vaccine in children has had a dramatic impact on epidemic pertussis in the United States [3]. In the mid-1990s, acellular pertussis vaccines were introduced that were immunogenic while having fewer adverse reactions than the whole cell vaccines that had been available. Recently, acellular pertussis vaccines aimed at adolescents and adults have been approved [11,12]. Use of these vaccines should reduce the transmission from older children and adults to young infants. All formulations of acellular vaccine are combined with diphtheria and tetanus toxoid components.

## References


1. Cherry JD. The epidemiology of pertussis: a comparison of the epidemiology of the disease pertussis with the epidemiology of *Bordetella pertussis* infection. *Pediatrics* 2005; 115:1422–1427.
2. Greenberg DP. Pertussis in adolescents: increasing incidence brings attention to the need for booster immunization of adolescents. *Pediatr Dis J* 2005; 24:721–728.
3. CDC. Pertussis—United States, 2001–2003. *MMWR* 2005; 54:1283–1286.
4. Celermajor JM and Brown J. The neurologic complications of pertussis. *Med J Aust* 1966; 1066–1069.
5. Jackson FE. Spontaneous spinal epidural hematomas coincident with whooping cough. *J Neurosurg* 1963; 20:715–717.
6. Southall DP, Thomas MG, and Lambert HP. Severe hypoxaemia in pertussis. *Arch Dis Child* 1988; 63:598–605.
7. Watts EC and Acosta C. Pertussis and bilateral subdural hematomas. *Am J Dis Child* 1969; 118:518–519.
8. Heininger U, Schmidt-Schlapfer G, Cherry JD, and Stehr K. Clinical validation of polymerase chain reaction assay for the diagnosis of pertussis by comparison with serology, culture and symptoms during a large pertussis vaccine efficacy trial. *Pediatrics* 2000; 105(3):E31.
9. American Academy of Pediatrics. Pertussis. In: Pickering LK, Baker CJ, Long SS, McMillan JA, eds: *Red Book: Report of the Committee on Infectious Diseases*, 27th ed. Elk Grove of Village, IL: American Academy of Pediatrics; 2006; 498–520.
10. CDC. Recommended antimicrobial agents for the treatment and post exposure prophylaxis of pertussis 2005 CDC Guidelines. *MMWR* 2005; 54 (No. RR-14):1–16.
11. CDC. Preventing tetanus, diphtheria, and pertussis among adolescents: Use of tetanus toxoid, reduced diphtheria toxoid and acellular pertussis vaccines. *MMWR* 2006; 55 (No.RR-3):1–34.
12. CDC. Preventing tetanus, diphtheria, and pertussis among adults: Use of tetanus toxoid, reduced diphtheria toxoid and acellular pertussis vaccine. *MMWR* 2006; 55 (No.RR-17):1–33.

# Chapter 17
# *Shigella* Species

**Barbara Stechenberg, M.D.**

## Shigella Infection

### *Introduction*

*Shigella* species are a common cause of bacterial gastroenteritis worldwide, especially in developing countries. Because the organism is acid stable, very few organisms can cause disease in a host. Shigella transmission occurs through direct person-to-person spread as well as from contaminated food or water.

### *Epidemiology*

There are approximately 14,000 laboratory-confirmed cases and an estimated 448,240 cases of shigellosis in the United States each year.

### *Pathogenesis*

*Shigella sonnei* is the predominant species (84%), with *S. flexneri* causing 12% of cases. In the developing world, *S. flexneri* is most common, with outbreaks of *S. dysenteriae* associated with a case fatality rate of 5 to 15%.

In the past, neurological complications were thought to be caused by circulating Shiga toxin produced by *S. dysenteriae*. However, that species is the least likely to be associated with seizures and recent studies have shown no association [1,2]. The etiology is not understood. The host response to lipopolysaccharide and specifically to the production of tumor necrosis factor-alpha may be involved.

L.L. Barton and N.R. Friedman (eds.), *The Neurological Manifestations of Pediatric Infectious Diseases and Immunodeficiency Syndromes.*

## Clinical Manifestations

Shigella is the cause of classic dysentery, infecting primarily the large bowel. The incubation period is 1 to 7 days. Patients typically present with fever, crampy abdominal pain, and bloody, mucoid diarrhea. Stools initially may be watery, small in volume, and frequent. Tenesmus is common.

Intestinal complications, although rare, may occur. They include proctitis or rectal prolapse, toxic megacolon, intestinal obstruction, or perforation.

## Neurological Manifestations

Seizures are the most common neurological complication of shigellosis. These are associated with fever, often higher than 39°C. For many children, fever and seizures may be the initial manifestations of the illness. These seizures are usually generalized, uncomplicated, nonrecurring, and not associated with neurological deficits or sequelae [3].

The reported prevalence of seizures in hospitalized children with shigellosis ranges from 10 to 45%. However, the incidence in outpatients with Shigella is much lower, less than 5%. The most common age group is between 6 months and 5 years [4].

Other than seizures, encephalopathy with lethargy, confusion, and headache has been noted in as many as 40% of hospitalized children. In the developing world, many of these patients also have dehydration and malnutrition [3,5]. Meningismus may precede the diarrhea and be misleading, making the diagnosis difficult. Rare findings include obtundation, coma, and posturing. A particularly fulminant form of encephalopathy with rapid development of seizures and coma, known as the Ekiri syndrome, was responsible for 15,000 deaths per year in Japan during the pre-World War II era [6].

## Diagnosis

The diagnosis of shigellosis is made by culture of feces. Children with seizures and Shigella infection are indistinguishable from children with febrile seizures. Results of analysis of cerebrospinal fluid typically are normal, although as many as 15% of these patients may have a mild pleocytosis with as many as 12 lymphocytes [3].

## Treatment

Most clinical infections with Shigella are self-limited. However, antimicrobial therapy may shorten the duration of diarrhea and eradicate the organism from feces. Because of resistance to antimicrobial agents, susceptibility testing of clinical isolates is indicated. If susceptible, ampicillin and trimethoprim-sulfamethoxazole are effective. Ceftriaxone, nalidixic acid, and azithromycin are therapeutic alternatives. Antimicrobials are administered for 5 days.

Acute symptomatic seizures should be treated with a benzodiazepine or fosphenytoin intravenously. Phenobarbital can also be used, however, associated sedation may limit its use if monitoring of mental status is important. More recently, an intravenous formulation of levetiracetam has become available, although its use in status epilepticus has not been studied. In the presence of seizures, it is important to check the glucose and electrolyte levels and correct these if they are abnormal. It is also important to institute fever control and maintain normothermia. Long-term maintenance with anticonvulsant therapy is usually not necessary. Supportive care with observation in a pediatric intensive care unit should be instituted in children with severe encephalopathy or coma.

## *Prognosis*

Prognosis is excellent. Shigella-related convulsions are not associated with an increased incidence of subsequent febrile or afebrile convulsions [7].

## References

1. Ashkenazi S, Cleary KR, Pickering LK, Murray BE, Cleary TG. The association of Shiga toxin and other cytokines with the neurologic manifestations of shigellosis. *J Infect Dis*. 1990 May; 161(5):961–965.
2. Noriega FR, Liao FM, Formal SB, Fasano A, Levine MM. Prevalence of Shigella enterotoxin 1 among Shigella clinical isolates of diverse serotypes. *J Infect Dis*. 1995 Nov; 172(5):1408–1410.
3. Ashkenazi S, Dinari G, Zevulunov A, Nitzan M. Convulsions in childhood Shigellosis. Clinical and laboratory features in 153 children. *Am J Dis Child*. 1987; 141:208–210.
4. Ashkenazi S, Dinari G, Weitz R, Nitzan M. Convulsions in Shigellosis: evaluation of possible risk factors. *Am J Dis Child*. 1983; 137:985–987.
5. Khan WA, Dhar U, Salam MA, Griffiths JK, Bennish ML. Central nervous system manifestations of childhood Shigellosis: prevalence, risk factors, and outcome. *Pediatr*. 1999; 103:E18.
6. Bennish ML. Potentially lethal complications of Shigellosis. *Rev Infect Dis*. 1991; 13 Suppl 4: S319–324.
7. Lahat E, Katz Y, Bistritzer T, Eshel G, Aladjem M. Recurrent seizures in children with Shigella-associated convulsions. *Ann.Neurol*. 1990; 28:393–395.

# Chapter 18
# *Campylobacter* Species

**Barbara Stechenberg, M.D.**

## Campylobacter Infection

### *Introduction*

*Campylobacter* species are common causes of diarrhea, particularly in industrialized countries. Campylobacter is usually a food-borne disease with uncommon acquisition from direct contact with animals or their products [1].

### *Epidemiology*

*Campylobacter* species are motile, comma-shaped, Gram-negative bacilli. *Campylobacter jejuni* and *Campylobacter coli* are the most common species that cause gastroenteritis. *Campylobacter fetus* predominately causes systemic illness in neonates and compromised hosts. The gastrointestinal tract of wild and domestic birds and animals is the reservoir of infection. Transmission usually occurs by ingestion of contaminated food, including unpasteurized milk and untreated water, or by direct contact with fecal material from infected animals or people.

### *Clinical Manifestations*

The incubation period averages 3 days (range, 1–7 days). Children often have diarrhea, fever, and abdominal pain. The pain can mimic appendicitis. Bloody stools occur in the majority of children [2]. Fever can be high; seizures may ensue.

L.L. Barton and N.R. Friedman (eds.), *The Neurological Manifestations of Pediatric Infectious Diseases and Immunodeficiency Syndromes.*

## *Neurological Manifestations*

Campylobacter is now recognized as the most commonly identified infection preceding Guillain-Barré syndrome (GBS). In a case–control study of patients with GBS, 26% had evidence of recent *C. jejuni* infections compared with 1% of age-matched controls [3]. Of those infected with *C. jejuni*, 70% had a history of diarrhea within 12 weeks before onset of GBS. In a cohort of persons with *C. jejuni* infection in Europe, the rate of GBS was 30.4 per 100,000 or a risk 100 times higher than in the general population [4].

The onset of GBS may be gradual or sudden, the latter often associated with pain and tenderness on palpation of muscles. Paresthesias are sometimes seen but often difficult to identify in young children. Weakness usually ascends progressively from the lower extremities to trunk and upper extremities and finally to bulbar muscles. Respiratory failure may ensue and require ventilatory support. The weakness is usually symmetrical but asymmetry is found in 9% of cases.

Autonomic involvement is not infrequent and is sometimes life threatening, especially cardiac arrhythmias. Additional manifestations include urinary retention, cardiac arrhythmias, blood pressure lability, and ileus.

The GBS variant, Miller–Fisher syndrome, which includes the classic triad of acute external ophthalmoplegia, ataxia, and areflexia, is also associated with Campylobacter infection. In some atypical cases, acute cranial motor neuropathies with ataxia may occur.

## *Neuropathology*

The main lesions are acute inflammatory polyradiculopathy and acute axonal degeneration producing flaccid paralysis. These changes may be caused by molecular mimicry, cross-reacting antibodies to GM1 ganglioside formed in response to similar epitopes expressed by the infecting Campylobacter strain [5]. Several studies suggest that GBS is more likely to follow infection with certain serotypes, such as 019 and 041. Host factors, particularly human lymphocyte antigen type, also seem to have a role in pathogenesis [6]. Cross-reacting antibodies to GQ1b ganglioside, which is present in cranial nerve myelin, have, in fact, been found in patients with Miller–Fisher syndrome [7].

## *Diagnosis*

An etiologic diagnosis of enteritis cannot be made on clinical grounds. Isolation from stool is the primary mode of diagnosis. Identification of the organism requires selective media, microaerophilic conditions, and an incubation temperature of 42°C.

The diagnosis of GBS is made by finding specific clinical features and classic cerebrospinal fluid (CSF) findings of elevated protein levels, normal glucose levels, and lack of pleocytosis. CSF findings are frequently normal, however, during the first week of the disease. Motor nerve conduction velocities are greatly reduced and typically show temporal dispersion and conduction block. Electromyography (EMG) shows acute denervation of muscles. In the very early stages of GBS, results of EMG and nerve conduction study findings may be normal or only show abnormal or absent H reflexes or F waves. As with the CSF findings, repeat studies may be needed to make the diagnosis if clinical doubt remains.

Antibodies to GM1 ganglioside in the case of GBS, or antibodies to GQ1b ganglioside in suspected cases of Miller–Fisher syndrome can be sought with commercially available tests [8]; however, the results take weeks to return and do not impact the immediate therapeutic decisions.

Results of stool cultures are rarely positive because the infection is self-limited; serologic testing for Campylobacter may establish the association.

## *Treatment*

Maintenance of hydration and correction of electrolyte imbalance are the cornerstones of treatment. Antimicrobial agents may, however, shorten the duration of clinical illness and prevent relapses. Erythromycin and azithromycin are commonly used.

The therapy of Campylobacter-associated GBS is primarily supportive. Close observation and monitoring for respiratory muscle involvement (vital capacity) and dysautonomia are essential. If the vital capacity falls below 20 ml/kg, or if there is bulbar involvement, the patient should be transferred to the pediatric intensive care unit (PICU) and elective intubation and ventilation considered before impending respiratory failure. All children should be placed on a cardiopulmonary monitor, and, if cardiac arrhythmias or blood pressure lability are detected, should also immediately be transferred to the PICU. Hypotension may require inotropic or fluid support, and hypertension should be treated with a short-acting drug, because swings in blood pressure are common. Urinary retention may require catheterization. Caution should be taken with oropharyngeal suctioning because the enhanced vagal response may cause a bradyarrhythmia.

In addition, immunomodulating agents are commonly used. Both intravenous gamma globulin (IVIG) and plasmapheresis appear to decrease the duration of the disease and improve neurological outcome [9,10]. Corticosteroids were shown, in one study in adults, to be detrimental. The prognosis for children who develop GBS is, however, generally excellent and better than that reported in older patients. In some cases, paraesthesias may persist for a number of months and may require treatment with a medication for neuropathic pain, such as amitriptyline, gabapentin, pregabalin, or carbamazepine.

## References


1. Allos BM. *Campylobacter jejuni* infections: Update on emerging issues and trends. *Clin Infect Dis*. 2001; 32:1201–1206.
2. Karmali MA, Fleming PC. Campylobacter enteritis in children. *J Pediatr*. 1979; 94:527–533.
3. Rees JH, Soudain SE, Gregson NA, Hughes RAC. *Campylobacter jejuni* infection and Guillain-Barré syndrome. *N Engl J Med*. 1995; 333:1374–1379.
4. McCarthy N, Giesecke J. Incidence of Guillain-Barré syndrome following infection with *Campylobacter jejuni*. *Am J Epidemiol*. 2001; 153:610–614.
5. Aspinall GO, Fujimoto S, McDonald AG, Pang H, et al. Lipopolysaccharides from *Campylobacter jejuni* associated with Guillain-Barré syndrome patients mimic human gangliosides in structure. *Infect Immun*. 1994; 62:2122–2125.
6. Sheikh KA, Nachamkin I, Ho TW, Willison HJ, et al. *Campylobacter jejuni* lipopolysaccharides in Guillain-Barré syndrome: molecular mimicry and host susceptibility. *Neurol*. 1998; 51:371–378.
7. Yuki, N, Ichikawa, H, Doi A. Fisher syndrome after *Campylobacter jejuni* enteritis: human leukocyte antigen and the bacterial serotype. *J Pediatr*. 1995; 126:55–57.
8. Jacobs BC, Hazenberg MP, van Doorn PA, Endtz HP, van der Meche FG. Cross-reacting antibodies against gangliosides and *Campylobacter jejuni* lipopolysaccharides in patients with Guillain-Barré or Miller-Fisher syndrome. *J Infect Dis*. 1997; 175:729–733.
9. Shahar E, Shorer Z, Roifman CM, Levi Y, et al. Immune globulins are effective in treatment of severe pediatric Guillain-Barré syndrome. *Pediatr Neurol*. 1997; 16:32
10. Khatri BO, Flamini JR, Baruah JK, Dobyns WB, Konkol RJ. Plasmapheresis with acute inflammatory polyneuropathy. *Pediatr Neurol*. 1990; 6:17–19.

# Chapter 19
# *Brucella* Species

**Barbara Stechenberg, M.D.**

## Brucella Infection

### *Introduction*

Brucellosis is an infection caused by one of the four species of Brucella that are pathogenic for humans: *B. abortus* (from cattle), *B. melitensis* (from goats and sheep), *B. suis* (from swine) and *B. canis* (from dogs).

### *Epidemiology*

The organism exists worldwide, especially in countries of the Mediterranean basin, the Arabian Gulf, the Indian subcontinent, as well as parts of Mexico and Central and South America.

#### Pathogenesis

The organism is a small, Gram-negative coccobacillus that is fastidious but can be grown on various laboratory media (e.g., chocolate and trypticase soy agars). The laboratory should be alerted because it may require incubation for at least 21 days to ensure growth.

Human brucellosis is a systemic infection that can affect any organ of the body and may be difficult to diagnose without a history of contact with animals or ingestion of animal or dairy products in or from an endemic area. Susceptibility to infection depends on several factors, including nutritional and immune status of host, size and route of inoculum, and the species of Brucella causing infection. *B. melitensis* and *B. suis* generally are more virulent [1].

The principal virulence factor of *Brucella* species seems to be the cell wall lipopolysaccharide. The organism is able to survive and multiply in phagocytic

L.L. Barton and N.R. Friedman (eds.), *The Neurological Manifestations of Pediatric Infectious Diseases and Immunodeficiency Syndromes.*

cells of the host. Localization of the organism in the reticuloendothelial system explains some of the manifestations, but the mechanism of involvement in the nervous system is not well studied.

## Clinical Manifestations

Symptoms may be acute or insidious and are often nonspecific, such as fever, weight loss, sweats, or depression. Arthralgias were seen in 73% of children in one large series [2]. On physical examination, the most frequent findings were arthritis (37%), splenomegaly (35%), and hepatomegaly (28%). Fever occurs in all patients but may wax and wane over weeks to months. Duration of symptoms for more than 30 days before diagnosis was a major risk factor for developing focal disease, a finding in 32% in one large series [3].

## Neurological Manifestations

Neurobrucellosis usually presents as meningitis, which is seen in 1 to 2% of patients [3]. Less common complications are papilledema, optic neuropathy, radiculopathy, stroke, and intracerebral hemorrhage, primarily in adults. Subdural empyema has also been reported [4]. Meningitis may be acute or chronic, mimicking meningeal involvement by other organisms.

More unusual neurological complications include optic neuropathy, radiculopathy, and meningovascular complications manifested by stroke or intracerebral hemorrhage from a presumed mycotic aneurysm. One child has been reported with a cerebellar syndrome without evidence of direct infection of the central nervous system [5] and another with a cerebellar abscess [6].

## Neuropathology

The pathology in neurobrucellosis demonstrates several different abnormalities: inflammation, particularly in the basal area with granuloma formation; white matter changes consistent with demyelination; and vascular insults, including inflammation of the small vessels causing lacunar infarcts, small hemorrhages, and venous thromboses [7].

## Diagnosis

Cerebrospinal fluid (CSF) analysis in neurobrucellosis typically demonstrates an elevated protein concentration, depressed glucose concentration, and lymphocytic pleocytosis [5,8]. CSF cultures are positive in a minority of patients with meningitis. One can increase the isolation of the organism from blood or other cultures by alerting the laboratory to hold the cultures for several weeks, to perform blind subcultures, or to use biphasic media (Ruiz-Castaneda) or lysis centrifugation cultures. Diagnosis is often made by serologic testing. The serum agglutination test is almost always positive. CSF agglutinins are also present [8].

## *Treatment*

Treatment requires prolonged antimicrobial therapy to prevent relapses. Oral doxycycline or tetracycline and rifampin for 4 to 6 weeks are used for older children. Children younger than 8 years of age may be treated with trimethoprim–sulfamethoxazole in combination with rifampin for 6 weeks with good results [9,10]. Streptomycin or gentamicin for the first 7 to 14 days may be a helpful adjunct in severe disease, such as meningitis.

The treatment of neurobrucellosis includes specific therapy, such as antibiotics (as above) or acute stroke or intracerebral hemorrhage management as appropriate, and generalized supportive care. Corticosteroids have been used in some cases of neurobrucellosis, but their role is not well delineated [5,8].

## *Prognosis*

Prognosis is variable in neurobrucellosis. In one series of 18 patients, only 11 patients had a complete recovery [5].

## References

1. Young EJ. An overview of human brucellosis. *Clin Infect Dis*. 1995; 21:283–289.
2. al-Eissa YA, Kambal AM, al-Nasser MN, al-Habib SA, al-Fawaz IM, al-Zamil FA. Childhood brucellosis: a study of 102 cases. *Pediatr Infect Dis J*. 1990; 9:74–79.
3. Colmenero JD, Reguera JM, Martos F, et al. Complications associated with *Brucella melitensis* infection: a study of 530 cases. *Medicine* (Baltimore). 1996; 75:195–211.
4. Shoshan Y, Maayan S, Gomori MJ, Israel Z. Chronic subdural empyema: a new presentation of neurobrucellosis. *Clin Infect Dis*. 1996; 23:400–401.
5. McLean DR, Russell N, Khan MY. Neurobrucellosis: clinical and therapeutic features. *Clin Infect Dis*. 1992; 15:582–590.
6. Ayala-Gaytan JJ, Ortega-Baquiero H, de la Maza M. *Brucella melitensis* cerebellar abscess. *J Infect Dis*. 1989; 160:730–732.
7. Al-Sous MW, Bohlega S, Al-Kawi MZ, Alwatban J, McLean DR. Neurobrucellosis: clinical and neuroimaging correlation. *AJNR*. 2004; 25:395–401.
8. al-Eissa YA. Clinical and therapeutic features of childhood neurobrucellosis. *Scand J Infect Dis*. 1995; 27:339–343.

9. Khuri-Bulos NA, Daoud AH, Azab SM. Treatment of childhood brucellosis: results of a prospective trial on 113 children. *Pediatr Infect Dis J.* 1993; 12:377–381.
10. Lubani MM, Dudin KI, Sharda DC, et al. A multicenter study of 1100 children with brucellosis. *Pediatr Infect Dis J.* 1989; 8:75–78.

# Chapter 20
# *Clostridium tetani*

**Barbara Stechenberg, M.D.**

## Tetanus

### *Introduction*

*Clostridium tetani* is the cause of tetanus. Still a major cause of morbidity and mortality in developing countries, tetanus is rare in the United States. Most cases occur in persons older than 60 years of age or in injection drug users; cases in children occur mainly in the unimmunized, often because of parental objection to vaccination. In developing countries, common forms are neonatal and maternal tetanus. In 2000, neonatal tetanus alone was responsible for 200,000 deaths [1].

### *Pathogenesis*

Tetanus is an acute, spastic paralytic illness caused by tetanus toxin or tetanospasmin. The neurotoxin is produced by *C. tetani,* a motile, Gram-positive, spore-forming obligate anaerobe that is ubiquitous in soil, dust, and in the gastrointestinal tract of some animals. Most non-neonatal cases are associated with a traumatic injury, often a penetrating wound by a dirty object. The wound may or may not show signs of inflammation. *C. tetani* is not an invasive organism.

Tetanus occurs after introduced spores germinate to vegetative forms in human tissue. They multiply in appropriate anaerobic milieu and produce two toxins, tetanolysin and tetanospasmin, the latter of which, a metalloprotease, is responsible for clinical tetanus. A prototype strain of *C. tetani* and tetanospasmin have been sequenced [2].

Although the pathway of entry into the nervous system has been debated, it most likely involves retrograde axonal transport [3]. The toxin binds tightly and irreversibly to receptors in the spinal cord and brainstem, blocking neurotransmission by the cleaving action on membrane proteins, disinhibiting neurons that modulate excitatory impulses from the motor cortex. Disinhibition of anterior horn cells and autonomic neurons results in increased muscle tone, spasms, and widespread autonomic instability.

L.L. Barton and N.R. Friedman (eds.), *The Neurological Manifestations of Pediatric Infectious Diseases and Immunodeficiency Syndromes.*

## Clinical and Neurological Manifestations

There are four clinical patterns of disease, generalized, neonatal, localized, and cephalic. The incubation period typically is 2 to 14 days, but may be much longer.

In generalized tetanus, trismus (or lock jaw) is the presenting symptom in approximately half of the cases. Headache, restlessness, and irritability are early symptoms, followed by stiffness, difficulty chewing, and neck spasms. The risus sardonicus facies or sardonic smile is caused by spasm of the facial and buccal muscles. As the paralysis spreads, the patient develops opisthotonos with severe hyperextension of the body. Laryngeal and respiratory muscle spasm can lead to airway compromise and asphyxiation. Painful tetanic seizures with sudden severe tonic contraction of muscles with fist clenching, flexion, and adduction of arms and hyperextension occur with the slightest environmental stimulus. Fever may occur because of the substantial metabolic energy generated by repeated spasms. Autonomic changes include tachycardia, arrhythmias, labile hypertension, and diaphoresis. The spasms progress over the first 2 weeks, plateau, and then slowly ameliorate over weeks.

Neonatal tetanus (tetanus neonatorum) typically presents 3 to 14 days after birth as increasing difficulty with feeding. It progresses to paralysis or decreased movement, stiffness to touch, spasms, and opisthotonos. It occurs in infants born to underimmunized mothers. The umbilical stump of the newborn becomes infected with the organism from poor obstetric technique or postnatal care or from cultural practices that include the application of cow dung or soil to the stump. There is a high mortality.

Localized tetanus results in painful spasms of muscles adjacent to a wound site. It may result from a lower inoculum of toxin, but it can progress to generalized tetanus.

Cephalic tetanus is a rare form, resulting from decreased neuromuscular transmission of lower cranial nerves. Manifestations usually occur 1 to 2 days after facial injury, with the development of facial palsy, dysphagia, paresis of extraocular muscles, trismus, and risus sardonicus.

## Diagnosis

The diagnosis of tetanus is established clinically in a setting of risk. The clinical picture is very dramatic and usually unmistakable. Differential diagnosis depends on the form of tetanus. Cephalic tetanus can be confused with Bell's palsy, trigeminal neuritis, or encephalitis. Trismus may be seen with dental problems, tonsillitis, peritonsillar abscess, temporal–mandibular joint dysfunction, and parotitis. Generalized tetanus may mimic rabies, strychnine poisoning, phenothiazine-induced dystonic reaction, and the tetany of hypocalcemia or hyperventilation. Results of routine laboratory studies and cerebrospinal fluid examination are normal. Electroencephalograms and electromyograms are neither characteristic nor necessary. Wound culture often does not yield the organism.

## *Treatment*

The goals of treatment are to decrease tetanic spasms and prevent complications by maintaining adequate airway and nutrition. Aggressive supportive care in an environment with a minimum of stimulation is essential. Survival is dependent on minimizing spasms until new presynaptic nerve endings are generated.

The child should be sedated and human tetanus immunoglobulin administered as soon as possible. Three thousand to 6,000 U is administered partly into the wound, with the rest administered intramuscularly.

Irrigation and debridement of the wound removes devitalized tissue. Antimicrobial therapy with penicillin G has been the treatment of choice; however, because of the possibility of penicillin acting as an agonist to tetanospasmin by inhibiting the release of GABA, metronidazole has become first line for treatment in many centers [4]. Antispasmodic agents, such as benzodiazepines, play an important role in decreasing spasms. If these agents are insufficient to control spasms, neuromuscular blockade with ventilatory support may be necessary.

Meticulous attention to supportive measures such as nutrition, hydration, prevention of decubitus ulcers, and avoidance of injuries during spasms help prevent complications.

## *Prognosis*

The average fatality rate associated with tetanus has been as high as 25 to 70% but can be reduced to 10 to 30% with modern intensive care. Newborns who survive often have evidence of brain damage. Poor prognostic signs are age younger than 10 days when admitted, symptoms of less than 5 days' duration, the presence of risus sardonicus, and fever.

## *Prevention*

Tetanus has decreased dramatically in countries with universal use of tetanus toxoid immunization and improved wound management. The use of tetanus prophylaxis in the evaluation of wounds in emergency departments also contributes to this decline in disease.

## References

1. Vandelaer J, Birmingham M, Gasse F, Kurian M, Shaw C, Garnier S. Tetanus in developing countries: an update on the Maternal and Neonatal Tetanus Elimination Initiative. *Vaccine.* 2003; 21:3442–3445.

2. Bruggemann H, Baumer S, Fricke WF, et al. The genome sequence of *Clostridium tetani*, the causative agent of tetanus disease. *Proc Natl Acad Sci U S A*. 2003; 100:1316–1321.
3. Farrar JJ, Yen LM, Cook T, et al. Tetanus. *J Neurol Neurosurg Psychiatry*. 2000; 69:292–301.
4. Ahmadsyah I, Salim A. Treatment of tetanus: an open study to compare the efficacy of procaine penicillin and metronidazole. *Br Med J (Clin Res Ed)*. 1985; 291:648–650.

# Chapter 21
# *Clostridium botulinum*

**Barbara Stechenberg, M.D.**

## Botulism

### *Introduction*

Botulism is a rare neuroparalytic syndrome resulting from the action of a neurotoxin produced by *Clostridium botulinum*. There are three naturally occurring forms of human botulism: 1) food-borne botulism from ingestion of food contaminated with preformed botulinum toxin; 2) wound botulism, infection of a wound with the organism, with subsequent in vivo toxin production; and 3) infant botulism, the most common, caused by ingestion of clostridial spores that then colonize the gastrointestinal tract and release toxin in vivo. A fourth man-made form, inhalational botulism, is a possible outcome of a bioterrorist attack.

### *Epidemiology*

An average of 110 cases of botulism are reported each year in the United States, of which, approximately 25% are food-borne; most of the rest are infant botulism. Wound botulism is rare, although there has been a recent upsurge among injection drug users. Food-borne cases are commonly recognized as small outbreaks. Although home-canned foods are the traditional sources, there have been cases from a variety of restaurant foods.

Infant botulism has been recognized as a separate disease entity since 1976. Although it has been associated with the ingestion of raw honey, this is most likely a minor environmental reservoir. There is no gender predilection. Most cases present between 6 weeks and 6 months of age. Almost all patients are younger than 1 year of age. Age at onset is younger in formula fed (7.6 weeks) than in breastfed infants (13.7 weeks), with the latter being a risk factor for the disease.

L.L. Barton and N.R. Friedman (eds.), *The Neurological Manifestations of Pediatric Infectious Diseases and Immunodeficiency Syndromes.*

## *Pathogenesis*

*C. botulinum* is a heterogeneous group of Gram-positive, rod-shaped, spore-forming anaerobic bacteria. They are ubiquitous in nature worldwide. The spores are heat resistant, but can be destroyed by heating to 120°C for 5 minutes. Germination and toxin production are most likely with conditions of restricted oxygen exposure, low acidity, and temperature between 25°C and 37°C. There are eight *C. botulinum* types, with A, B, E, and, rarely, F and G causing human disease. *Clostridium butyricum* and *C. baratii* are distinct species that also can produce type E and F toxins [1].

Regardless of the route of entry into the body, the toxin is carried through the bloodstream to peripheral cholinergic synapses, where it binds irreversibly to the presynaptic terminals [2]. This blocks acetylcholine release and causes impaired neuromuscular and autonomic transmission. Return of synaptic function requires sprouting of a new presynaptic terminal, a process that may require 6 months.

## *Clinical and Neurological Manifestations*

Symptoms of descending symmetric paralysis progress over hours to days before recognition. The function of cranial nerves is affected before others. Parents often note subtly flat facial expression, weak cry, and decreased suck. Constipation is typically seen early, but may, rarely, be absent [3]. The infant rapidly develops floppiness, gurgling, drooling, and poor feeding [4]. Rare cases may present with acute onset of weakness, progressing rapidly to respiratory and/or cardiorespiratory arrest [2].

Cranial nerve dysfunction is associated with severe disease. Signs include poor suck, new onset strabismus, ptosis, and head and facial weakness. These infants should be monitored closely for pooling of secretions and poor upper airway tone.

Autonomic dysfunction is under-recognized and may include decreased tearing and salivation, and fluctuations of blood pressure, pulse, and skin tone.

The onset of symptoms in food-borne botulism usually is 12 to 36 hours after ingestion of the preformed toxin. Prodromal symptoms often include nausea, vomiting, abdominal pain, diarrhea, and dry mouth. Disease presentation can be very variable, from mild to fulminant, with findings similar to those seen in infants.

## *Diagnosis*

The diagnosis of botulism requires a high index of suspicion in a patient with acute onset of flaccid paralysis with clear sensorium, without fever and paresthesias. Differential diagnosis often includes bacterial or viral sepsis, dehydration, pneumonia, hypothyroidism, cerebrovascular accident, genetic metabolic disorder (such as an amino acid disorder or medium-chain acyl-CoA dehydrogenase deficiency), congenital myopathy, myasthenia gravis, meningitis or encephalitis, anterior horn cell disease, heavy metal poisoning, anticholinergic poisoning, poliomyelitis, and Guillain-Barré syndrome.

Routine laboratory tests are not useful for diagnosis. Definitive diagnosis requires isolation of the organism or physiologic detection of toxin in stool; coordination of this sampling should be performed with reference laboratory, state health department, or the Centers for Disease Control and Prevention (CDC). Toxin is detected in 46% of serum or stool specimens of clinically diagnosed cases [5].

The electromyographic abnormalities consistent with infant botulism may be absent early in the disease and are not pathognomonic. However, certain findings are strongly supportive in the appropriate clinical scenario: 1) brief, small, abundant motor unit action potentials (BSAP) in clinically weak muscles; 2) facilitation (potentiation) of the evoked muscle action potential at high-frequency stimulation; and 3) absence of posttetanic exhaustion [6].

## *Treatment*

The mainstay of management is meticulous supportive care with anticipation of potential complications, particularly respiratory failure and autonomic dysfunction. Prophylactic endotracheal intubation may be necessary. Careful monitoring is imperative and should be in an intensive care unit. Nutritional support may be achieved via nasogastric feedings or parenteral alimentation. Breast-feeding seems to be protective against sudden death [7].

Antibiotics do not play a role in therapy and, in fact, have been associated with serious complications. Bacterial cell wall lytic agents increase the release of neurotoxin; aminoglycosides potentiate toxin-induced neuromuscular blockade. For food-borne or wound botulism, an equine serum trivalent (A, B, E) antitoxin has been shown to reduce mortality and is available through the CDC.

For infant botulism, specific treatment is now available with a human-derived botulinum antitoxin (BIG-IV) developed by the California Health Department. In a 5-year randomized, double-blind, placebo-controlled trial, it was demonstrated to be safe and to decrease mean hospital stay [8]. A subsequent 6-year open-label study of 382 laboratory-confirmed cases of infant botulism treated with BIG-IV confirms its safety and efficacy [8].

## *Prognosis*

With attentive care to reduce complications, recovery should be complete with restoration of neuromuscular transmission by new regenerated motor end plates. Relapses of infant botulism have been rarely reported; reinfection has not been observed.

## References

1. Barash JR, Tang TWH, Arnon SS. First case of infant botulism caused by Clostridium baratti Type F in California. *J Clin Microgiol.* 2005; 43:4280–4282.
2. Black JD, Dolly JO. Interaction of I-125 labeled botulinum neurotoxins with nerve terminal. II. Autoradiographic evidence for its intake into motor nerves by acceptor-mediated endocytosis. *J Cell Biol.* 1986; 103:535.
3. Mitchell WG, Tseng-Ong L. Catastrophic presentation of infant botulism may obscure or delay diagnosis. *Pediatrics.* 2005; 116:e436–438.
4. Schreiner MS, Field E, Ruddy R. Infant botulism: a review of 12 years' experience at the Children's Hospital of Philadelphia. *Pediatrics.* 1991; 87:159–165.
5. Shapiro RL, Hthaway C, Swerdlow DL. Botulism in the United States: a clinical and epidemiologic review. *Ann Intern Med.* 1998; 129:221–228.
6. Guiterrez AR, Bodensteiner J, Gutmann L. Electrodiagnosis of infantile botulism. *J Child Neurol.* 1994; 9:362–365.
7. Arnon SS, Damus K, Thompson B, et al.: Protective role of human milk against sudden death from infant botulism. *J Pediatr.* 1982; 100:568–573.
8. Arnon SS, Schecter R, Maslanka SE, et al: Human botulism immune globulin for the treatment of infant botulism. *N Engl J Med.* 2006; 354:462–471.

# Chapter 22
# *Corynebacterium diphtheriae*

**Barbara Stechenberg, M.D.**

## Diphtheria

### *Introduction*

Diphtheria is an acute toxic infection caused by *Corynebacterium diphtheriae*. Although a rarity in the Western hemisphere, there have been outbreaks in many areas of the world, most recently in the newly independent states of the former Soviet Union [1].

### *Pathogenesis*

*C. diphtheriae* is an aerobic, non-encapsulated, Gram-positive bacillus. Although not fastidious in growth requirements, its isolation is enhanced by using cystine-tellurite blood agar to inhibit growth of other organisms. There are three biotypes, mitis, gravis, and intermedius, all of which can cause diphtheria when infected with a lysogenic bacteriophage carrying the gene for production of exotoxin [2].

Humans are the only reservoir for *C. diphtheriae*. Asymptomatic carriers are important in transmission because immunity does not prevent carriage. Spread is primarily by airborne droplets, or direct contact with respiratory secretions or exudate from skin lesions.

### *Clinical Manifestations*

Respiratory diphtheria classically involves the tonsils or pharynx in more than 90% of cases, with the nose and larynx being the next two most common sites. After an incubation period of 2 to 5 days, local signs and symptoms of inflammation develop. Infection of the anterior nares, more common among infants, produces

L.L. Barton and N.R. Friedman (eds.), *The Neurological Manifestations of Pediatric Infectious Diseases and Immunodeficiency Syndromes.*

purulent, serosanguinous, erosive rhinitis with membrane formation. Shallow ulcerations of the upper lip and external nares are seen. In tonsillar and pharyngeal disease, sore throat is an early symptom, but only half of patients have fever, which may be low grade. Mild pharyngeal infection is followed by unilateral or bilateral membrane formation, which may extend proximally or distally. Underlying soft tissue edema and lymphadenopathy can produce the typical bull-neck appearance. Morbidity and mortality are caused by airway compromise or toxic complications, including cardiomyopathy and neuropathy.

## *Neurological Manifestations*

The neurological complications parallel the extent of the primary infection [3,4]. They are multiphasic in onset. Acutely or within 2 to 3 weeks after onset of the oropharyngeal inflammation, local paralysis and hypesthesia of the soft palate occur commonly. Weakness of the posterior pharyngeal, laryngeal, and facial nerves may follow, causing difficulty swallowing and a nasal voice. In the fifth week, cranial neuropathies, leading to oculomotor and ciliary paralysis, cause strabismus, blurred vision, and problems with accommodation.

Peripheral neuropathy follows weeks to months later. This symmetric polyneuropathy can descend, or more commonly, ascend, and may be indistinguishable clinically from Guillain-Barré syndrome. It can be mild or severe enough to cause total paralysis. The severity is related to the time between onset of symptoms and antitoxin administration as well as to the intensity of inflammation at the initial primary site.

## *Neuropathology*

In general, the most prominent pathologic features are necrosis and toxic hyaline degeneration of various tissues and organs. A toxic neuritis with fatty degeneration and interstitial fibrosis of paranodal myelin can be seen early in the disease; segmental demyelination occurs later [5].

## *Treatment*

The cornerstones of treatment are antitoxin administration, antimicrobial therapy, and supportive care. Specific antitoxin administration is the mainstay; it should be administered on clinical grounds as quickly as possible to neutralize any free toxin. An equine antitoxin is available from the Center for Disease Control and Prevention (CDC) [6]. A single empiric dose of 20,000 to 120,000 units is administered intravenously based on the degree of toxicity, site and size of the membrane, and duration of illness. Penicillin or erythromycin [7] is administered to halt toxin production and treat local infection.

Careful attention to respiratory status is important because these patients are at risk from both obstruction and aspiration. Treatment of the neuropathy is supportive and requires extensive rehabilitation with physical and occupational therapy.

## *Prognosis*

Recovery from neurological complications is usually slow but complete.

## *Prevention*

Diphtheria is prevented primarily by universal immunization with diphtheria toxoid.

## References


1. Vitek CR, Wharton M. Diphtheria in the former Soviet Union: re-emergence of a pandemic disease. *Emerg Infect Dis.* 1998; 4:539–550.
2. Nakao H, Pruckler JM, Mazurova IK, et al. Heterogeneity of diphtheria toxin gene, tox, and its regulatory element, dtxR, in *Corynebacterium diphtheriae* strains causing epidemic diphtheria in Russia and Ukraine. *J Clin Microbiol.* 1996; 34:1711–1716.
3. Naiditeh MJ, Bower AG. Diphtheria: a study of 1433 cases observed during a ten-year period at Los Angeles County Hospital. *Am J Med.* 1954; 17:229–245.
4. Kadirova R, Kartoglu HU, Strebel PM. Clinical characteristics and management of 676 hospitalized diphtheria cases, Kyrgyz Republic, 1995. *J Infect Dis.* 2000; 181 Suppl:S110–115.
5. Baba M, Gilliatt RW, Harding AE, Reiners K. Demyelination following diphtheria toxin in the presence of axonal atrophy. *J Neurol Sci.* 1984; 64:199–211.
6. Centers for Disease Control and Prevention (CDC). Availability of diphtheria antitoxin through an investigational new drug protocol. *MMWR.* 1997; 46:380.
7. Kneen R, Pham NG, Solomon T, et al. Penicillin vs. erythromycin in the treatment of diphtheria. *Clin Infect Dis.* 1998; 27:845–850.

# Chapter 23
# *Bartonella* Species

**Andrew M. Margileth, M.D., F.A.A.P., F.A.C.P.**
**and Mobeen H. Rathore, M.D., C.P.E., F.A.A.P.**

## Cat Scratch Disease

### *Introduction*

Cat scratch disease (CSD), caused by *Bartonella henselae*, *quintana*, and *clarridgeiae*, is the most common cause of chronic (≥3 weeks) benign, infectious lymphadenopathy in children and young adults. Approximately 22,000 cases occur each year in the United States. Lymphadenopathy usually develops after cat contact and/or a cat scratch [1,2]. Rarely, in approximately 2% of cases, CSD develops after dog contact or flea bites [3,5,7]. CSD is usually self-limited, resolving in 2 to 4 months [3].

### *Epidemiology*

CSD is rare in patients younger than age 2 years; however, 80% of cases occur in patients younger than age 21 years. It occurs in all races; male patients (55%) outnumber female patients in most reports. The incidence is highest in southern states, lowest in arid, western states; CSD occurs worldwide [1,3,4,6,7].

### *Pathogenesis*

The domestic cat and human flea are the major reservoirs for *B. henselae* and *B. quintana* as well as the major vectors for transmission of *B. henselae* to humans [7]. Asymptomatic *B. henselae* bacteremia occurs in 41 to 70% of healthy kittens and young cats [5]. CSD is transmitted by cutaneous, ocular, or mucous membrane inoculation; 95% of 2,000 patients had cat contact, 77% had cat scratches and/or a bite. A primary inoculation papule or pustule occurred in 54%, an ocular granuloma or conjunctivitis in 6%, and a mucous membrane ulcer was noted in 4% of

L.L. Barton and N.R. Friedman (eds.), *The Neurological Manifestations of Pediatric Infectious Diseases and Immunodeficiency Syndromes.*

patients [3]. Most patients develop CSD in fall and winter. Seasonality may relate to feline reproduction in summer, with high flea infestation of kittens. Kittens scratch more often and intimate contact with children is frequent. CSD is a sporadic illness, with no evidence of person-to-person transmission. Multiple cases have occurred in families [1,3].

## *Clinical Presentation*

In 90% of patients with CSD, typical clinical manifestations occur, i.e., lymphadenopathy with fever, malaise, anorexia, fatigue, and headache. However, systemic symptoms may be absent. Atypical CSD develops in 10 to 14% of patients [1,3]. Parinaud's oculoglandular syndrome is the most common, followed by encephalopathy, severe chronic systemic disease, and neuroretinitis. Less common clinical presentations are hepatosplenitis, pulmonary or thoracic disease, osteomyelitis, erythema nodosum, and Guillain Barré Syndrome (Table 23.1) [2,3,6,8,9].

## *Neurological Manifestations*

Children and adolescents with nervous system involvement (2% of 3,355 patients [1,3]) may develop encephalopathy, neuroretinitis, meningitis, radiculitis, polyneuritis, or myelitis with paraplegia [8,13]. The onset of blindness or neurological symptoms is usually sudden and occurs within 1 to 8 weeks of the onset of adenopathy

**Table 23.1** Cat scratch disease: clinical presentation of 2,104 patients observed over 39 years

| Clinical features | Number | Percentage of patients |
|---|---|---|
| Typical presentation | 1,793 | 85.3% |
| Inoculation lesion (skin, eye, mucous membrane) | 1,277 | 61% |
| Unusual manifestations | 311 | 14.8% |
| Parinaud's oculoglandular syndrome | 125 | 6.0% |
| Encephalopathy | 60 | 2.8% |
| Peripheral neuritis | 14[a] | 0.6% |
| Systemic disease, severe, chronic | 48 | 2.3% |
| Neuroretinitis | 33 | 1.6% |
| Erythema nodosum | 15 | 0.7% |
| Thrombocytopenic purpura | 7 | 0.3% |
| Hepatosplenomegaly | 7 | 0.3% |
| Osteomyelitis | 8 | 0.3% |
| Primary atypical pneumonia | 3 | 0.1% |
| Breast tumor | 3 | 0.1% |
| Angiomatoid papules | 2 | 0.1% |

[a]Complication in 12 patients with typical CSD, 2 with neuroretinitis.

Data from Margileth [3] and Margileth and Baehrens [6].

**Table 23.2** Clinical and laboratory characteristics in 82 patients with CSD encephalopathy

| Characteristic | Percentage of patients |
|---|---|
| Lymphadenopathy (≥3 weeks) | 100% |
| Headache, generalized, persistent | 80% |
| Lethargy and malaise | 73% |
| Coma, 1 to 5 d average | 63% |
| Convulsions, generalized or status | 60% |
| Fever (≥38.3–40°C) | 49% |
| Combative behavior | 40% |
| Ataxia, persistent, 7–21 d | 9% |
| Sedimentation rate (>20 mm/h) | 54% |
| CSF, elevated protein and leukocytes | 37% |
| EEG slow waves | |
| Focal transient | 3% |
| Generalized | 68% |
| CT or MRI scan results normal | 98% |
| Focal temporoparietal changes, transient | 2% |

[3,11,13]. Rarely, symptoms or signs precede adenopathy or occur in its absence. The frequency of major symptoms and signs found in 129 patients with nervous system involvement was neuroretinitis in 33, encephalopathy in 82, radiculitis in 12 and Bell's palsy in 2 patients [1,3,13]. Of the 82 patients with CSD encephalopathy in Table 23.2, 65% were male. The age range was 1 to 66 years (mean, 11.6 years). The commonest neurological symptom was headaches in 80%, followed by coma in 63%, convulsions in 60%, combative behavior in 40%, and ataxia in 9% of patients. Although generalized seizures and status epilepticus were described in these patients, additional reports have included patients with varying seizure types, including focal and brief, self-limited seizures (Fig. 23.1). Lethargy and malaise occurred in 73% and fever in 49% of patients. In 37% of 68 patients tested, cerebrospinal fluid (CSF) pleocytosis, elevated protein levels, or both were detected. Glucose levels were normal.

Electroencephalograms (EEG) in 66 patients revealed transient, nonfocal, slow waves for one to several months. Results of computed tomographic (CT) or magnetic resonance imaging (MRI) scan studies were normal in 48 (98%) of 49 patients studied. An MRI scan in a 7-year-old patient with status epilepticus revealed transient focal left temporoparietal localization consistent with cerebritis. Her EEG also showed transient epileptiform discharges on the left. Severe manifestations usually lasted 1 to 2 weeks, with gradual recovery to normal status in 1 to 12 months in all patients [3,13].

## Encephalopathy

Encephalopathy caused by CSD may be caused by *B. henselae* or *B. quintana* [9,14–16]. In four patients in three reports, encephalopathy was caused by *B. quintana* [14,15].

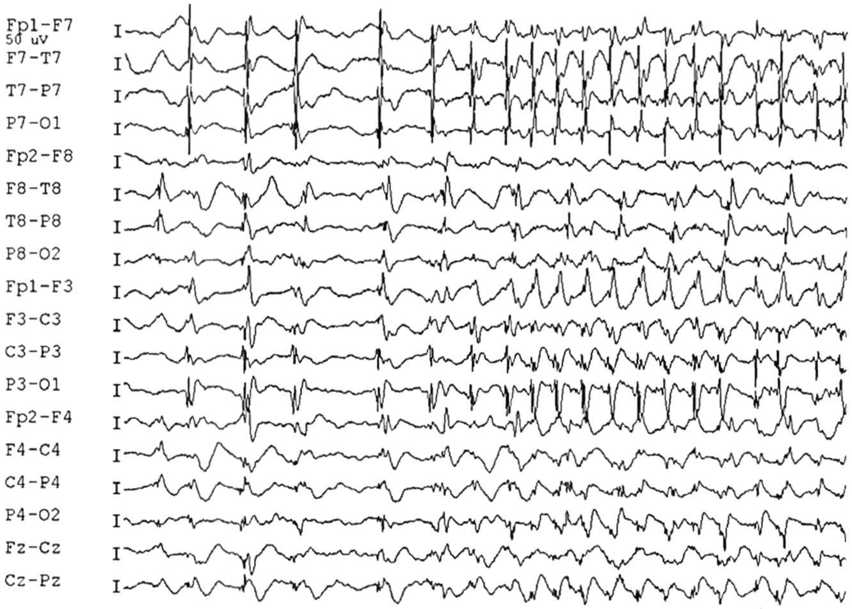


**Fig. 23.1** EEG of a teenage girl with CSD showing a focal left hemispheric seizure (EEG courtesy of Deepak Lachhwani, M.D.).

One 19-year-old patient had a granulomatous process of the thalamus and adjacent tissues. *B. quintana* was identified in CSF by polymerase chain reaction (PCR) in both patients [13]. A 10-year-old patient presented with frontal headaches and paresthesias of the mouth and face. Headache and fever (40°C) and paresthesias persisted, with abdominal pains and hepatomegaly. A gallium scan revealed an intracranial mass at the base of the brain. Brain biopsy revealed chronic inflammation and cat scratch bacilli by a Warthin-Starry silver stain. Convalescent titers were positive (>1:1,024) for both *B. henselae* and *B. quintana*. Treatment with trimethoprim–sulfamethoxazole and rifampin for 6 weeks was associated with rapid improvement in 5 days [15].

Recurrent CSD encephalopathy occurred in a 14-year-old girl and was caused by *B. quintana* [16]. Two separate seizure episodes with combative behavior occurred during a 3-month period after kitten exposure. Recovery was complete after 4 months. In two patients with unexplained, refractory seizures, diffusion-weighted MRI scan abnormalities directed a search for Bartonella encephalitis [17]. In New Zealand, a 30-year-old patient presented with headaches and unilateral decreased visual acuity with papilledema. Results of an abnormal MRI brain scan and positive antibodies to *B. henselae* confirmed two diagnoses: encephalopathy and neuroretinitis caused by CSD. Recovery occurred 1 week after therapy with ceftriaxone and rifampicin [18].

## Neuroretinitis

Optic neuritis or neuroretinitis (Fig. 23.2) with sudden onset of painless, usually unilateral, blindness occurred in 33 of the patients in Table 23.1; 7 children and 26 adults. Ages ranged from 5 to 65 years (mean, 28 years). Papilledema was seen with macular exudates in a star formation. Other types of inflammation of the retina and anterior and posterior segment cells are reported [19]. Adenopathy was present in 30 of 33 patients. Many patients (73%) presented with a viral prodrome that typically included throbbing headaches, malaise, fever (≥101 °F), chills, arthralgias, and myalgias. The prodrome lasted several days to 2 weeks. Visual loss usually occurred a few days after the initial systemic symptoms, and often was complete at onset. Of 33 patients, 32 had cat contact; 19 were exposed to kittens, 26 reported a cat scratch. Visual acuity returned to normal (20/25–30) in the majority (> 67%) of patients within a few weeks to 6 months, and 90% by 1 year.

Diagnosis of neuroretinitis caused by CSD in a previously healthy child or young adult is suggested by the sudden onset of painless blindness in one eye coupled with lymphadenopathy, exposure to a kitten or cat and/or a kitten or cat scratch, a viral prodrome, and presence of papilledema (76%) and/or a macular star (1 to 2 weeks; 86%) [19]. Tests excluding syphilis, tuberculosis, toxoplasmosis, Epstein Barr Virus (EBV), cytomegalovirus (CMV), toxocariasis, and leptospirosis with a

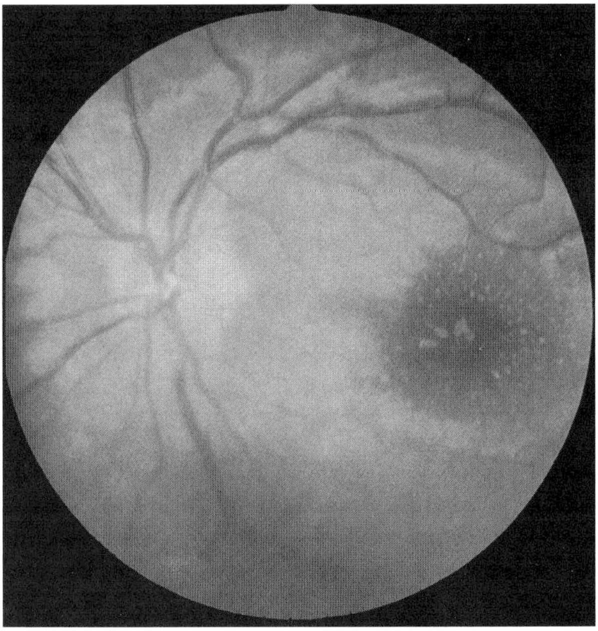

**Fig. 23.2** Stellate neuroretinitis associated with CSD in the left eye of a child (photograph courtesy of Robert W. Hered, M.D.).

positive (≥1:64) *B. henselae* titer result confirm the diagnosis. Spontaneous return of normal visual acuity in 1 to 12 months is usual. Rarely, disciform keratitis caused by *B. henselae* occurs; PCR analysis of corneal material may be positive [20].

Transient dysfunction of cranial and/or peripheral nerves occurred in 16 of 2,104 patients; two patients with neuroretinitis had radiculitis [3,15]. Two children aged 18 months and 8 years had temporary facial nerve paresis (Bell's palsy) associated with CSD oculoglandular syndrome lasting 4 to 5 weeks [3,10]. Of 14 patients with peripheral neuritis, 13 were adults and one was a 12-year-old girl with persistent radiating neck pain for 3 months. Tender postauricular, lymphadenitis with fever occurred after kitten scratches. CT scan results of the head and neck were normal.

## *Diagnosis*

Diagnostic criteria for CSD are enumerated in Table 23.3. When indicated by clinical features, serologic tests for EBV, CMV, toxoplasmosis, syphilis, and antistreptolysin O should also be performed to exclude these infections [9,10]. Results of cultures of blood, CSF, and lymph node aspirates, if performed, should be negative except if cultured for *Bartonella spp*. Serologic tests to detect antibodies to *B. henselae* are the most sensitive modality to confirm the diagnosis of CSD [10,11,12].

## *Treatment*

Management of encephalopathy, neuroretinitis, and peripheral neuritis is primarily supportive because typical and atypical CSD are usually self-limited, resolving spontaneously in 1 to 12 months. Over-treatment (anticonvulsants, corticosteroids)

**Table 23.3** Diagnosis of CSD[a]

| Criteria[b] |
|---|
| 1. Cat or flea contact with or without a scratch mark or a regional inoculation lesion (skin papule, eye granuloma, mucous membrane) |
| 2. Laboratory/radiology: negative purified protein derivative or serology for other infectious causes of adenopathy; sterile pus aspirated from node; PCR assay positive for *Bartonella henselae*, *B. quintana*, or *B. clarridgeiae*. CT scan: liver/spleen abscesses |
| 3. Positive enzyme immunoassay or indirect fluorescent antibody assay serology test >1:64 for *B. henselae* or *B. quintana* or *B. clarridgeiae*; fourfold rise in titer between acute and convalescent specimens is definitive |
| 4. Biopsy of node, skin, liver, bone, or eye granuloma showing granulomatous inflammation compatible with CSD; positive Warthin–Starry silver stain |

[a]Lymphadenopathy (≥10 mm) present ≥3 weeks.
Data from Margileth [3] and Margileth and Baehrens [6].
[b]Three of four criteria confirm the diagnosis; in an atypical case, all four criteria may be needed.

has been associated with poor outcome [1,3,13,21]. There is little evidence of the usefulness of antibiotic therapy in shortening or altering the course in immunocompetent patients. However, seriously ill or immunocompromised patients may be treated with azithromycin or ciprofloxacin or gentamicin and trimethoprim–sulfamethoxazole or rifampin and clarithromycin [2,3,10,15,22,23]. The role of high-dose corticosteroids in treatment of CSD encephalopathy requires further study [24]. Corticosteroids have also been used to treat retinitis: this should always be performed in consultation with an ophthalmologist.

## *Prevention*

The suspect cat need not be destroyed because it is invariably well and only 5% of family members scratched by the same cat develop CSD. The patient with CSD does not require isolation or quarantine, because there is no evidence of disease spread from human to human. Rigorous control of flea infestation in pets is essential, especially for immunocompromised subjects [3,7,23,25]. Preventive measures include declawing and regular nail clipping of young cats and dogs, keeping cats indoors, flea control, proper handling of pets and the litter box, washing hands after close contact with a cat, especially a kitten, and washing bites and scratches from dogs and cats with soap and water [25].The potential role of dogs and/or ticks that harbor and perhaps transmit *Bartonella* to humans, needs further investigation [25].

## References


1. Carithers HA. Cat Scratch Disease: an overview based on a study of 1200 patients. *Am J Dis Child.* 1985; 139:1124–1133.
2. English R. Cat Scratch Disease. *Pediatr Rev*. 2006; 27:123–128.
3. Margileth AM. Cat Scratch Disease. In: Rudolph CD, Rudolph AM, Hostetter MK, Lister G, Siegel NJ, eds. *Rudolph's Pediatrics*. 21st Ed. New York, NY: McGraw Hill; 2003; 926–928.
4. Murakami K, Tsukahara M, Tsuneoka H, et al. Cat scratch disease: analysis of 130 seropositive cases. *J Infect Chemother*. 2002; 8:349–3452.
5. Kordick D, Brown TT, Shin K, Breitschwerdt EB. Clinical and pathological evaluation of chronic Bartonella henselae or Bartonella clarridgeiae infection in cats. *J Clin Microbiol.* 1999; 37:1536–1547.
6. Margileth AM, Baehren DF. Chest wall abscess due to cat scratch disease (CSD) in an adult with antibodies to Bartonella clarridgeiae: case report and review of the thoracopulmonary manifestations of CSD. *Clin Infect Dis*. 1998; 27:353–357.
7. Rolain JM, Bourry O, Davoust B, Raoult D. Bartonella quintana and Rickettsia felis in Gabon. *Emerg Infect Dis*. 2005; 11:1742–1744.
8. Massei F, Gori L, Taddeucci G, Macchia P, Maggiore G. Bartonella henselae infection associated with Guillain–Barré syndrome. *Pediatr Infect Dis J*. 2006; 25:90–91.
9. Mantadakis E, Spanaki A.M, Psaroulaki A, et al. Encephalopathy complicated by Guillain-Barré Syndrome and hyrdocephalus and associated with Acute *Bartonella quintana* infection. *Pediatr Infect Dis J*. 2007; 26:860–862.

10. Slater LN, Welch DF. Bartonella infections including Cat-Scratch Disease. In: Scheld WM, Whitley RJ, Durack DT, eds. *Infections of the Central Nervous System.* 2nd Ed. Philadelphia, PA; Lippincott-Raven Publishers: 1997.
11. Schutze GE. Diagnosis and Treatment of Bartonella henselae Infections. *Pediatr Infect Dis J.* 2000; 19:1185–1187.
12. Frandson JM, Rawlings J, Burgess CR, Hendricks KA. Cat-Scratch Disease in Texas. *Infect Med.* 2000; 17:690–694.
13. Carithers HA, Margileth AM. Cat-Scratch Disease: acute encephalopathy and other neurologic manifestations. *Am J Dis Child.* 1991; 145:98–101.
14. Parrott JH, Dure L, Sullender W, et al. Central nervous system infection associated with Bartonella quintana: a report of two cases. *Pediatrics.* 1997; 100:403–408.
15. Grossman M, Azimi PH. Your Diagnosis, Please. *Pediatr Infect Dis J.* 1995; 14:725–728.
16. Noyola DE, Holder DL, Fishman MA, Edwards M. Recurrent Encephalopathy in Cat-Scratch Disease. *Pediatr Infect Dis J.* 1999; 18:567–568.
17. Singhal AB, Newstein MC, Budzik R, et al. Diffusion-weighted magnetic resonance imaging abnormalities in Bartonella encephalopathy. *J Neuroimaging.* 2003; 13:79–82.
18. McGrath N, Wallis W, Ellis-Pegler R, Morris AJ, Taylor W. Neuroretinitis and encephalopathy due to B. henselae infection. *Aust N Z J Med.* 1997; 27:454.
19. Ormerod LD, Skolnick KA, Menosky MM, Pavan PR, Pon DM. Retinal and choroidal manifestations of cat-scratch disease. *Ophthalmology.* 1998; 105:1024–1031.
20. Lohmann CP, Gabler B, Kroher G, Spiegel D, Linde HJ, Reischl U. Disciforme keratitis caused by Bartonella henselae: an unusual ocular complication in cat scratch disease. *Eur J Ophthalmol.* 2000; 10:257–258.
21. Jordan L, Kossoff E. Status epilepticus in a preadolescent: a ball of twine unravels. (Pediatric Puzzler). *Contemp Pediatr.* 2002; 19:27–39.
22. Bass JW, Freitas BC, Freitas AD, et al. Prospective randomized double blind placebo-controlled evaluation of azithromycin for treatment of cat-scratch disease. *Pediatr Infect Dis J.* 1998; 17:447–452.
23. Foucault C, Brouqui P, Raoult D. Bartonella quintana Characteristics and Clinical Management. *Emerg Infect Dis.* 2006; 12:217–223.
24. Weston KD, Tran T, Kimmel KN, Maria BL. Possible role of high-dose corticosteroids in the treatment of cat-scratch disease encephalopathy. *J Child Neurol.* 2001; 16:762–763.
25. Chomel BB, Boulouis HJ, Maruyama S, Breitschwerdt EB. Bartonella Spp. in pets and effect on human health. *Emerg Infect Dis.* 2006; 12:389–394.

# Chapter 24
# *Mycobacterium tuberculosis*

**Barbara Stechenberg, M.D.**

## Tuberculosis

### *Introduction*

Infection with *Mycobacterium tuberculosis* continues to cause significant worldwide morbidity and mortality. The World Health Organization (WHO) estimates that each year there are more than 8 million new cases and 2 million people die of the disease [1]. More than one third of the world's population is infected with this organism. In the United States, an estimated 15 million people are infected. Tuberculosis occurs disproportionately among disadvantaged populations, such as the homeless, malnourished, and overcrowded. The spread of human immunodeficiency virus (HIV) and immigration of persons from areas of high incidence has resulted in an increased number of cases in the United States.

### *Epidemiology*

Tuberculosis is spread from person to person via airborne droplets, 1 to 5 μm in diameter. The chance of transmission increases when the patient has an acid-fast positive smear of sputum; extensive upper lobe disease, especially with cavitation; copious, thin secretions; and severe, forceful cough. Young children rarely infect other children or adults.

### *Pathogenesis*

After inhalation, a single tubercle bacillus can initiate infection. The primary complex in the lungs includes the primary focus, lymphangitis, and regional adenopathy. The incubation period from infection to the development of cutaneous sensitivity is 3 weeks to 3 months. For most patients, the infection becomes latent.

L.L. Barton and N.R. Friedman (eds.), *The Neurological Manifestations of Pediatric Infectious Diseases and Immunodeficiency Syndromes.*

Tuberculosis of the central nervous system is the most serious complication or extrapulmonary manifestation in children and is fatal without effective treatment. Tuberculous meningitis usually arises from lymphohematogenous dissemination of the primary infection, which forms metastatic lesions in the cerebral cortex or meninges. This initial lesion increases in size and discharges small numbers of organisms into the subarachnoid space. The resulting exudate infiltrates vessels, producing inflammation and infarction of the cerebral cortex. The brainstem is often involved, leading to associated cranial nerve dysfunction [2]. Communicating hydrocephalus is common.

## *Clinical Manifestations*

Most children infected with *M. tuberculosis* remain asymptomatic and do not develop signs or symptoms at any time. Occasionally, infection is marked by low-grade fever and cough. Rarely, there are flu-like symptoms that resolve within a week. Primary pulmonary disease is the most common form of tuberculosis or active disease caused by this organism. Approximately 25 to 30% of children with tuberculosis have an extrapulmonary presentation.

## *Neurological Manifestations*

Tuberculous meningitis is seen in approximately 0.3% of untreated infections in children, particularly between 6 months and 4 years of age. Occasionally, it occurs many years after initial infection from rupture of one or more subependymal tubercles discharging bacilli into the subarachnoid space.

The clinical presentation of central nervous system disease can be acute or chronic. Infants and young children are more likely to have rapid progression with only several days before the onset of hydrocephalus with seizures and cerebral edema.

More commonly, signs and symptoms progress over several weeks and can be divided into three stages [3]. The first stage, typically lasting 1 to 2 weeks, is characterized by nonspecific symptoms, including fever, irritability, headache, malaise, and drowsiness. There may be a loss or plateauing of developmental milestones. The second stage may begin abruptly, with lethargy, nuchal rigidity, seizures, positive Kernig or Brudzinski signs, hypertonia, cranial nerve palsies, and other focal signs. This is often associated with the development of hydrocephalus. Some children do not have signs of meningeal irritation but are encephalopathic, with speech impairment, movement disorders, or disorientation. The third stage denotes severe deterioration, with coma, hemiplegia or paraplegia, hemodynamic instability, decerebrate posturing, and, eventually, death. Prognosis correlates with the stage at presentation. A high index of suspicion is imperative in a child presenting with basilar meningitis, hydrocephalus, cranial nerve palsy, or stroke with no apparent etiology.

Tuberculoma, another central nervous system manifestation of tuberculosis, may be silent or present clinically as a space-occupying mass or a brain tumor. In India and China, tuberculomas account for 20 to 30% of brain tumors in children, but are rare in North America and Europe [4]. In adults, they are most often supratentorial, but, in children, are often infratentorial and located at the base of the brain. The most common symptoms are headache, fever, seizures, and signs and symptoms of intracranial hypertension.

An extremely rare form of tuberculosis in children is spinal tuberculous arachnoiditis [5]. It is produced by gradual encasement of the spinal cord by gelatinous exudate. Symptoms develop slowly over weeks to months. Patients present with nerve root and cord compression signs: spinal or radicular pain; hyperesthesias or paresthesias; lower motor neuron paralysis; and bladder or rectal sphincter dysfunction.

## *Neuropathology*

Meningeal involvement is most marked at the base of the brain. The intense hypersensitivity reaction to the spillage of tubercular protein into the arachnoid space produces a strong inflammatory response. A gelatinous mass may extend from the pons to the optic nerves. The mass produced by this proliferative arachnoiditis may involve several cranial nerves and penetrating vessels. Vasculitis with resulting thrombosis and infarction may occur. Communicating hydrocephalus may result from the extension of the inflammatory process.

## *Diagnosis*

The diagnosis of tuberculous meningitis can be difficult. Up to 50% of patients will have a nonreactive tuberculin skin test result, and 20 to 50% will have a normal chest radiograph result. In addition to the tuberculin skin test, a new in vitro test, QuantiFERON®-TB Gold, an enzyme-linked immunosorbent assay (ELISA) that detects the release of interferon-gamma, has been approved as an aid in diagnosing tuberculosis disease and latent infection [6]. Use in children (particularly younger than 5 years) is not well studied.

Examination of the CSF usually demonstrates a leukocyte count of 10 to 500 cells/$mm^3$; polymorphonuclear leukocytes may be present early, but lymphocytes usually predominate. The CSF glucose level is usually less than 40 mg/dl, but may initially be normal. The protein is generally elevated and may be markedly so secondary to hydrocephalus and spinal block. It is important to obtain 5 to 10 ml of CSF for acid-fast stain and culture to maximize the yield. If an adequate quantity of CSF is obtained, up to 30% of smears of the sediment will demonstrate acid-fast bacilli, and culture results will be positive in 50 to 70% of cases. Culture of other fluids, such as gastric aspirates, may be useful, both for organism identification and determination of susceptibility to antimicrobials. Polymerase chain reaction (PCR) and antigen detection in clinical specimens for diagnosis have limited usefulness at this time.

Results from radiographic studies, such as contrast-enhanced computed tomographic (CT) or magnetic resonance imaging (MRI) scans may be normal early in the disease but may later show basilar enhancement and communicating hydrocephalus. There may be signs of cerebral edema or focal ischemia, as well as clinically silent tuberculomas.

In patients with tuberculomas, the tuberculin skin test result is usually positive, but the chest radiograph result may be normal. On CT or MRI scan, tuberculomas usually appear as discrete lesions with surrounding edema. With contrast, there may be significant ring enhancement. In spinal tuberculous arachnoiditis, the diagnosis is based on abnormal CSF protein levels and MRI scan changes, combined with tissue biopsy.

## *Treatment*

Treatment of tuberculous infection is determined by the stage of the disease. Latent infection is treated with one agent, usually isoniazid, for 9 months. The goal of treating tuberculosis is achievement of sterilization of the lesion in the shortest period. A 6-month regimen of isoniazid, rifampin, and pyrazinamide for the first 2 months and isoniazid and rifampin for the remaining 4 months is recommended for treatment of drug-susceptible disease.

Chemotherapy should be initiated as soon as possible in patients with probable tuberculous meningitis. A four-drug regimen with isoniazid, rifampin, pyrazinamide, and ethambutol should be started for the initial 2 months [7]. Isoniazid and rifampin, as well as the aminoglycosides, capreomycin, and the fluoroquinolones are available in parenteral forms for patients who cannot take oral medications.

After 2 months, if the infection strain is susceptible, therapy can be continued with isoniazid and rifampin for an additional 7 to 10 months, although optimal duration is not defined and some experts treat for up to 2 years.

A number of investigators have examined the role of adjunctive corticosteroid therapy in tuberculous meningitis [8,9]. Six of eight controlled trials noted benefit on the basis of limited data. Corticosteroid therapy with dexamethasone is recommended [7]. In children, the initial dose is 8 mg/d for children less than 25 kg and 12 mg/d for children greater than 25 kg and for adults. This dose is administered for 3 weeks and then tapered over 3 weeks.

Careful attention to supportive care is paramount. Many patients have inappropriate secretion of antidiuretic hormone and need careful monitoring of fluids and electrolytes (especially hyponatremia). Repeated lumbar punctures may be necessary to monitor CSF findings. Surgical intervention may be necessary to decompress the ventricles in patients with hydrocephalus.

In patients with tuberculomas, surgical removal is not necessary because most resolve with medical management and removal has been associated with severe fatal meningitis. Corticosteroids may be helpful adjuncts. Treatment for spinal arachnoiditis has not been studied extensively: however, similar regimens as for tuberculous meningitis may be used.

## *Prognosis*

Even with prompt treatment, neurological sequelae are common in tuberculous meningitis, although prognosis is dependent on early recognition and treatment. Patients presenting in late stage II or stage III, with obtundation or coma, have the greatest risk of sequelae.

## *Prevention*

Prevention of tuberculous meningitis is closely aligned with campaigns to eliminate tuberculosis globally. Three meta-analyses have confirmed the efficacy of BCG vaccine in the prevention of serious forms of TB, particularly tuberculous meningitis [10–12].

## References

1. World Health Organization. Fact Sheet 104. Tuberculosis. WHO, Geneva, Switzerland 2002.
2. Auerbach O. Tuberculous meningitis: correlation of therapeutic results with the pathogenesis and pathologic changes. II. Pathologic changes in untreated and treated cases. *Am Rev Tuberc*. 1951; 64:419–429.
3. Kennedy DH, Fallon RJ. Tuberculous meningitis. *JAMA*. 1979; 241:264–268.
4. Harder E, Al-Kawi MZ, Carney P. Intracranial tuberculoma: conservative management. *Am J Med*. 1983; 74:570–576.
5. al-Deeb SM, Yaqub BA, Sharif HS, Motaery KR. Neurotuberculosis: a review. *Clin Neurol Neurosurg*. 1992; 94 Suppl:S30–33.
6. Mazurek GH, Jereb J, Lobue P, et al. Division of Tuberculosis Elimination, National Center for HIV, STD, and TB Prevention, Centers for Disease Control and Prevention (CDC). Guidelines for using QuantiFERON®-TB Gold test for detecting *Mycobacterium tuberculosis* infection, United States. *MMWR*. 2005; 54 (RR-15):49–55.
7. Blumberg HM, Burman WJ, Chaisson RE, et al. American Thoracic Society/Centers for Disease Control and Prevention/Infectious Diseases Society of America: treatment of tuberculosis. *Am J Respir Crit Care Med*. 2003; 167:603–662.
8. Dooley DP, Carpenter JL, Rademacher S. Adjunctive corticosteroid therapy for tuberculosis: a critical reappraisal of the literature. *Clin Infect Dis*. 1997; 25:872–887.
9. Girgis NI, Farid Z, Kilpatrick ME, Sultan Y, Mikhail IA. Dexamethasone adjunctive treatment for tuberculous meningitis. *Pediatr Infect Dis J*. 1991; 10:179–183.
10. Colditz GA, Brewer TF, Berkey CS, et al. Efficacy of BCG vaccine in the prevention of tuberculosis. Meta-analysis of the published literature. *JAMA*. 1994; 271:698–702.
11. Rodrigues LC, Diwan VK, Wheeler JG. Protective effect of BCG against tuberculous meningitis and miliary tuberculosis: a meta-analysis. *Int J Epidemiol* 1993; 22:1154–1158.
12. Trunz BB, Fine P, Dye C. Effect of BCG vaccination on childhood tuberculous meningitis and miliary tuberculosis worldwide: a meta-analysis and assessment of cost-effectiveness. *Lancet*. 2006; 367:1173–1180.

# Chapter 25
# *Mycobacterium leprae*

**Barbara Stechenberg, M.D.**

## Mycobacterium Leprosy

### *Introduction*

Leprosy (Hansen disease) is a chronic infectious disease, known since the time of the Old Testament, that primarily involves the skin, upper respiratory tract, testes, eyes, and superficial segments of peripheral nerves.

### *Epidemiology*

The major mode of transmission seems to be contact by humans with some forms of untreated disease. A long period of exposure, such as with a household contact, is common; however, a large number of cases in endemic areas have no history of known exposure. A major source may be infected nasal secretions. In the United States, 90% of cases are imported. The highest prevalence of disease is found in tropical Africa, South America, and Southeast Asia, with India and Brazil leading the list of countries with endemic disease [1]. The discovery of naturally acquired leprosy-like disease in armadillos, chimpanzees, a mangabey monkey, and a macaque make consideration of leprosy as a zoonosis possible [2]. The incubation period is usually 2 to 5 years, but can range from one to many years.

### *Pathogenesis*

Leprosy is caused by *Mycobacterium leprae,* a Gram-positive, obligate intracellular, acid-fast bacillus (AFB). The bacillus grows very slowly, and grows best at 27°C to 33°C, which correlates with its predilection for cooler areas of the human body. It does not grow on artificial media.

L.L. Barton and N.R. Friedman (eds.), *The Neurological Manifestations of Pediatric Infectious Diseases and Immunodeficiency Syndromes.*

*M. leprae* causes disease by its ability to survive and multiply in macrophages. This survival depends on the immune response of the patient. The clinical syndromes of leprosy represent a spectrum that reflects the cellular immune response to the organism and the unique tropism for peripheral nerves. The role of immunologic processes in the nerve damage of leprosy remains undefined. It has been suggested that antineural antibodies may develop, especially in lepromatous disease, and may be related to the damage [3]. Tumor necrosis factor, TNF-α, has been associated with macrophage infiltration of peripheral nerves, during reversal reactions [4].

## *Clinical and Neurological Manifestations*

The two poles of the clinical spectrum are the tuberculoid and lepromatous forms.

Tuberculoid leprosy is characterized by a single or few well-demarcated, hypopigmented or erythematous anesthetic macules or plaques, often with raised borders and central clearing. The lesions can arise de novo or from indeterminate macules. Lesions vary greatly in size. Sensory loss with impaired sweating and eventual hair loss is common. Peripheral nerve involvement occurs; cutaneous nerves can often be palpated adjacent to or within lesions. Nerves become enlarged and tender. Cell-mediated immune responses are intact.

Borderline leprosy (dimorphous) has features of both tuberculoid and lepromatous disease and represents a continuous spectrum between the two. It is often subdivided into borderline-tuberculoid, borderline, and borderline-lepromatous leprosy. In borderline-tuberculoid leprosy, the lesions are more numerous and less well defined than in tuberculoid leprosy. In borderline-lepromatous leprosy, widespread nodular infiltration or plaques may occur. Damage to nerves and resultant deformities develop early and are often widespread. The disease is unstable and can change character from borderline-tuberculoid to borderline-lepromatous and back.

In lepromatous leprosy, bacilli multiply freely and disease disseminates widely with numerous, ill-defined, hypopigmented or erythematous macules that progress to papules and nodules. Hypoesthesia is late occurring. Dermal infiltration of the face, hands, and feet may be dramatic. Specific cell-mediated immunity is diminished.

Indeterminate is an early form of leprosy that is typified by hypopigmented macules without distinct edges or hypoesthesia. It is often overlooked but may develop into any of the other forms.

Serious consequences of leprosy result from immune reactions and nerve damage, with resultant anesthesia. This can lead to repeated unrecognized trauma, ulcerations, fractures, and bone reaction. This is particularly a problem in borderline cases, in which the disease tends to be relatively unstable immunologically. A reversal or type I reaction may occur; this is a delayed hypersensitivity reaction often associated with additional motor and sensory loss if not treated promptly. Cutaneous lesions become erythematous and edematous, frequently associated with neuritis and ulceration. Erythema nodosum leprosum may develop after a few months of therapy in patients with lepromatous leprosy. It resembles the Arthus reaction, with the development of tender, erythematous subcutaneous nodules.

Ocular manifestations are varied. Neuropathy of cranial nerves V and VII can result in lid abnormalities and corneal hypoesthesia, resulting in exposure keratopathy. Uveitis is seen in 7% of patients [5]. Acute anterior iridocyclitis is uncommon, developing during therapy or at cessation of therapy. A chronic, low-grade uveitis, with minimal or no symptoms until late in the disease, is more common. If not aggressively treated, it may result in pinpoint pupils, glaucoma, iris atrophy, cataracts, and ciliary body damage. Iris pearls, which are white to yellow clusters on the anterior surface of the iris, are pathognomonic of leprosy.

## *Neuropathology*

The neuropathology varies with the immune response of the patient, which determines the clinical presentation. Patients with tuberculoid leprosy have a high level of cell-mediated immunity to the organism and this is reflected in the exuberant cellular reaction with granuloma formation. Damage to nerves is a distinctive feature. In early disease, Schwann cells are increased in number and nerves are invaded by mononuclear cells; this process progresses to total destruction of cutaneous nerves in advanced disease. Typical tuberculoid infiltrates may replace entire nerve trunks. In borderline leprosy, pathology is variable; nerves are usually less damaged and more recognizable than in tuberculoid leprosy. Lepromatous leprosy is associated with anergy to *M. leprae*. Bacilli-laden macrophages (Virchow cells) are the predominant cells. They become vacuolated as they age and often hold large numbers of organisms. Large nerve trunks may show typical infiltration by these cells. Mild inflammation is seen in indeterminate leprosy.

## *Diagnosis*

The cardinal signs of leprosy are hypoesthetic lesions of the skin with associated enlargement of peripheral nerves. Careful history of exposure or travel to endemic areas, as well as adoption from endemic areas, is important. Physical examination should evaluate for sensory changes, damage to hands and feet, abnormal sweating, and tenderness and/or enlargement of nerves. Obtaining and examining smears for AFB or the use of other diagnostic modalities, including enzyme-linked immunosorbent assays for the measurement of antibodies, as well as DNA probes and polymerase chain reaction examination of tissue specimens, should be performed in consultation with the National Hansen's Disease Program (Baton Rouge, LA; 800-642-2477; www.bphc.hrsa.gov/nhdp).

## *Treatment*

Therapy for patients with leprosy should be undertaken with consultation with the national program. Multidrug therapy is necessary for all patients. Dapsone, rifampin, and clofazimine are often used. Prompt corticosteroid therapy is necessary to prevent complications if a reversal reaction is present.

With specific chemotherapy and control of reactions, prognosis is good in nearly all patients. Started early, therapy can prevent mutilation and deformity. However, after chemotherapy, some patients continue to suffer significant neuritis and loss of peripheral nerve function. Patients have to recognize limb insensitivity to avoid trauma, ulcerations, and infections. Appropriate monitoring and rehabilitation, such as physical therapy or surgery may also be necessary.

## *Prevention*

Prevention of leprosy depends on prompt therapy for identified patients and surveillance of contacts to detect early leprosy. Chemoprophylaxis is not recommended for contacts. Bacillus Calmette Guérin (BCG) vaccination seems to have a protective effect against the disease. A single dose seems to be 50% protective, and two doses increase protection further [6,7]. The World Health Organization does not recommend BCG for prevention of leprosy at this time. It may be used in certain high-risk situations.

## References

1. WHO, Leprosy Fact Sheet 101, January 2003.
2. Meyers WM, Gormus BJ, Walsh GP. Nonhuman sources of leprosy. *Int J Lepr.* 1992; 60:477–481.
3. Park JY, Cho SN, Youn JK, et al. Detection of antibodies to human nerve antigens in sera from leprosy patients by ELISA. *Clin Exp Immunol.* 1992; 87:368–372.
4. Khanolkar-Young S, Rayment N, Brickell PM, et al. Tumour necrosis factor-alpha (TNF-alpha) synthesis is associated with the skin and peripheral nerve pathology of leprosy reversal reactions. *Clin Exp Immunol.* 1995; 99:196–202.
5. Dana MR, Hochman MA, Viana MA, Hill CH, Sugar J. Ocular manifestations of leprosy in a noninstitutionalized community in the United States. *Arch Ophthalmol.* 1994; 112:626–629.
6. Bertolli J, Pangi C, Frerichs R, Halloran ME. A case-control study of the effectiveness of BCG vaccine for preventing leprosy in Yangon, Myanmar. *Int J Epidemiol.* 1997; 26:888–896.
7. Randomised controlled trial of single BCG, repeated BCG, or combined BCG and killed *Mycobacterium leprae* vaccine for the prevention of leprosy and tuberculosis in Malawi. Karonga Prevention Trial Group. *Lancet* 1996; 348:17–24.

# Section III
# Rickettsia and Spirochetes

# Chapter 26
# *Rickettsia rickettsii*

**Abeer Khayat M.D. and Mobeen H. Rathore, M.D., C.P.E., F.A.A.P.**

## Rocky Mountain Spotted Fever

### *Introduction*

Rocky Mountain spotted fever (RMSF) is the most common and one of the most virulent rickettsial illnesses in the United States [1,2]. The disease begins with an abrupt onset of fever, headache, and generalized myalgia followed by rash. Because of its diverse clinical features, RMSF can be exceptionally difficult to diagnose in its early stages, and, without prompt and appropriate treatment, can be fatal [2].

### *Epidemiology*

RMSF occurs throughout the Western Hemisphere. In the United States, RMSF has been reported in almost every state with more than half (56%) of reported cases from only five states: North Carolina, South Carolina, Tennessee, Oklahoma, and Arkansas [3]. Approximately 250 to 1,200 cases are reported annually, with two thirds in children younger than 15 years of age; the peak age is between 5 and 9 years of age [2,3]. Most reported cases are in white males and more than 90% occur from April through September, mirroring the period with increased numbers of *Dermacentor* ticks [2,4,5]. However, a history of a tick bite may be absent in 30 to 40% of patients with RMSF [4,6].

### *Pathogenesis*

*Rickettsia rickettsii*, the etiologic agent of RMSF, is a small, weakly Gram-negative, obligate intracellular coccobacillus, transmitted to humans by an Ixodid tick [4,7]. The vectors for *R. ricketsii* include several Ioxidid ticks; *Dermacentor variabilis*

L.L. Barton and N.R. Friedman (eds.), *The Neurological Manifestations of Pediatric Infectious Diseases and Immunodeficiency Syndromes.*

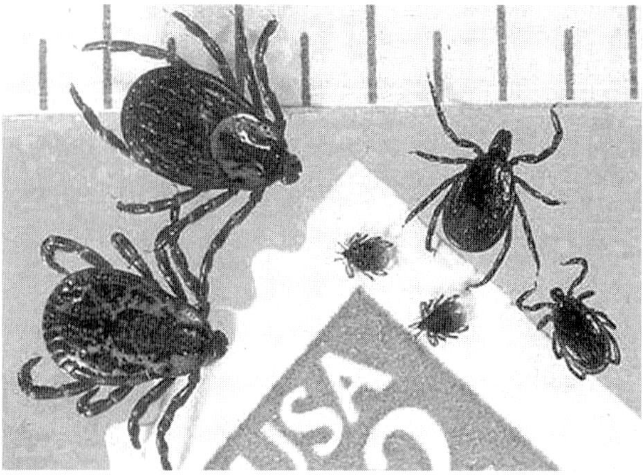


**Fig. 26.1** To the right of the postage stamp are two black-legged ticks (*Ixodes scapularis*). The two small specimens on the stamp itself are nymphal black-legged ticks. The two ticks to the left are American dog ticks (*Dermacentor variablis*). Photo by Jim Occi.

(dog tick) is the main vector in the eastern United States and *Dermacentor andersoni* (wood tick) is the primary vector in the western United States and Canada (Fig. 26.1) [4]. In 2005, the brown dog tick (*Rhipicephalus sanguineus*), a vector of RMSF in Mexico, was implicated as a vector of this disease in a confined geographic area in Arizona [8]. The tick must be attached to the host for at least 6 to 10 hours before it is able to transmit the organism [5].

RMSF is characterized by a vasculitis, which can occur in virtually all organs and leads to cutaneous vasculitis, interstitial pneumonitis, hepatic portal triaditis, interstitial nephritis, interstitial myocarditis, and meningoencephalitis [9].

## Clinical Manifestations

After an incubation period of 2 to14 days, patients develop an abrupt onset of fever, myalgias, headache, and weakness. Rash develops in 80 to 90% of cases, and is considered the hallmark of RMSF. In most patients, rash appears by the second or third day and begins as a maculopapular exanthem that evolves into a petechial or purpuric rash in half of the cases. It appears first on the wrists and ankles and spreads centripetally. Palms and soles are usually involved [1,4,7]. Ten percent of patients with RMSF do not have a rash (Rocky Mountain spotless fever). Many children experience initial gastrointestinal complaints including nausea, vomiting, and abdominal pain [6,10]. Hepatosplenomegaly and liver dysfunction with jaundice as well as shock and multiple organ failure may ensue [6,11].

## *Neurological Manifestations*

RMSF often presents with central nervous system (CNS) symptoms (Table 26.1) [12]. Almost 60% of children with RMSF have CNS involvement [13]. Neurological manifestations are attributed to the effect of vasculitis on tissue. Of the less serious neurological symptoms, headache is the most common [6,9,10]. The headache is frontal and severe, and unresponsive to analgesics [9–11]. Patients with RMSF may be restless, irritable, and photophobic, and may complain of insomnia. The neurological examination generally lacks focality, although a variety of findings have been reported, including hyperreflexia, Babinski sign, cranial nerve palsies (especially the sixth nerve), aphasia, dysphagia, deafness, severe vertigo, neurogenic bladder, complete paralysis, and ataxia [9–11]. Alteration of the sensorium, ranging from lethargy to coma, with evidence of encephalitis, is seen in approximately 25% of patients with RMSF [9–11]. Focal motor and generalized tonic–clonic seizures can occur occasionally in the acute phase of the illness, but in the absence of coma, seizures are not considered a significant prognostic indicator of long-term neurological sequelae. The Guillain-Barré syndrome and acute disseminated encephalomyelitis (ADEM) have also been associated with RMSF [14,15].

Most patients who survive RMSF with neurological involvement regain all or almost all neurological function [12]. Major neurological long-term sequelae, such as seizures, ataxia, peripheral neuropathy, paraplegia, and urinary and fecal incontinence are unusual in pediatric patients after RMSF [9]. However, children with severely impaired consciousness and coma during the acute phase of the disease are at risk for persistent neurological sequelae [13,16]. Behavioral and personality disturbances occur most frequently and may present as emotional liability, hyperactivity, memory loss, and depression [12,16]. These children are also at risk for intellectual deterioration, which may manifest as a learning disability. Any patient with an abnormal neurological examination during the course of the acute illness should be followed closely until residual signs and symptoms resolve completely or remain stable. Children with severely impaired states of consciousness during the acute phase of RMSF should undergo

**Table 26.1** The most common neurological manifestations of RMSF in children (approximate percentage)

| Neurological manifestation | Percentage |
|---|---|
| Headache | 91% |
| Nausea/vomiting | 60% |
| Agitation/stupor | 17% |
| Coma | 9% |
| Meningismus | 18% |
| Seizures | 8% |
| Hearing deficit | 3% |

Adapted from reference 6.

psychological testing to exclude any behavioral problems or/and learning disabilities [17]. Patients with suspected hearing deficit should have baseline audiometric examinations and serial examinations if abnormalities are found [17].

## Neuropathology

The pathologic hallmark of RMSF is a vasculitis with a monocellular cell infiltrate around blood vessels. *R. rickettsii* can infect several different cell types, preferentially the endothelia of small arteries, veins, and capillaries of all major tissues and organs. *R. rickettsii* proliferate in the cytosol and the nucleus of the infected cells, and spread centripetally from cell to cell. Endothelial damage leads to increased vascular permeability, formation of microthrombi, recruitment of mononuclear inflammatory cells, and, occasionally, luminal destruction and microinfarctions [5,9,18].

The pathologic findings of RMSF in the CNS are similar to those seen in other organ systems. Gross inspection of the brain at necropsy shows variable degrees of cerebral and meningeal edema; punctuate hemorrhages are often seen. Focal lesions are usually present in patients dying after the 10th day of illness [12]. Microscopically, these lesions are of three general types: perivascular inflammation, arteriolar thrombonecrosis with microinfarcts that are mainly seen in the white matter, and glial nodules that consist of accumulations of macrophages and lymphocytes in the brain parenchyma [10,12,19].

## Diagnosis

The diagnosis of RMSF is initially based on clinical findings and epidemiologic clues. Confirmation of the diagnosis is made serologically and by immunostaining of skin biopsies [5,7,20]. The recommended serologic test is the indirect immunofluorescence antibody test (IFA). This test is widely available, has a sensitivity of greater than 90%, and detects IgM and IgG antibodies. Antibodies generally appear 10 to 14 days after infection [3,7]. A probable diagnosis can be established by a single convalescent serum titer of 1:64 or greater by IFA. Testing of acute- and convalescent-phase sera is recommended to demonstrate a fourfold or greater rise in titer. Limitations of the IFA test include the retrospective confirmation of the diagnosis, and cross-reaction of *R. rickettsii* and other members of the spotted fever group, unless cross-absorption with selected antigens is performed. The diagnosis of RMSF may also be achieved by the demonstration of rickettsia in the endothelial cells of blood vessels in skin biopsies by immunofluorescent microscopy. This method has a sensitivity of 70% and specificity of 100% [5,20]. Polymerase chain reaction (PCR) can be used for detection of rickettsial DNA in whole blood or biopsy specimens; this test demonstrates a varying level of sensitivity and is available only in research laboratories [1,3,5,20]. Other diagnostic tests (including enzyme immunoassays,

Western blot, and cultures) that can be used to confirm *R. rickettsii* infection are also not widely available.

Results of routine laboratory tests reveal normal, low, or elevated total white blood count with a left shift, thrombocytopenia, persistent hyponatremia, and elevated liver enzymes with hyperbilirubinemia [1,9].

The cerebrospinal fluid (CSF) in RMSF may be normal, but, more commonly, there is a mild pleocytosis with either lymphocytic or polymorphonuclear predominance and a modest increase in protein levels [3,4,9]. Imaging studies may reveal evidence of infarcts, edema, meningeal enhancement, and prominent perivascular spaces. After treatment, resolution of symptoms occurs in most patients who had normal imaging findings and only in two thirds of those who had abnormal imaging findings [21].

### Differential Diagnosis

Diseases to consider in the differential diagnosis of a patient with fever, headache, and/or a petechial rash include meningococcemia, thrombotic thrombocytopenic purpura, immune complex vasculitis, ehrlichiosis, leptospirosis, infectious mononucleosis, and bacterial sepsis [5].

## *Treatment*

RMSF is a life-threatening disease; appropriate antimicrobial therapy must be started immediately on the basis of clinical and epidemiologic suspicion and should never be delayed pending laboratory confirmation. Optimal outcome is achieved when treatment is initiated within the first 5 days of symptoms [5,10,22,23]. Untreated RMSF will slowly progress to multisystem involvement, with pulmonary hemorrhage, encephalitis, severe thrombocytopenia, acute renal failure, hypovolemic shock, and death. Doxycycline is the preferred agent for the treatment of RMSF in adults and children of any age [23–26]. The duration of therapy is generally 7 to 10 days, and should be continued for at least 2 to 3 days after the patient becomes afebrile. Chloramphenicol or a fluoroquinolone are acceptable alternatives when tetracyclines are contraindicated (e.g., pregnancy, hypersensitivity) [23]. However, chloramphenicol is associated with potentially serious side effects and requires monitoring of blood indices; it is no longer available in the oral form in the United States. Epidemiologic studies in which the Centers for Disease Control and Prevention (CDC) case report data have been used have suggested that patients with RMSF treated with chloramphenicol have a higher risk of dying than those who received a tetracycline [26].

All patients with neurological symptoms, elevated creatinine, vomiting, or unstable vital signs should be admitted to the hospital if RMSF is suspected. Supportive care and fluid maintenance should be provided as indicated. Glucocorticoids have been administered to severely ill patients without proof of efficacy, and are not recommended. When meningococcemia is also a diagnostic consideration, initial therapy should include both ceftriaxone and doxycycline to provide coverage for both organisms [5].

The case–fatality rate for RMSF is 2 to 3% for patients aged younger than 10 years with RMSF and is 3 to 5% for all age groups [7,17,22]. Avoidance of tick-infested areas is the best preventive measure. Protective clothing and insect repellents may provide protection when entering tick-infested areas. There is no role for prophylactic antimicrobial agents in preventing RMSF. No licensed *R. rickettsii* vaccine is available in the United States [23].

## References

1. Bennett NJ, Domachowske J, Abuhammour W, Salman R. Rocky Mountain Spotted Fever. In: Romero JR, Windle ML, Lutwick LI, Tolan RW Jr, Steele R, eds. eMedicine Specialties. *Pediatrics*. Infectious Diseases. Available at: http://www.emedicine.com/ped/topic2709.htm.
2. Centers for Disease Control and Prevention. National Center for Infectious Diseases. Division of Viral and Rickettsial Diseases. Viral and Rickettsial Zoonoses Branch. Rocky Mountain spotted fever. Available at: http://www.cdc.gov/ncidod/dvrd/rmsf.
3. Chapman AS, Bakken JS, Folk SM, et al. Diagnosis and management of tickborne rickettsial diseases: Rocky Mountain spotted fever, ehrlichiosis, and anaplasmosis—United States: a practical guide for physicians and other healthcare and public health professionals. *MMWR* 2006; 55(RR-4):1–27.
4. Sexton DJ, Kaye KS. Rocky Mountain spotted fever. *Med Clin N Am* 2002; 86:351–360, vii–viii.
5. Thorner AR, Walker DH, Petri WA Jr. Rocky mountain spotted fever. *Clin Infect Dis*. 1998; 27:1353–1359.
6. Helmick CG, Bernard KW, D'Angelo LJ. Rocky Mountain spotted fever: clinical, laboratory, and epidemiological features of 262 cases. *J Infect Dis*. 1984; 150:480–488.
7. Gayle A, Ringdahl E. Tick-borne diseases. *Am Fam Physician*. 2001; 64:461–466.
8. Demma LJ, Traeger MS, Nicholson WL, et al. Rocky Mountain spotted fever from an unexpected tick vector in Arizona. *N Engl J Med*. 2005; 353:587–594.
9. Kirk JL, Fine DP, Sexton DJ, Muchmore HG. Rocky Mountain spotted fever. A clinical review based on 48 confirmed cases, 1943-1986. *Medicine (Baltimore)*. 1990; 69:35–45.
10. Miller JQ, Price TR. The nervous system in Rocky Mountain spotted fever. *Neurology*. 1972; 22:561–566.
11. Roos KL. Nonviral Infections. In: Goetz CG, Pappert EJ, eds. *Textbook of Clinical Neurology* 2nd ed. Philadelphia, PA: W. B. Saunders Company; 2003; 935–936.
12. Horney LF, Walker DH. Meningoencephalitis as a major manifestation of Rocky Mountain spotted fever. *South Med J*. 1988; 81:915–918.
13. Massey EW, Thames T, Coffey CE, Gallis HA. Neurologic complications of Rocky Mountain spotted fever. *South Med J* 1985; 78:1288–1290, 1303.
14. Toerner JG, Kumar PN, Garagusi VF. Guillain-Barré syndrome associated with Rocky Mountain spotted fever: case report and review. *Clin Infect Dis*. 1996; 22:1090–1091.
15. Wei TY, Baumann RJ. Acute disseminated encephalomyelitis after Rocky Mountain spotted fever. *Pediatr Neurol*. 1999; 21:503–505.
16. Gorman RJ, Saxon S, Snead OC 3rd. Neurologic sequelae of Rocky Mountain spotted fever. *Pediatrics*. 1981; 67:354–357.
17. Archibald L, Sexton D. Long-term sequelae of Rocky Mountain spotted fever. *Clin Infect Dis*. 1995; 20:1122–1125.

18. Walker DH, Mattern WD. Rickettsial vasculitis. *Am Heart J*. 1980; 100:896–960.
19. McAdam AJ, Sharpe AH. Infectious Diseases. In: Cotran R, Collins T, Kumar V, eds. *Robbins Pathologic Basis of Disease*. 7th ed. Philadelphia, PA: W.B. Saunders Company; 2005: 395–397.
20. Paddock CD, Childs JE. *Rickettsia rickettsii* (Rocky Mountain Spotted Fever). In: Long SS, Pickering LK, Prober CG. *Principles and Practice of Pediatric Infectious Diseases* 2003. 2nd ed. Philadelphia, PA: Churchill Livingstone; 2003; 942–945.
21. Bonawitz C, Castillo M, Mukherji SK. Comparison of CT and MR Features with clinical outcome in patients with Rocky Mountain spotted fever. *AJNR Am J Neuroradiol*. 1997; 18:459–456.
22. Kirkland KB, Wilkinson WE, Sexton DJ. Therapeutic delay and mortality in cases of Rocky Mountain spotted fever. *Clin Infect Dis*. 1995; 20:1118–1121.
23. American Academy of Pediatrics. Rocky Mountain Spotted Fever. In: Pickering LK, Baker CJ, Long SS, McMillan JA, eds. *Red Book: Report of the Committee on Infectious Diseases*. 27th ed. American Academy of Pediatrics. Elk Grove Village, IL: American Academy of Pediatrics. 2006; 570–572.
24. Purvis JJ, Edwards MS. Doxycycline use for rickettsial disease in pediatric patients. *Pediatr Infect Dis J*. 2000; 19:871–874.
25. Cale DF, McCarthy MW. Treatment of Rocky Mountain spotted fever in children. *Ann Pharmacother*. 1997; 31:492–494.
26. Holman RC, Paddock CD, Curns AT, Krebs JW, McQuiston JH, Childs JE. Analysis of risk factors for fatal Rocky Mountain spotted fever: evidence for superiority of tetracyclines for therapy. *J Infect Dis*. 2001; 184:1437–1444.

# Chapter 27
# *Ehrlichia* and *Anaplasma* Species

**Abeer Khayat, M.D. and Mobeen H. Rathore, M.D., C.P.E., F.A.A.P.**

## Ehrlichiosis and Anaplasmosis

### *Introduction*

The ehrlichioses are infections of white blood cells that affect various mammals [1]. Human ehrlichioses represent a group of clinically similar, yet epidemiologically and etiologically diverse, illnesses [2,3]. Two main types of human ehrlichiosis have been identified in the United States: human monocytotropic ehrlichiosis (HME), and human granulocytotropic anaplasmosis (HGA), formerly known as human granulocytotropic ehrlichiosis (HGE) [1,2].

### *Epidemiology*

#### Human Monocytotropic Ehrlichiosis

Human ehrlichiosis caused by *Ehrlichia chaffeensis* was first described in 1987 [4,5]. The disease occurs primarily in the southeastern and south central regions of the United States [1,6–8]. Serologic evidence of *E. chaffeensis* infection has been reported in Africa, South America, Mexico, Russia, and Asia; however, the majority of cases are recognized in the United States [9]. HME is primarily transmitted by *Amblyomma americanum* (the lone star tick) [1,2,6,10,11], and possibly *Dermacentor variabilis* (the dog tick) [2,10,11]. Most cases are rural or suburban, and most patients have a history of tick bite or tick exposure [4,12]. Similar to other tick-borne diseases, most HME cases occur sporadically; however, clusters of cases have been reported [6]. HME is seasonal, with most cases occurring between April and September [4,8,10]. More than 75% of HME patients are male [1,2,11,12]. Unlike Rocky Mountain spotted fever, in which most reported cases are in children, most reported HME cases are in adults [2].

L.L. Barton and N.R. Friedman (eds.), *The Neurological Manifestations of Pediatric Infectious Diseases and Immunodeficiency Syndromes.*

**Human Granulocytotropic Anaplasmosis**

HGA represents the second recognized ehrlichial infection of humans in the United States, and was first described in 1994 [6]. The causative agents are *Anaplasma phagocytophilum* (which include organisms formerly called the "HGE agent" and "*E. equi*") and *E. ewingii* that is responsible for ewingii ehrlichiosis [6]. The vector responsible for its transmission in the eastern and midwestern United States is *Ixodes scapularis* [1,2,6,10,11]. In California, *I. pacificus* has been implicated as a vector, and *I. ricinus* is the vector in Europe [1,9,11]. Most cases of HGA occur in southern New England, the upper Midwestern states, and the mid-Atlantic states, mainly in rural areas and suburban settings [6]. HGA, similar to HME, occurs in male patients more frequently than female patients (3:1 ratio) [1,2,9]. As with most tick-borne diseases, the highest incidence of HGA occurs during the peak months of human exposure to ticks, from April to September [9,10]. Simultaneous infection with other tick-borne diseases, such as Lyme disease and babesiosis, has been reported [6,13].

## *Pathogenesis*

Ehrlichiosis is caused by obligate intracellular bacteria, which were largely ignored as important human pathogens until 1987 [6,9]. The taxonomy of the bacteria that cause ehrlichiosis recently has been revised, based on genetic sequences of the 16S rRNA gene [7]. Thus, under the new classification, the five human pathogens described to date have been reassigned into three genera within the family Rickettsiaceae [6]. The organism of most importance in the first genogroup, *Anaplasma*, is *A. phagocytophilum*, the cause of HGA in humans [5,6]. The second genogroup, *Ehrlichia*, contains *E. chaffeensis*, which causes HME in humans; *E. ewingii,* which invades granulocytes; and *E. canis,* which causes ehrlichiosis in dogs [5,6]. Another genogroup, *Neorickettsia*, includes *E. sennetsu*, the cause of sennetsu fever in Japan [5,6].

The main target cells of HME and HGA are mononuclear phagocytes and neutrophils, respectively [6,14]. Ehrlichial organisms are seen as intracytoplasmic, basophilic inclusions (called morulae) [1,6]. Ehrlichia infections are characterized by a lack of severe inflammatory response, pyogenic reaction, and tissue necrosis [4,14]. However, a response in the lymphoreticular system affecting the liver, lungs, lymph nodes, and spleen is seen in infections with *Ehrlichia* species [4,6]. Perivascular lymphohistiocytic infiltrates may be observed in many organs, including the central nervous system (CNS) in HME [6]. Hemorrhage may occur and is most likely related to the severe thrombocytopenia that may be present [6].

## *Clinical Manifestations*

The human ehrlichioses have a wide clinical spectrum, ranging from inapparent infection to severe life-threatening disease [7,8,15]. The incubation period is 1 to

21 days [8]. Children with HME usually present with nonspecific symptoms, such as fever, chills, headache, myalgia, and anorexia or nausea [4,9,12,15–17]. Rash, more common in children than in adults, may be macular, maculopapular, vesicular, or petechial, and the usual distribution is on the trunk and extremities [4,9,15,16]. Gastrointestinal symptoms, including abdominal pain and tenderness, vomiting, and diarrhea, are common [18]. Pulmonary manifestations, including pleural effusion and pulmonary edema, have been reported [4,9]. The prognosis of ehrlichiosis is excellent. The illness is occasionally prolonged and rarely fatal [9].

## *Neurological Manifestations*

CNS involvement is relatively common in patients with HME and less frequent in patients with HGA [17,20]. Headache, nuchal rigidity, photophobia, lethargy, confusion, and delirium are common in children with HME [4,6,9,17]. Meningitis and meningoencephalitis have been described, with a cerebrospinal fluid (CSF) profile suggesting aseptic meningitis [6,7,9,17,19]. Other reported neurological manifestations include ataxia, vertigo, hyperreflexia, and coma [4,6]. Seizures are unusual [9].

Long-term neurological sequelae in children after HME have been reported, including decrease in cognitive and neurological performance, which manifest as speech impairment, and decreased reading, writing, and fine motor skills [9,12].

## *Diagnosis*

The diagnosis of HME and HGA is clinical and is confirmed serologically [8]. The most widely available antibody test is the indirect immunofluorescence assay (IFA). IFA can be used to detect IgG or IgM antibodies in a patient's serum or plasma that are reactive with *E. chaffeensis* or *E. phagocytophila* antigens. Confirmation of the diagnosis of ehrlichiosis can be made in a person with a compatible illness and a fourfold change in antibody titer between acute- and convalescent-phase samples [6,11,12,21]. Other available serological assays, which include enzyme-linked immunosorbent assay (ELISA) and immunoblotting, are only available in research laboratories. Polymerase chain reaction (PCR) is a valuable adjunct in the diagnosis of HME and HGE, especially during the acute phase of the disease, and has been shown to be rapid, sensitive, and specific; however, PCR testing is not widely available [7,11]. Identification of intraleukocytic morulae in blood smears, CSF sediment, or bone marrow aspirates has the advantages of being specific, rapid, and simple to perform, but the sensitivity of this test is low [7,11,14,19,20].CSF examination in children with HME often shows lymphocytic pleocytosis, elevated protein, and, less frequently, borderline low CSF glucose concentrations [17,20]. In both forms of human ehrlichiosis, a high percentage of patients develop leukopenia, thrombocytopenia, elevated hepatic transaminases, and, less frequently, anemia

[4,7,9,13,14,16,22,23]. The differential diagnosis of the ehrlichioses includes Rocky Mountain spotted fever, meningococcemia, and viral syndromes such as those caused by enteroviruses, Epstein-Barr virus, and cytomegalovirus.

## *Treatment*

Doxycycline is the drug of choice for treatment of human ehrlichiosis in children of any age [9,15]. The recommended dose of doxycycline is 4 mg/kg per day, every 12 hours intravenously or orally (maximum, 100 mg/dose) [11,15]. Initiation of therapy early in the course of illness helps minimize complications [11]. Current data recommend continuation of treatment until the patient has been afebrile for at least 3 days and for a minimum total course of 5 to 10 days. Severe or complicated disease may require longer treatment courses [11].

Treatment of neurological manifestations is supportive, directed at managing the headache, encephalopathy, and seizures, when they occur.

## References

1. Bennett NJ, Domachowske J, Abuhammour W: Ehrlichiosis. Editors: Nissen MD, Windle ML, Domachowske J, Tolan RW, Steele RW. *emedicine* 2006. *www.emedicine.com/.*
2. Cunha B: Ehrlichiosis. Editors: Marrie TJ, Talavera F, Bronze MF, Mylonakis E, Zevits ME. *emedicine* 2006. *www.emedicine.com/.*
3. Byrd RP,Jr, Roy TM, Faul JL, Ruoss SJ. Ehrlichiosis in the United States. *Chest.* 2000; 117:1524–1525.
4. Standaert SM, Yu T, Scott MA, et al. Primary isolation of *Ehrlichia chaffeensis* from patients with febrile illnesses: clinical and molecular characteristics. *J Infect Dis.* 2000; 181:1082–1088.
5. Rathore MH. Infection due to *Ehrlichia canis* in children. *South Med J.* 1992; 85:703–705.
6. Lantos P, Krause P. Ehrlichiosis in children. *Semin Pediatr Infect Dis.* 2002; 13:249–256.
7. Paddock CD, Childs JE. *Ehrlichia chaffeensis*: a prototypical emerging pathogen. *Clin Microbiol Rev.* 2003; 16:37–64.
8. Jacobs R. Human monocytis ehrlichiosis: similar to Rocky Mountain Spotted Fever but different. *Pediatric Ann.* 2002; 31:180–4.
9. Fritz CL, Glaser CA. Ehrlichiosis. *Infect Dis Clin North Am.* 1998; 12:123–136.
10. Nochimson G. Tick-Borne Diseases, Ehrlichiosis. Editors: Keim SM, Talavera F, Hirshon JM, Halamka J, Pollack CV. *eMedicine* 2006. *www.emedicine.com/.*
11. *Ehrlichia* and *Anaplasma* Infections. *Red Book. Report of the Committee on Infectious Diseases.* 27th edition. American Academy of Pediatrics. Elk Grove Village, IL. 2006; 281–284.
12. Schutze GE, Jacobs RF. Human monocytic ehrlichiosis in children. *Pediatrics.* 1997; 100(1): E10.
13. Barton LL, Dawson JE, Letson GW, Luisiri A, Scalzo A. Simultaneous ehrlichiosis and Lyme disease. *Pediatr Infect Dis J.* 1990; 9:127–129.
14. Dumler JS, Dawson JE, Walker DH. Human ehrlichiosis: hematopathology and immunohistologic detection of *Ehrlichia chaffeensis. Hum Pathol.* 1993; 24:391–396.
15. Dumler JS, Dey C, Meier F, Lewis LL. Human monocytic ehrlichiosis: a potentially severe disease in children. *Arch Pediatr Adolesc Med.* 2000; 154:847–849.

16. Tieman S. Residents Column: Spots and Stripes. *Pediatr Ann*. 2002; 31:207–208.
17. Ratnasamy N, Everett ED, Roland WE, McDonald G, Caldwell CW. Central nervous system manifestations of human ehrlichiosis. *Clin Infect Dis*. 1996; 23:314–319.
18. Gershel J. Experience and reason: human granulocytic ehrlichiosis presenting as abdominal pain. *Pediatrics*. 2000; 106:602–604.
19. Fordham LA, Chung CJ, Specter BB, Merten DF, Ingram DL. Ehrlichiosis: findings on chest radiographs in three pediatric patients. *AJR Am J Roentgenol*. 1998; 171:1421–1424.
20. Berry DS, Miller RS, Hooke JA, Massung RF, Bennett J, Ottolini MG. Ehrlichial meningitis with cerebrospinal fluid morulae. *Pediatr Infect Dis J*. 1999; 18:552–555.
21. Bakken JS, Krueth J, Wilson-Nordskog C, Tilden R, Asanovich K, Dumler JS. Clinical and laboratory characteristics of human granulocytic ehrlichiosis. *JAMA* 1996; 275:199–205.
22. Williams CV, Van Steenhouse JL, Bradley JM, Hancock SI, Hegarty BC, Breitschwerdt EB. Naturally occurring *Ehrlichia chaffeensis* infection in two prosimian primate species: ring-tailed lemurs (Lemur catta) and ruffed lemurs (Varecia variegata). *Emerg Infect Dis*. 2002; 8:1497–1500.
23. Barton LL, Rathore MH, Dawson JE. Infection with Ehrlichia in childhood. *J Pediatr*. 1992; 120:998–1001.

# Chapter 28
# *Borrelia burgdorferi*

**Abeer Khayat, M.D. and Mobeen H. Rathore, M.D., C.P.E., F.A.A.P.**

## Lyme Disease

### *Introduction*

Lyme disease was recognized in 1977 when arthritis was observed in a cluster of children in Lyme, Connecticut [1]. It is the most common vector-borne zoonosis in the United States. Although the disorder was initially described as a multisystem, rheumatologic illness, the nervous system is appreciated as a major target for the etiologic agent, *Borrelia burgdorferi* [2].

### *Epidemiology*

Lyme disease has a highly focal, worldwide distribution. It is acquired by the transmission *of B. burgdorferi* to humans through the bite of an infected tick of the *Ixodes* species. *Ixodes scapularis*, the deer tick, in the Northeast and Midwest, and *Ixodes pacificus*, in the far west, are the predominant tick vectors of Lyme disease in the United States [3,4]. Although most cases occur during the summer months, Lyme disease is seen throughout the year [3,5]. In the United States, approximately 20,000 cases per year have been reported to the Centers for Disease Control and Prevention (CDC) [6].

Although infection affects both sexes and all ages, the highest reported rates of Lyme disease occur in children 5 to 19 years of age (25% of reported cases) and in persons older than 30 years of age (45% of reported cases) [6,7].

The principal risk factors for Lyme disease are periresidential exposure to infected ticks by persons engaged in recreational or property maintenance activities, and outdoor occupations in endemic areas [8,9].

L.L. Barton and N.R. Friedman (eds.), *The Neurological Manifestations of Pediatric Infectious Diseases and Immunodeficiency Syndromes.*

## *Pathogenesis*

*B. burgdorferi* is a cylindrical, microaerophilic bacterium with a motile flagella and an outer membrane. There are three genospecies of *B. burgdorferi* that are known to cause disease in humans. *B. burgdorferi sensustricto* is the only known etiologic agent of human borreliosis in the United States [3,9]. *B. garinii* and *B. afzelii* are more dominant species in Europe, Eastern Russia, and Japan. Biological differences in these strains are responsible for differences in clinical manifestations of the disease [3–5]. Transmission of *B. burgdorferi* from an infected tick bite, usually during the nymph stage, requires prolonged duration of attachment (>48 hours). Once inoculated, *B. burgdorferi* spreads locally and subsequently systemically via blood vessels or lymphatics to other sites, including eyes, muscles, bones, central nervous system (CNS), synovial tissues, and heart [5].

## *Clinical Manifestations*

Lyme disease is generally categorized into three clinical stages punctuated by relatively silent periods. These stages are: early localized disease, early disseminated, and late-stage infection. The major clinical features of each stage are shown in Table 28.1 [6]. Approximately 20% of infections are thought to be asymptomatic [5,9].

Early localized disease presents with erythema migrans (EM), the pathognomonic clinical marker of Lyme disease, in approximately two thirds of children with

**Table 28.1** Clinical manifestations of Lyme disease in children

| Stage of disease | Clinical findings | |
|---|---|---|
| Early localized disease (3–30 days) | Skin | Erythema migrans (single) |
| | Constitutional symptoms | Fever, fatigue, myalgia, arthralgia, headache |
| | Lymphadenopathy | Regional |
| Early disseminated disease (3–10 weeks) | Skin | Erythema migrans (multiple) |
| | Nervous system | Headaches |
| | | Cranial neuropathies |
| | | Meningitis |
| | | Radiculoneuritis |
| | Cardiac | Carditis (heart block) |
| | Constitutional symptoms | Fever, fatigue, myalgia, arthralgia, headache |
| | Lymphadenopathy | Generalized |
| Late disseminated disease (2–12 months) | Musculoskeletal | Arthritis (monoarticular or pauciarticular) |

Adapted from reference 6.

symptomatic infection (Fig. 28.1). This characteristic rash develops as an expanding erythematous, macular–papular lesion at the site of tick bite after an incubation period of 7 to 14 days (range, 1–32 days). It generally resolves spontaneously in approximately 1 to 2 weeks. Regional lymphadenopathy is common and is often associated with flu-like symptoms including fever, malaise, chills, and fatigue [2,4,9–11].

Early disseminated disease is identified by the appearance of multifocal secondary EM lesions after hematogenous spread of *Borrelia*. Usually, these lesions are smaller than the primary lesion (1–3 cm), and they occur several days or weeks after the first lesion (3–10 weeks). This stage of Lyme disease can include cardiac and/or neurological manifestations. Late disseminated disease is predominantly a musculoskeletal disorder, mainly arthritis [6,9–13].

## *Neurological Manifestations*

Nervous system involvement is more common in European than in North American disease and presents a broad clinical spectrum [9]. Most patients develop neurological complications within 12 months of the infection, rarely later.

### Headaches

Headaches are reported in 70% of children with Lyme disease. They may occur at the onset of the disease, months later, or may be recurrent. They are frontal or occipital in location and less frequently bitemporal or vertex. The headaches are not

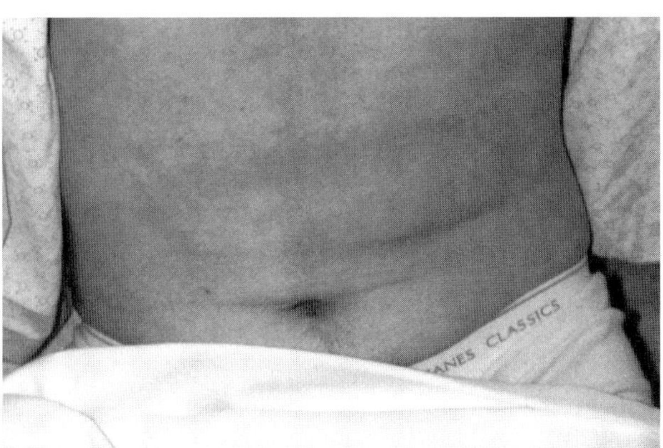

**Fig. 28.1** Classic erythema migrans rash in the early stage of Lyme disease (photograph courtesy of Johanna Goldfarb, M.D.).

usually associated with nausea or vomiting [9]. However, they are often concurrent with arthritis, arthralgias, and myalgias [14].

### Cranial Nerve Palsies

Facial nerve palsy is one of the most commonly reported neurological manifestations of Lyme disease among children [15,16]. It occurs in 3 to 5% of symptomatic patients days or weeks after EM, or with or after other manifestations of systemic dissemination [4]. Up to one third of patients have bilateral facial nerve involvement [9,17]. When Lyme disease is suspected in a child with seventh cranial nerve palsy, cerebrospinal fluid (CSF) examination is indicated to exclude occult CNS involvement, even in the absence of meningeal signs [16,18]. Facial nerve palsy caused by Lyme disease carries an excellent prognosis; complete recovery usually occurs within a few months. Residual facial weakness is rare [9,19]. The second most commonly involved cranial nerve is the optic nerve. Both optic neuritis and increased intracranial pressure are reported pathophysiologic mechanisms for loss of visual acuity [20]. Patients with Lyme disease may also develop diplopia caused by ocular motor nerve palsies. Involvement of other cranial nerves is rare [21].

### Lyme Meningitis

*B. burgdorferi* may spread to the meninges and produce a syndrome that mimics viral (aseptic) meningitis. Meningitis is the presenting manifestation of Lyme disease in 1% of pediatric cases. Nonspecific symptoms, including headache, neck pain, and malaise, are similar to those seen in viral meningitis. However, the duration of these symptoms is significantly longer, lasting for 3 to 4 weeks. Fever and vomiting are infrequent [22]. Clues to Lyme meningitis are associated EM, cranioneuropathy (especially peripheral facial nerve palsy), and papilledema [9,22].

### Pseudotumor Cerebri-Like Syndrome

This syndrome is unique in children and adolescents with Lyme disease. It is characterized by increased intracranial pressure and papilledema [14]. In contrast to classic pseudotumor cerebri, obesity and female sex are not associated factors [21]. This syndrome has been described even in the absence of CSF pleocytosis, indicating the possibility of an immune-mediated process.

### Acute Painful Radiculoneuritics (Bannwarth's Syndrome)

This syndrome is characterized by symptoms of meningeal irritation associated with striking lancinating intrascapular or extremity pains. It occurs most commonly in adults with the European Lyme disease variant and is very rare in children [15,19,21].

### Other

Behavioral and mood disturbances have been reported in children with Lyme disease, including irritability, emotional liability, and listlessness [23]. These symptoms are often temporally related to constitutional symptoms of fever, myalgia, and arthralgia [13,21,23]. Sleep disturbances have also been described in some children; daytime sleepiness is the most common complaint [14].

A wide range of other neurological abnormalities related to *B. burgdorferi* infection have been reported in children, such as ataxia, seizures, progressive encephalomyelitis, vertigo, chronic myelitis, and the Guillain-Barré-like syndrome [4,14,17]. All are rare in children.

## *Neuropathology*

Neuropathologic studies are limited because Lyme disease is almost never fatal. *B. burgdorferi* have been detected primarily in the leptomeninges and nerve roots, but not in the CNS parenchyma or peripheral nerves. *B. burgdorferi* produces inflammation out of proportion to the number of organisms, causing meningeal and perivascular mononuclear infiltrates, microglial nodules, and, rarely, obliterative vasculopathy, demyelination, or granulomatous changes [9,24]. Nerve biopsy studies from patients with peripheral nervous system complications of Lyme borreliosis showed epineurial, perineural, and perivascular infiltrations, angiopathy of the vasa nervorum, and axon damage [9,25].

## *Diagnosis*

The diagnosis of Lyme disease is clinical; laboratory tests are supportive [4]. The CDC surveillance criteria are strict and are recommended only for epidemiologic and formal clinical studies [21]. Currently, a two-step test approach is recommended, beginning with a sensitive serologic screening test, either enzyme-linked immunosorbent assay (ELISA) or immunofluorescent assay (IFA) [3–6,26]. ELISA sensitivity is 40 to 60% in the first few weeks and later increases to 90%; its specificity is 70 to 90%. Second generation antibody tests have been developed to improve the specificity of ELISA; these tests are only available in research laboratories and are not approved by the US Food and Drug Administration (FDA) [8,9,27].

If the result of the initial screening antibody test is positive or equivocal, a Western immunoblot should be obtained to confirm the diagnosis. A Western immunoblot is considered positive if 2 of 3 IgM bands or 5 of 10 IgG bands are positive. IgM antibody levels rise approximately 2 to 4 weeks after the onset of EM, peak at approximately 6 to 8 weeks, and become nondetectable 4 to 6 months after EM. Persistence of IgM may be an indicator of persistent infection or re-infection.

IgG antibody levels rise 6 to 8 weeks after EM, peak at 4 to 6 months after EM, and remain elevated for life [4,28]. Diagnostic tests based on identifying the genome (DNA polymerase chain reaction) of *B. burgdorferi* lack sufficient specificity and sensitivity to be of routine diagnostic use [8–10,27]. Detection of *B. burgdorferi* antigen in urine, although available in some commercial laboratories, is neither specific nor sensitive and is not approved by the FDA [9].

CSF findings in neuroborreliosis include mononuclear pleocytosis and increased protein level [1,9,17,18]. The detection of antibodies to *B. burgdorferi* in CSF does not constitute proof of the CNS invasion by the spirochete. Meningeal or parenchymal involvement is better assessed by the measurement of intrathecal anti-*B. burgdorferi* antibody production [8,9,14,17,21,27]. This test is indicated in patients with Lyme disease who have nonfocal symptoms suggestive of CNS involvement, but normal CSF findings. Magnetic resonance imaging (MRI) scanning may be a helpful adjunct in evaluating pediatric patients with neuroborreliosis. Brain MRI scan findings may include small, punctate, linear areas of increased signal intensity that are suggestive of vascular involvement, and, more commonly, small, nodular, hyperintense lesions in the deep white matter [21,29].

The differential diagnosis of neuroborreliosis includes aseptic meningitis including enteroviral, mycobacterial, and fungal; leptospirosis; multiple sclerosis; and sarcoidosis.

## *Treatment*

Children with Lyme disease respond exceedingly well to appropriate antimicrobial therapy; the earlier initiated the better. The CDC (Table 28.2) recommendations for the treatment of Lyme disease are primarily based on studies performed in adults [3,6].

Doxycycline is the therapy of choice for children older than 8 years of age for early, localized disease (EM, multiple EM). Amoxicillin may be used for children younger than 8 years of age. Cefuroxime, [26,30] erythromycin, or azithromycin are alternative agents for patients who can take neither doxycycline nor amoxicillin [3,26].

Intravenous ceftriaxone is the antimicrobial of choice for neurological disease [9,26]. It is superior to penicillin because of higher serum levels, better CSF penetration, and *in vitro* activity against *B. burgdorferi*. Patients with isolated facial nerve palsy without evidence of CNS involvement can be successfully treated with an oral regimen of antibiotics as used in localized disease [9,26]. Corticosteroids appear to offer no additional benefit. Antibiotic therapy for facial nerve palsy is used to prevent progression to late stage of neuroborreliosis. However, with or without antimicrobials, facial nerve palsy generally resolves within 4 to 6 weeks.

## *Prognosis*

The clinical course of Lyme disease is usually milder and shorter in children, and neuroborreliosis seems to have a better long-term prognosis than in adults [22].

**Table 28.2** Recommended treatment for Lyme disease in children

| Disease category | Drug regimen |
|---|---|
| Early localized disease | |
| ≥8 years | 100 mg doxycycline orally twice daily for 14–21 days |
| All ages | 50 mg/kg/d amoxicillin divided in three doses for 14–21 days |
| | If allergic: |
| | Cefuroxime axetil |
| | Erythromycin |
| Early disseminated disease and late disease | |
| Multiple erythema migrans | Oral regimen |
| Facial nerve palsy (without evidence of neurological involvement) | Oral regimen |
| Arthritis | Oral regimen, but for 28 days |
| Carditis | Same as for neurological disease (see below) |
| Neurological disease | 75–100 mg/kg ceftriaxone IV or IM once daily (maximum, 2 g/d) |
| | If allergic: |
| | 300,000 U/kg/d penicillin IV, divided into six doses (maximum, 20 million U/d) for 14–21 days |

IV, intravenous; IM, intramuscular.
Adapted from reference 6.

Neurocognitive function after treatment for childhood Lyme disease seems to be excellent [22,31]. Occasionally, neurological and constitutional symptoms such as headache and fatigue persist for a few weeks after treatment, but usually resolve in approximately 2 months [19]. There is no evidence that persistence of these symptoms indicates inadequate treatment or persistent infection [19]. Chronic fatigue and fibromyalgia syndromes caused by Lyme disease are infrequent in children [32].

## Prevention

Measures for the prevention of Lyme disease include the avoidance of tick-infested areas, the use of protective clothing and insect repellents, tick checks, and full and careful removal of ticks [9,33–35]. Routine use of antibiotic prophylaxis after a tick bite for those living in hyperendemic areas is not recommended [26]. Some experts recommend a single 200-mg dose of doxycycline for people 12 years of age and older who have been bitten in an area with hyperendemic infection who have found an engorged deer tick, especially if the suspected period of attachment is longer than 72 hours [26,36]. Primary prevention of Lyme disease with a vaccine is the only feasible strategy. No vaccine is currently commercially available [26,34,37,38].

## References


1. Roos KL. Nonviral Infections. In: Goetz CG, Pappert EJ, eds. *Textbook of Clinical Neurology*. 2nd ed. Philadelphia, PA: W. B. Saunders Company; 2003; 933–934.
2. Hedayati H. Lyme disease. *J Am Osteopath Assoc*. 1992; 92(6):755–760, 763–765.
3. Shapiro ED. *Borrelia burgdorferi* (Lyme Disease). In: Long SS, Pickering LK, Prober CG, eds. *Principles and Practice of Pediatric Infectious Diseases*. 2nd ed. Philadelphia, PA: Churchill Livingstone, Inc; 2003; 965–969.
4. Rahn DW. Lyme disease: clinical manifestations, diagnosis, and treatment. *Semin Arthritis Rheum*. 1991; 20(4):201–218.
5. Steere AC. *Borrelia burgdorferi* (Lyme Disease, Lyme Borreliosis). In: Mandell GL, Bennett JE, Dolin R, eds. *Principles and Practice of Infectious Diseases*. 6th ed. Philadelphia, PA: Churchill Livingstone, Inc; 2005; 2798–2807.
6. Centers for Disease Control and Prevention. Division of Vector-Borne Infectious Diseases. Lyme disease. Available at: *http://www.cdc.gov/ncidod/dvbid/lyme/index.htm*.
7. Centers for Disease Control and Prevention. Lyme disease-United States, 2001–2002. *MMWR* 2004; 53(17):365–369.
8. Marques AR. Lyme disease: an update. *Curr Allergy Asthma Rep*. 2001; 1:541–549.
9. Coyle PK, Schutzer SE. Neurologic aspects of Lyme disease. *Med Clin North Am*. 2002; 86(2):261–284.
10. Donta ST. Late and chronic Lyme disease. *Med Clin North Am*. 2002; 86(2):341–349, vii.
11. Sigal LH. Toward a more complete appreciation of the clinical spectrum of *Borrelia burgdorferi* infection: early Lyme disease without erythema migrans. *Am J Med*. 2003; 114(1):74–75.
12. Coyle PK. Lyme disease. *Curr Neurol Neurosci Rep*. 2002; 2(6):479–487.
13. Logigian EL, Kaplan RF, Steere AC. Chronic neurologic manifestations of Lyme disease. *N Engl J Med*. 1990; 323(21):1438–1444.
14. Belman AL, Iyer M, Coyle PK, Dattwyler R. Neurologic manifestations in children with North American Lyme disease. *Neurology*. 1993; 43(12):2609–2614.
15. Bingham PM, Galetta SL, Athreya B, Sladky J. Neurologic manifestations in children with Lyme disease. *Pediatrics*. 1995; 96(6):1053–1056.
16. Millner M. [Neurologic manifestations of Lyme borreliosis in children.] *Wien Med Wochenschr*. 1995; 145(7-8):178–182.
17. Garcia-Monco JC, Benach JL. Lyme neuroborreliosis. *Ann Neurol*. 1995; 37(6):691–702.
18. Belman AL, Reynolds L, Preston T, Postels D, Grimson R, Coyle PK. Cerebrospinal fluid findings in children with Lyme disease-associated facial nerve palsy. *Arch Pediatr Adolesc Med*. 1997; 151(12):1224–1228.
19. Shapiro ED, Seltzer EG. Lyme disease in children. *Semin Neurol*. 1997;17(1):39–44.
20. Rothermel H, Hedges TR III, Steere AC. Optic neuropathy in children with Lyme disease. *Pediatrics*. 2001; 108:477–481.
21. Coyle PK. Neurologic complications of Lyme disease. *Rheum Dis Clin North Am*. 1993; 19(4):993–1009.
22. Eppes SC, Nelson DK, Lewis LL, Klein JD. Characterization of Lyme meningitis and comparison with viral meningitis in children. *Pediatrics*. 1999; 103(5 pt 1):957–960.
23. Fallon BA, Nields JA, Burrascano JJ, Liegner K, DelBene D, Liebowitz MR. The neuropsychiatric manifestations of Lyme borreliosis. *Psychiatr Q*. 1992; 63(1):95–117.
24. Cadavid D, O'Neill T, Schaefer H, Pachner AR. Localization of *Borrelia burgdorferi* in the nervous system and other organs in a nonhuman primate model of Lyme disease. *Lab Invest* 2000; 80(7):1043–1054.
25. Meier C, Grahmann F, Engelhardt A, Dumas M. Peripheral nerve disorders in Lyme-Borreliosis. Nerve biopsy studies from eight cases. *Acta Neuropathol (Berl)*. 1989; 79(3):271–278.
26. American Academy of Pediatrics. Lyme Disease (Lyme borreliosis, *Borrelia burgdorferi* Infection). In: Pickering LK, Baker CJ, Long SS, McMillan JA, eds. *Red Book: 2006 Report*

*of the Committee on Infectious Diseases*. 27th ed. American Academy of Pediatrics. Elk Grove Village, IL: American Academy of Pediatrics; 2006; 428–433.
27. Bunikis J, Barbour AG. Laboratory testing for suspected Lyme disease. *Med Clin North Am*. 2002; 86(2):311–340.
28. Ravel R. Spirochetal and Rickettsial Infections. In: Ravel R, ed. *Clinical Laboratory Medicine*. 6th ed. St. Louis, MO: Mosby Inc.; 1995; 232–233.
29. Belman AL, Coyle PK, Roque C, Cantos E. MRI findings in children infected by *Borrelia burgdorferi*. *Pediatr Neurol*. 1992; 8(6):428–431.
30. Eppes SC, Childs JA. Comparative study of cefuroxime axetil versus amoxicillin in children with early Lyme disease. *Pediatrics*. 2002; 109(6):1173–1177.
31. Adams WV, Rose CD, Eppes SC, Klein JD. Cognitive effects of Lyme disease in children: a 4 year followup study. *J Rheumatol*. 1999; 26(5):1190–1194.
32. Gerber MA, Shapiro ED, Burke GS, Parcells VJ, Bell GL. Lyme disease in children in southeastern Connecticut. Lyme Disease Study Group. *N Engl J Med*. 1996; 335(17):1270–1274.
33. Orloski KA, Hayes EB, Campbell GL, Dennis DT. Surveillance for Lyme disease—United States, 1992–1998. *MMWR CDC Surveill Summ*. 2000; 49(3):1–11.
34. American Academy of Pediatrics. Committee on Infectious Diseases. Prevention of Lyme Disease. *Pediatrics*. 2000; 105:142–147.
35. American Academy of Pediatrics. Prevention of Tickborne Infections. In: Pickering LK, Baker CJ, Long SS, McMillan JA, eds. *Red Book: Report of the Committee on Infectious Diseases*. 27th ed. American Academy of Pediatrics. Elk Grove Village, IL: American Academy of Pediatrics; 2006: 195–197.
36. Nadelman RB, Nowakowski J, Fish D, et al. Prophylaxis with single-dose doxycycline for the prevention of Lyme Disease after an *Ixodes* scapularis tick bite. *N Engl J Med*. 2001; 345(2):79–84.
37. Hayes EB, Piesman J. How can we prevent Lyme disease? *N Engl J Med*. 2003; 348(24): 2424–2430.
38. Wormser GP, Dattwyler RJ, Shapiro ED, et al. The clinical assessment, treatment, and prevention of Lyme disease, human granulocytic anaplasmosis, and babesiosis: clinical practice guidelines by the Infectious Diseases Society of America. *Clin Infect Dis*. 2006; 43(9): 1089–1134.

# Chapter 29
# *Treponema pallidum*

**Abeer Khayat, M.D. and Mobeen H. Rathore, M.D., C.P.E., F.A.A.P.**

## Neurosyphilis

### *Introduction*

Syphilis is a systemic venereal disease with protean clinical presentations [1]. Although early symptoms generally resolve without treatment, late complications of neurosyphilis, cardiovascular syphilis, or both may occur [2]. Untreated or inadequately treated infection in pregnant women may also result in congenital syphilis [2–5].

### *Epidemiology*

Syphilis occurs throughout the world, more frequently in large urban areas, and in young people between 20 and 30 years of age [1,2,6,7]. Congenital syphilis is the most frequently recognized syphilitic disease in children. The prevalence of seroreactivity in pregnant women approaches 10 to 15% in some areas of the world; in the United States it is below 1% [5,7,8]. Reported cases of syphilis remained at low levels in the United States until 1986, when the incidence of both acquired and congenital syphilis increased dramatically, with the epidemic peaking in 1990. The rate of primary and secondary syphilis decreased throughout the 1990s, and, in 2000, reached an all-time low. However, between 2000 and 2004, the rate of syphilis in the United States increased [2,9]. The increase in cases was observed only among men, primarily in men who have sex with men, and was associated with high rates of human immunodeficiency virus (HIV) co-infection and high-risk sexual behavior [2,9–12]. In 2004, for the first time in more than 10 years, the rate among women did not decrease. The rate of congenital syphilis, however, decreased between 2003 and 2004, likely reflecting the substantial reduction in syphilis among women that had occurred during the preceding decade [2,9], This overall positive trend seen in the United States has not been mirrored worldwide; increases in the number of cases of syphilis have been seen in South Africa, South America, and Southeast Asia [13]. In the pre-antibiotic era, tabes dorsalis was the most common form of neurosyphilis [14]. However, during the past decade, an increasing

L.L. Barton and N.R. Friedman (eds.), *The Neurological Manifestations of Pediatric Infectious Diseases and Immunodeficiency Syndromes.*

number of cases of early neurosyphilis and syphilitic eye disease have been reported, particularly, in individuals with HIV infection [14,15].

## Pathophysiology

The causative agent of syphilis, *Treponema pallidum*, belongs to the family *Spirochaetaceae* [1,16,17]. It is a thin helical bacterium that can neither be cultivated *in vitro* nor seen on Gram stain [16,18]. However, it can be detected by silver stain, dark field examination, and immunofluorescent techniques [1]. Soon after penetration, *T. pallidum* enters the lymphatics or blood stream and disseminates throughout the body. Any organ may be invaded, especially the central nervous system (CNS) [19].

## Clinical Manifestations

Acquired syphilis is transmitted almost exclusively by sexual contact [20]. When untreated, syphilis is a life-long infection that evolves in three clear stages: primary syphilis, secondary and latent syphilis, and tertiary syphilis [16,18,20]. Primary syphilis occurs in approximatlely 30% of exposures [7,13,16]. It is characterized by a single painless papule at the site of inoculation that appears after an incubation period of 1 to 4 weeks [7]. The papule becomes eroded and forms an ulcer (the chancre) that heals completely in 3 to 6 weeks [7,18]. Painless enlargement of regional lymph nodes accompanies the chancre in 50% of cases [16,18].

Secondary syphilis develops 6 to 12 weeks after infection [1,7,18–20]. This stage is associated with widespread multiorgan disease [16,19]. Mucocutaneous lesions are the commonest manifestation of the disease and involve most of the body, including the palms and soles [7,16,20]. Condylomata lata and mucous membranes lesions are detected in 10% of patients [7,18]. Generalized lymphadenopathy occurs in 85% of patients [7,19]. Renal, hepatic, neurological, and ophthalmologic manifestations may be present [7,16,18]. Without treatment, complete resolution of secondary syphilis occurs in 3 to 12 weeks, followed by asymptomatic latency [7,18].

Tertiary syphilis occurs in 30% of untreated infected individuals [7,13,14,18,20]. It is exceedingly rare in the pediatric population [13]. Manifestations consist of destructive lesions in the CNS (late neurosyphilis), cardiovascular system (aortic aneurysm), and skeletal system and skin (gummatous syphilis) [7,13,14,16,18,20].

## Neurological Manifestations

### Neurosyphilis

CNS involvement may occur any time throughout the course of the disease [16,21]. Early neurosyphilis is limited to the involvement of meninges and vessels. It includes asymptomatic neurosyphilis, acute syphilitic meningitis, and cerebrovascular syphilis [17]. Late neurosyphilis is characterized by parenchymatous involvement and is seen decades after infection. Thus, it is extremely rare in the pediatric population. Clinical manifestations include tabes dorsalis, dementia paralytica, and CNS gummata [17]. Neurosyphilis should be considered in the differential diagnosis of any neurological disease in HIV-infected patients.

### Asymptomatic Neurosyphilis

Asymptomatic neurosyphilis can be seen anytime after infection, with a peak during the second year. It occurs in approximately 30 to 40% of patients with secondary syphilis [1,18,22]. Although signs and symptoms of CNS involvement are absent, cerebrospinal fluid (CSF) abnormalities, including a reactive nontreponemal test (Venereal Disease Research Laboratory test [VDRL]), elevated protein level, and pleocytosis may be detected [1,14,17]. Spontaneous resolution of these abnormalities occurs in 7% of patients; the remaining untreated individuals are at risk for progression to symptomatic neurosyphilis.

### Acute Syphilitic Meningitis

Acute syphilitic meningitis occurs in the first few years of infection in 1 to 2% of patients with secondary syphilis [7,14,17–19,23]. It is more common in young adults and may also be a feature of congenital syphilis [16]. Patients usually have signs of meningeal irritation, including stiff neck, headache, nausea, and vomiting [1,14,16–18]. Fever is unusual. Cranial neuropathy is common, involving, in descending order of frequency, cranial nerves VII, VIII, VI, and II, resulting in facial weakness, hearing loss, and visual disturbances [1,7,13,14,17,18,23]. This form of meningitis, if untreated, may progress to a more severe form of neurosyphilis [1,6,17,18].

### Meningovascular Syphilis

Meningovascular syphilis is a chronic meningitis involving the base of the brain but may also involve the cerebral convexities and the spinal leptomeninges [24]. This form of neurosyphilis occurs in untreated individuals 4 to 10 years after infection, with an average of 7 years [1,14,16,17,23]. Affected patients usually have an abrupt onset of neurological deficits [1,7,14,16–18]. The middle cerebral artery is the most commonly involved, clinically manifested by "luetic hemiplagia." [7,14]. Localized or diffuse cerebral involvement may occur and lead to seizures, cranial neuropathies, psychological, and intellectual abnormalities (e.g., personality changes, emotional lability, insomnia, and decreased memory) [1,7,13,17,18,21]. Syphilitic arteritis can also develop in any spinal artery and may result in paraplegia, sensory level, and loss of sphincter control [14]. Computed tomographic scan of the brain may reveal multiple areas of infarction [1,14,21]. Cerebral angiography may demonstrate a nonspecific pattern of diffuse narrowing of intracranial arteries [1,21].

### Tabes Dorsalis

Tabes dorsalis is a slowly progressive degenerative disease involving the sensory nerves and ganglia in the dorsal columns (demyelination) and sensory roots (inflammatory changes with fibrosis) of the spinal cord [1,14,17,18]. No spirochetes have been found in the posterior columns [6]. This form of neurosyphilis occurs 20 to 30 years after the initial infection [1,6]. Clinically, it is characterized by loss of pain sensation, leading to skin and joint damage (Charcot joints), paresthesias, impaired joint position sense and resultant ataxia (locomotor ataxia), and diminished deep tendon reflexes [1,24]. Painful dysesthesias, particularly the characteristic lancinating pain (lightning like, appearing suddenly, spreading rapidly, and disappearing) often occur early and require treatment [1,16,18,24]. Bowel and bladder dysfunction and loss of sexual function are common [1,17,21]. The Argyll-Robertson pupillary abnormality, miotic pupils that demonstrate normal constriction to accommodation but fail to constrict further to light, may be present [1,17,21].

### Dementia Paralytica (General Paresis)

Dementia paralytica (general paresis) represents chronic progressive frontotemporal encephalitis with resultant ongoing loss of cortical function [1,17]. This form of neurosyphilis typically occurs 20 to 30 years after the initial infection, and is caused by the invasion of the brain by *T. pallidum* [1,24]. Clinically, it is characterized by deterioration in cognitive functioning, with impaired memory, loss of judgment, language abnormalities, tremors of the hands and tongue, and loss of bowel or bladder control [1,14,16].

### Gummatous Neurosyphilis

Gummatous neurosyphilis is characterized by gummata located in the leptomeninges or within the parenchyma. They produce local neurological deficits and cranial nerve palsies [14]. Ear and eye involvement occur during any stage of disease [19,23]. Uveitis, retinitis, and optic and acoustic neuritis, when detected early, may respond to antimicrobial therapy [13,23].

## Congenital Syphilis

Congenital syphilis is usually acquired in utero and only rarely during delivery [13,16,18]. The rate of transmission varies according to maternal disease stage, and ranges from 90% in untreated maternal primary or secondary syphilis to less than 10% in late, latent syphilis [7,16,19]. Perinatal death caused by congenital syphilis may occur in 40% of affected untreated pregnancies [9,18].

Among survivors, clinical manifestations range from benign to life-threatening [18]. In early onset disease, detected before 2 years of age, initially asymptomatic infants develop symptoms before 3 months of age [7]. Clinical findings include snuffles, diffuse rash involving the palms and soles, and hepatosplenomegaly [7,13,16–19]. Skeletal involvement is common and affects multiple long bones with a painful periostitis, resulting in pseudoparalysis [7,13,16,18]. Severely symptomatic newborns are usually born prematurely and hydropic, with hepatosplenomegaly, rash, anemia, thrombocytopenia, and, occasionally, consolidated pneumonia [7,16,18,19]. Neurological involvement is thought to occur in 60% of these infants, particularly in those with abnormal clinical, laboratory, or radiographic findings [7,25]. If untreated, congenital neurosyphilis can result in cranial nerve palsies, hydrocephalus, cerebral infarction, seizure disorder, and mental retardation.

Late-onset disease, detected after 2 years of age, is manifested by interstitial keratitis, deafness, Hutchinson teeth, and musculoskeletal abnormalities [7,13,16,18,19]. Asymptomatic neurosyphilis is more common in these children than symptomatic disease, but, if untreated, may progress to a more severe form, resembling neurosyphilis disease in adults [7,18].

## *Neuropathology*

The histologic hallmark of all syphilitic lesions is an obliterative endarteritis with plasma cell-rich mononuclear infiltrates [1,14,19,21,22]. Luminal narrowing secondary to fibroblastic proliferation of the intima, thinning of the media, and fibrosis and inflammation in the adventitia can lead to cerebrovascular thrombosis, ischemia, and infarctions [1,14]. There is often an associated hydrocephalus with damage to the ependymal lining and proliferation of the subependymal glia (granular ependymitis) in patients with dementia paralytica (general paresis) [6].

## *Diagnosis*

The diagnosis of syphilis is suggested by clinical findings and confirmed by serologic testing [13,18]. Definitive diagnosis is achieved by identifying spirochetes by microscopic dark field examination or direct fluorescent antibody tests of lesion exudate or tissue [7,16,18,20,26]. Serologic testing is the preferred diagnostic modality. Nontreponemal tests, including rapid plasma reagin (RPR) and VDRL, are used for initial screening and serial follow-up [7,16,18,20,26,27]. False-positive tests occur in 1 to 2% of the general population [13,16,18]. Therefore, a positive nontreponemal reaginic test must be confirmed by a treponemal-specific test. These tests include fluorescent treponemal antibody absorption (FTA-abs) and microhemagglutination assay for *T. pallidum* (MHA-TP) [7,16,18,20]. Both tests are very reactive in secondary, latent, and tertiary syphilis. False-positive results rarely occur, especially with other spirochetal infections [7,18]. Once reactive, *Treponema*-specific tests remain positive indefinitely [7,16,18,26]. Cerebrospinal fluid (CSF) examination is recommended in all patients with untreated syphilis of unknown duration or duration longer than 1 year, all patients with HIV infection, adults and adolescents with clinical evidence of neurological or ophthalmic involvement (cognitive dysfunction, motor and sensory deficits, ophthalmic or auditory symptoms, cranial nerve palsies, and symptoms and signs of meningitis), patients with treatment failure, unconfirmed treatment, and all children who are evaluated for congenital syphilis [1,16,26]. The CSF-VDRL, the only test approved for testing reactivity of CSF, is highly specific but not sensitive [16,18,25,26]. The diagnosis of neurosyphilis is usually made in the presence of a reactive serologic test with either neurological manifestations consistent with neurosyphilis or abnormalities of CSF (elevated white blood cell [WBC] count or protein level), and/or a positive CSF-VDRL result [14,26]. The polymerase chain reaction (PCR) test for *T. pallidum* in the CSF is very specific, but does not distinguish live from dead organisms, and it is not widely available [13,20,23].

All infants in whom congenital syphilis is suspected should undergo a comprehensive evaluation that includes quantitative nontreponemal titers in mother and infant, long-bone radiography, complete blood count, liver function tests, and lumbar puncture [18,25]. A definitive diagnosis of congenital syphilis requires the direct identification of spirochetes in the placenta, umbilical cord, mucocutaneous lesions, or mucous discharge by dark-field examination or direct fluorescent antibody tests [7]. Serologic diagnosis of congenital syphilis is often difficult in asymptomatic infants because of transplacental transfer of maternal antibodies, and because, in an infected infant, nontreponemal tests may be reactive or nonreactive depending on the timing of maternal and fetal infection [7,18,26]. However, congenital syphilis is probable in an infant with a quantitative nontreponemal titer that is fourfold greater than the mother's titer [18,26]. The CSF should be examined for increased protein concentration and WBC and CSF-VDRL [18]. Because of the wide range of normal values in the newborn infants, interpretation of CSF findings is often difficult. A negative CSF-VDRL test result does not exclude congenital neurosyphilis, nor does a positive result absolutely confirm it. Cerebrospinal fluid FTA-abs, although lacking in specificity, has greater sensitivity than CSF-VDRL and is preferred by some experts. Recently, IgM immunoblotting and PCR assay of blood and CSF have been used to identify infants with CNS infection [7,13,23,25].

## Treatment

Parenteral penicillin G is the drug of choice for treatment of syphilis at any stage, and is the only documented effective therapy for neurosyphilis, congenital syphilis, and syphilis during pregnancy [13,26,28].

Primary, secondary, and early latent syphilis are treated with a single dose of intramuscular benzathine penicillin G [7,18,23,26]. Acquired syphilis of more than 1 year duration (without neurosyphilis) is treated with benzathine penicillin G administered intramuscularly weekly for 3 successive weeks [7,23,26,28]. Follow-up quantitative nontreponemal tests should be performed at 3, 6, and 12 months (and at 24 months in patients with syphilis for longer than 1 year) after the conclusion of treatment [7]. With successful treatment, the quantitative RPR test usually becomes nonreactive after 1 year in primary syphilis, 2 years in secondary syphilis, and 5 years in late syphilis [6,13,23].

Children with neurosyphilis should receive intravenous aqueous crystalline penicillin G for 10 to 14 days [7]. Some experts recommend following this regimen with a single dose of intramuscular benzathine penicillin G administered weekly for 3 weeks. If CSF pleocytosis was present initially, CSF examination should be repeated every 6 months, until the WBC count is normal. The CSF examination can also be used to evaluate changes in CSF-VDRL and protein level; however, change in these two parameters is slower. If the WBC count has not decreased after 6 months, or if the CSF is not normal after 2 years, retreatment is indicated [6].

Because of the serious sequelae of congenital syphilis, and because CNS involvement cannot be reliably excluded during the neonatal period, all newborns with a presumed or established diagnosis of congenital syphilis generally should be treated with intravenous aqueous crystalline penicillin G for 10 to 14 days [18,23,26]. Some experts recommend procaine penicillin G for the treatment of congenital syphilis. However, adequate CSF treponemicidal concentration (≥0.018 μg/ml) may not always be achieved by this regimen [7,29]. Asymptomatic infants, whose mothers received appropriate penicillin treatment for syphilis more than 4 weeks before delivery and responded with a documented fourfold or greater decrease in their titers, are at minimal risk for syphilis. These infants may not require a full workup, and may be treated with a single dose of intramuscular benzathine penicillin [13,26]. However, these infants should be examined carefully and followed closely until their nontreponemal serologic test results are negative [26]. Infants older than 4 weeks of age with possible congenital syphilis or who have neurological involvement should be treated with intravenous, aqueous penicillin G for 10 to 14 days [26]. This regimen is used for previously untreated congenital syphilis in children older than 1 year of age and may be followed by three weekly doses of intramuscular benzathine penicillin [28].

Both symptomatic and asymptomatic infants should undergo repeated clinical and serologic evaluations. If titers fail to decline, increase or persist at 12 months of age, the infant should be evaluated and retreatment should be considered [26]. Treated infants with congenital neurosyphilis and initially reactive CSF-VDRL test results or an abnormal or uninterpretable results of the initial CSF examination should undergo repeated CSF examinations at 6 month intervals until the WBC count is normal and CSF-VDRL is nonreactive [18,26]. A reactive CSF-VDRL at 6 months and/or a persistently abnormal CSF WBC count or protein level at 2 years warrant evaluation and retreatment [18].

## References

1. Knudsen R, Sotero de Menezes M. Neurosyphilis. Pruitt AA. Talavera F. Thomas FP. Benbadis SR. Lorenzo N. *eMedicine*. 2005. *www.emdicine.com.*
2. Centers for Disease Control and Prevention. Trends in Reportable Sexually Transmitted Diseases in the United States, 2004. *Sexually Transmitted Diseases Surveillance, 2004*. 2005. *www.cdc.com.*
3. Centers for Disease Control and Prevention. Congenital Syphilis—United States, 2000. *MMWR*. 2001; 50(27):573–577.
4. Gust D, Levine WC, St. Louis ME, Braxton J, Berman SM. Mortality associated with congenital syphilis in the United States, 1992–1998. *Pediatrics*. 2002; 109(5):e79.
5. Walker DG, Walker GJ. Forgotten but not gone: the continuing scourge of congenital syphilis. *Lancet Infect Dis*. 2002; 2(7):432–436.
6. Hook EW. Syphilis. *Cecil Textbook of Medicine*. 22nd ed. 2004. Goldman L and Bennett JC. W.B. Saunders Company, Philadelphia, PA. 1923–1932.
7. Rawstron SA. *Treponema pallidum* (syphilis). *Principles and Practice of Pediatric Infectious Diseases*. 2nd ed. 2003. Long SS, Pickering LK, Prober CG. Churchill Livingstone, Inc., Philadelphia, PA. 954–962.
8. Dorfman DH, Glaser JH. Congenital syphilis presenting in infants after the newborn period. *N Engl J Med*. 1990; 323:1299–1302.
9. Centers for Disease Control and Prevention. Syphilis Surveillance Report. *Sexually Transmitted Disease Surveillance 2004 Supplement*. 2005. *www.cdc.gov.*
10. Centers for Disease Control and Prevention. Primary and Secondary Syphilis—United States, 2003–2004. *MMWR*. 2006; 55:269–273.
11. Centers for Disease Control and Prevention. Syphilis Surveillance Report. *Sexually Transmitted Disease Surveillance 2001 Supplement*. 2003. *www.cdc.gov.*
12. Centers for Disease Control and Prevention. Syphilis Surveillance Report. *Sexually Transmitted Disease Surveillance* 2002 Supplement. 2004. *www.cdc*.gov.
13. Goldenberg RL, Culhane JF, Johnson DC. Maternal infection and adverse fetal and neonatal outcomes. *Clin Perinatol*. 2005; 32(3):523–559.
14. Roos KL. Non-viral infections. *Goetz: Textbook of Clinical Neurology*. 2nd ed, 2003. Goetz CG. Pappert EJ. W. B. Saunders Company, Philadelphia, PA. 931–933.
15. Marra CM. Syphilis and human immunodeficiency virus infection. *Semin Neurol*. 1992; 12:43–50.
16. Sung L, MacDonald NE. Syphilis: a pediatric perspective. *Pediatr Rev*. 1998; 19(1):17–22.
17. Estanislao LB, Pachner AR. Spirochetal infection of the nervous system. *Neurol Clin*. 1999; 17(4):783–800.
18. Darville T. Syphilis. *Pediatr Rev*. 1999; 20(5):160–164.
19. Waseem M. Syphilis. Tolan RW. Windle ML. Barton LL. Rauch D. Steele R W. *eMedicine*. 2006. *www.emdicine.com.*
20. Weir E, Fishman D. Syphilis: Have we dropped the ball? *Can Med Assoc*. 2002; 167(11): 1267–1268.
21. Brightbill TC, Ihmeidan IH, Post MJ, Berger JR, Katz DA. Neurosyphilis in HIV-positive and HIV-negative patients: neuroimaging findings. *Am J Neuroradiol*. 1995; 16(4):703–711.
22. McAdam AJ. Sharpe AH. Infectious diseases: syphilis. *Robbins and Cotran Pathologic Basis of Disease*. 7th ed. 2005. Cotran R, Collins T, Kumar V. W. B. Saunders Company, Philadelphia, PA. 388–391.
23. Tramont EC. *Treponema pallidum* (syphilis). *Principles and Practice of Infectious Diseases*. 6th ed. 2005. Mandell GL, Bennett JE, Dolin R. Churchill Livingstone, Inc. Philadelphia, PA. 2768–2783.
24. De Girolami U. Anthony DC. Forsch MP. Central nervous system. *Robbins and Cotran Pathologic Basis of Disease*. 7th ed. 2005. Cotran R, Collins T, Kumar V. W. B. Saunders Company, Philadelphia, PA. 1372.

25. Michelow IC, Wendel GD Jr, Norgard MV, Zeray F, Leos NK, Alsaadi R, Sanchez PJ. Central nervous system infection in congenital syphilis. *N Engl J Med*. 2002; 346(23):1792–1798.
26. Centers for Disease Control and Prevention. Sexually transmitted Diseases Treatment Guidelines 2006. *www.cdc.gov/std*.
27. Roos KL. What I have learned about infectious diseases with my sleeves rolled up. *Semin Neurol*. 2002; 22(1):9–15.
28. Syphilis. *Red Book. Report of the Committee on Infectious Diseases*. 27th edition. American Academy of Pediatrics. Elk Grove Village, IL. 2006; 631–644.
29. Azimi PH, Janner D, Berne P, Fulroth R, Lvoff V, Franklin L, Berman SM. Concentrations of procaine and aqueous penicillin in the cerebrospinal fluid of infants treated for congenital syphilis. *J Pediatr*. 1994; 124(4):649–653.

# Section IV
# Fungi

# Chapter 30
# *Candida* Species

**Barbara Stechenberg, M.D.**

## Candidiasis

### *Introduction and Epidemiology*

Members of the genus *Candida* are ubiquitous. *Candida albicans*, the most common species, is present on the skin and in the mouth, intestinal tract, and vagina of immunocompetent persons, with changes in the local flora caused by antibiotic use or other factors. It may cause annoying but easily treatable mucocutaneous infection. However, *C. albicans* and other species including *C. parapsilosis*, *C. glabrata*, and *C. krusei* cause serious infections in immunocompromised hosts. Most at risk are children with congenital or acquired immunodeficiency (human immunodeficiency virus [HIV]/ acquired immunodeficiency syndrome [AIDS]), extreme prematurity, neutropenia, diabetes mellitus, and treatment with corticosteroids or chemotherapy. Patients on broad-spectrum antibiotics or undergoing intravenous hyperalimentation are also at risk.

Primary candidiasis of the brain or meninges is rare. Central nervous system involvement in disseminated candidiasis is frequent, and is increasing [1–3]. In a report of 12 children with candidal meningitis and cancer, risk factors included prolonged neutropenia and fever, antibiotic therapy, and total parenteral nutrition [3]. In a study of premature infants with systemic candidiasis, almost one fourth had meningitis, often manifested by respiratory decompensation [4].

### *Pathogenesis*

The pathogenesis of candidal infection involves a cascade of events including adhesion, colonization, and invasion. Epithelial cells in the oropharynx, the gastrointestinal tract, and the genitourinary tract have carbohydrates or proteins that facilitate adhesion of the yeast to human tissue [5]. Once attached, the yeast can replicate and colonize the host. Virtually all humans become colonized with

L.L. Barton and N.R. Friedman (eds.), *The Neurological Manifestations of Pediatric Infectious Diseases and Immunodeficiency Syndromes.*

*C. albicans* during the first month of life; the initial colonization is acquired from the mother by vertical transmission. When host defenses are impaired, such as in the neonate, colonizing yeast can invade from endogenous sites. Intact integument is particularly important in the defense against invasive disease. Virtually every aspect of the host defense system is operative in combating candidal infection.

## *Clinical and Neurological Manifestations*

The clinical features are not well defined and vary from the usual signs and symptoms of meningeal inflammation or encephalitis to no discernible signs referable to the central nervous system. Cranial nerve palsies and seizures rarely occur. Brain abscesses may occur in immunocompromised hosts and can involve any lobe. Depending on location, focal neurological signs or symptoms of intracranial hypertension may result. *Candida* endophthalmitis is common in patients, especially low birth weight infants and other high-risk children receiving parenteral hyperalimentation.

## *Diagnosis*

Even with meningeal involvement, only half of the patients will have cerebrospinal fluid pleocytosis or hypoglycorrhachia. In a large multicenter study of candidiasis in extremely low birth weight infants, only approximately half of those with meningitis had positive blood cultures [6]. Organisms can be seen on Gram stain and are easily cultured from cerebrospinal fluid. Computed axial tomography and magnetic resonance imaging scanning may be helpful in revealing typical, well-demarcated lesions in the brain.

## *Neuropathology*

The neuropathologic lesions include microabscesses and macroabscesses, non-caseating granulomas, diffuse glial nodules, vasculitic thrombosis, meningitis, ependymitis, mycotic aneurysm, balls of pseudohyphae, demyelination, and transverse myelitis [2].

## *Treatment*

Amphotericin B deoxycholate (0.7–1.0 mg/kg/d) plus 25 mg/kg flucytosine four times a day is appropriate initial therapy [7]. Premature infants with disseminated candidiasis, including meningitis, respond well to amphotericin B monotherapy, with an excellent outcome [4]. The response in other immunocompromised patients often depends on control of the underlying problem. Practice guidelines for treatment of candidiasis have been developed [7]. The reduction of *Candida* infections during neonatal intensive care of extremely premature infants is an area of intense study [8].

## References

1. Hughes WT. Systemic candidiasis. A study of 109 fatal cases. *Pediatr Inf Dis J*. 1982; 1:11–18.
2. Lipton SA, Hickey WF, Morris JH, Loscalzo J. Candidal infection in the central nervous system. *Am J Med*. 1984; 76:101–108.
3. McCullers JA, Vargas S, Flynn PM, Razzouk BI, Shenep JL. Candidal meningitis in children with cancer. *Clin Infect Dis*. 2000; 31:451–457.
4. Fernandez M, Moylett EH, Noyola DE, Baker CJ. Candidal meningitis in neonates: a 10-year review. *Clin Infect Dis*. 2000; 31:458–463.
5. Hostetter MK. Adhesins and ligands involved in the interaction of Candida spp. With epithelial and endothelial surfaces. *Clin Microbiol Rev*. 1994; 7:29–42.
6. Benjamin DK Jr, Stoll BJ, Fanaroff AA, et al. Neonatal candidiasis among extremely low birth weight infants: risk factors, mortality rates, and neurodevelopmental outcomes at 18 to 22 months. *Pediatrics*. 2006; 117:84–92.
7. Pappas PG, Rex JH, Sobel JD, et al. Guidelines for the treatment of candidiasis. *Clin Infect Dis*. 2004; 38:161–189.
8. Long SS, Stevenson DK. Reducing Candida infections during neonatal intensive care: management choices, infection control and fluconazole prophylaxis. *J Pediatr*. 2005; 147:135–141.

# Chapter 31
# *Cryptococcus neoformans*

**Barbara Stechenberg, M.D.**

## Cryptococcosis

### *Introduction and Epidemiology*

Cryptococcosis is a life-threatening systemic, sporadic fungal infection caused by *Cryptococcus neoformans*, a monomorphic yeast. It occurs worldwide. *C. neoformans* is isolated from soil, especially in areas enriched with bird droppings. It is an encapsulated yeast that grows at 37°C. The organism becomes airborne and is inhaled, although most pulmonary involvement is subclinical. There is no person-to-person spread. Cryptococcosis occurs in 5 to 10% of adults with acquired immunodeficiency syndrome (AIDS), but is less common in children with human immunodeficiency virus (HIV) infection.

### *Pathogenesis*

Primary infection acquired by inhalation is usually mild or asymptomatic; disease is usually identified after hematogenous dissemination. Spread can occur to the central nervous system, bones and joints, skin, and mucous membranes. Cryptococcal meningitis is the most common manifestation; in a study of 171 cases of cryptococcosis, meningitis accounted for 76% [1]. Dissemination is rare in children without defects in cellular immunity, such as those undergoing transplantation, those with malignancies, collagen vascular disease, HIV infection, sarcoidosis, or requiring long-term corticosteroid therapy.

### *Clinical and Neurological Manifestations*

Meningitis is the most serious manifestation of *C. neoformans* infection. There is tremendous variability in the clinical presentation, but it often assumes an indolent course, especially in patients without HIV infection. Headache and fever are

L.L. Barton and N.R. Friedman (eds.), *The Neurological Manifestations of Pediatric Infectious Diseases and Immunodeficiency Syndromes.*

common. Stiff neck also is commonly noted in nonimmunocompromised patients, but not in those with AIDS. Other findings include behavioral changes, alteration of consciousness, and impaired mental function, which typically develop over 2 to 4 weeks. Less frequent findings are cranial nerve lesions, visual deficits, papilledema, seizures, diplopia, focal neurological deficits, photophobia, and abnormal cerebellar signs. The duration of symptoms before diagnosis can be as short as a few days to as long as several months.

## *Diagnosis*

Diagnosis is made by lumbar puncture. The opening pressure is often very elevated. Results of the cerebrospinal fluid (CSF) analysis may show a variable pleocytosis, often low in AIDS patients but moderate (20–200 cells/mm$^3$) in other patients. There is a mononuclear predominance. The protein level is normal or mildly elevated and the glucose concentration is low in 75% of patients without AIDS.

Definitive diagnosis is made by isolating the organism. India ink preparations or CSF cryptococcal antigen assays can offer rapid diagnosis. The latter is a highly sensitive and specific tool.

Results of computed tomographic (CT) or magnetic resonance imaging (MRI) scan findings may be normal or reveal diffuse atrophy, cerebral edema, hydrocephalus, or focal mass lesions. Multiple nonenhancing lesions may be present, most often in the basal ganglia and thalamus. The gelatinous pseudocysts seen on histopathologic specimens are thought to correspond to these findings [2]. Parenchymal nonenhancing cryptococcomas, as well as enhancing nodules in the subarachnoid space and parenchyma may also be present [3].

## *Treatment*

The combination of 0.7 to 1.0 mg/kg/d amphotericin B with 100 mg/kg/d flucytosine is administered as induction therapy, followed by 6 to 12 mg/kg/d fluconazole for a minimum of 10 weeks [4,5]. Alternatively, the initial combination may be continued for 6 to 10 weeks. A lumbar puncture should be performed after 2 weeks of therapy, at which time, 60 to 70% will have sterile fluid. Patients without sterile fluid may need prolonged combination therapy. Rarely, intraventricular or intrathecal amphotericin B is necessary in refractory cases. Lipid formulations of amphotericin B may be substituted in children with renal dysfunction. Children with HIV require lifelong suppressive therapy with fluconazole.

Some patients present with increased intracranial pressure, which may require repeated lumbar punctures, ventricular shunts, or lumbar drains. Communicating hydrocephalus may necessitate ventricular shunting.

## *Prognosis*

The most important prognostic factor for an individual with cryptococcal meningitis is the nature of the underlying illness. Patients without underlying immunosuppression can expect to be cured of the infection, with excellent survival rates. Immunosuppressed children without HIV also have a favorable response to treatment [6]. Risk factors for relapse include persistently low CSF glucose level, low initial CSF white blood cell count, post-treatment CSF or serum antigen titer of more than 1:8, and post-treatment therapy with corticosteroids [7].

## References

1. Rozenbaum R, Goncalves AJ. Clinical epidemiologic study of 171 cases of cryptococcosis. *Clin Infect Dis*. 1994; 18:369–380.
2. Popovich MJ, Arthur RH, Helmer E. CT of intracranial cryptococcosis. *AJR*. 1990; 154:603–606.
3. Miszkiel KA, Hall-Craggs MA, Miller RF, et al. The spectrum of MRI findings in CNS cryptococcosis in AIDS. *Clin Radiol*. 1996; 51:842–850.
4. Bennett JE, Dismukes WE, Duma RJ, et al. A comparison of amphotericin B alone and combined with flucytosine in the treatment of cryptococcal meningitis. *N Engl J Med*. 1979; 301:126–131.
5. Saag MS, Graybill RJ, Larsen RA, et al. Practice guidelines for the management of cryptococcal disease. Infectious Diseases Society of America. *Clin Infect Dis*. 2000; 30:710–718.
6. Leggiadro RJ, Barrett FF, Hughes WT. Extrapulmonary cryptococcosis in immunocompromised infants and children. *Pediatr Inf Dis J* 1992; 11:43–47.
7. Diamond RD, Bennett JE. Prognostic factors in cryptococcal meningitis. A study in 111 cases. *Ann Intern Med* 1974; 80:176–181.

# Chapter 32
# *Histoplasma capsulatum*

**Barbara Stechenberg, M.D.**

## Histoplasmosis

### *Introduction*

Histoplasmosis is the most common pulmonary and systemic mycosis in the world today. However, it causes symptoms that reach medical attention in fewer than 5% of infected persons. For many, it causes a self-limited, flu-like illness without sequelae. The only residual findings are incidental radiographic demonstration of typical granulomata in the lungs. Symptomatic disease may be acute or chronic; pulmonary, extrapulmonary, or disseminated.

### *Epidemiology*

*Histoplasma capsulatum* is a dimorphic fungus that grows in soil as a spore-bearing mold with macroconidia. At body temperature, it converts to a yeast phase. It is acquired in environments contaminated with bird droppings and bat guano, which contain the organism. The spores become aerosolized and inhaled.

In the United States, it is endemic in Eastern and Central regions, particularly in Mississippi, Ohio, and Missouri River Valleys. Outbreaks have occurred during activities that promote dispersal of spores. The degree of illness is dependent on the size of the inoculum inhaled, strain virulence, and the immune status of host. Person-to-person transmission does not occur.

### *Pathogenesis*

After inhalation, microconidia germinate in the distal bronchioles and pulmonary alveoli. Acute inflammation ensues. The transition from the mycelial to the yeast

L.L. Barton and N.R. Friedman (eds.), *The Neurological Manifestations of Pediatric Infectious Diseases and Immunodeficiency Syndromes.*

phase of the organism is one of the most crucial determinants for the establishment of infection [1]. After the early transformation to yeasts, lymphohematogenous spread occurs, even in self-limited disease. The yeasts grow very readily in resting macrophages. Activation of cellular immunity is necessary for restricting growth, although latent infection does develop. Lesions heal by fibrous encapsulation and may calcify. In progressive disseminated disease, granulomas may be poorly formed or absent.

## *Clinical Manifestations*

Most symptomatic disease is acute pulmonary histoplasmosis. Progressive disseminated histoplasmosis (PDH) can develop in otherwise healthy infants, usually younger than 1 year of age. The illness is usually subacute, with symptoms of 1 to 12 weeks duration at presentation [2,3]. Early symptoms include fever, failure to thrive, and hepatosplenomegaly. If untreated, malnutrition, oropharyngeal ulcerations, diffuse adenopathy, pneumonia, pancytopenia, disseminated intravascular coagulopathy (DIC), and bleeding may develop. Central nervous system (CNS) abnormalities, primarily meningitis, are common; 62% in one large series from Costa Rica [3].

Immunocompromised children, especially those with depressed cellular immunity from organ transplantation, aggressive therapy for malignancies, or acquired immunodeficiency syndrome, may develop PDH. In its acute form, persistent fever is common. Hepatosplenomegaly and interstitial pneumonitis may ensue, as well as pancytopenia and DIC. CNS involvement is rare, but may be seen in a more subacute presentation observed primarily in adults.

## *Neurological Manifestations*

CNS manifestations occur in 10 to 29% of adults with disseminated histoplasmosis, but may also occur as chronic meningitis without other findings [4]. Meningitis accounts for 60% of CNS disease, with focal mass lesions, either single or multiple stroke syndromes, and encephalitis making up the balance. Symptoms include chronic headache, confusion, decreased level of consciousness, and cranial nerve deficits. Seizures also may occur.

The entity called presumed ocular histoplasmosis syndrome consists of a triad of discrete atrophic choroidal scars in the macula or midperiphery (histo spots), peripapillary atrophy, and choroidal neovascularization that can lead to loss of central vision [5]. This syndrome does not seem to occur in children younger than 10 years of age.

## Neuropathology

The neuropathology consists of granulomatous basilar meningitis and vascular inflammation, perineural inflammatory changes in the cranial nerves, and many organisms at the periphery of mass lesions [4].

## Diagnosis

The cerebrospinal fluid (CSF) findings in meningitis associated with histoplasmosis are nonspecific, with a mild pleocytosis (10–500 cells/$mm^3$), elevated protein level, and depressed glucose concentration. Neuroimaging may show evidence of hydrocephalus, or single or multiple granulomatous lesions.

Diagnosis is confirmed by the isolation of the organism from the CSF, which is difficult, demonstrating the presence of antibodies in the CSF, or by detection of histoplasma antigen in the CSF. The organism grows on standard mycologic media in 1 to 6 weeks; it is important to culture at least 10 ml of CSF. Multiple specimens may be necessary [6]. A DNA probe for *H. capsulatum* permits rapid identification of growth. Demonstration of typical intracellular yeast forms with Gomori methenamine silver or other stains strongly supports the diagnosis in the appropriate clinical and epidemiologic situation. Both mycelial and yeast phase antigens are used in serologic testing by complement fixation. A fourfold rise in yeast-phase titers, or a single titer of 1:32 or greater is presumptive evidence of active infection. In the immunodiffusion test, H bands, although rare, are indicative of acute infection. Serologic diagnosis of meningitis is problematic because of false-positive results with other fungal infections. The mycelial-phase complement-fixing antibody seems to be the most sensitive and specific. The use of semiquantitative histoplasma antigen detection in serum or urine provides a sensitive tool for diagnosis and for monitoring response to therapy in patients with progressive disseminated disease [7]. Newer antigen tests used on CSF specimens may demonstrate higher antigen values in the CSF samples compared with serum or urine samples and confirm the diagnosis of CNS histoplasmosis [6].

## Treatment

Amphotericin B is the mainstay of therapy for disseminated histoplasmosis. In children with PDH of infancy, even with meningitis, the prognosis is excellent with amphotericin B therapy for 4 to 6 weeks [8]. Some experts use a shorter course for CNS involvement. For treatment beyond infancy, Amphotericin B often is recommended for 3 to 4 months, followed by 9 to 12 months of an oral azole, especially in cases of recurrence. Liposomal amphotericin B reaches higher concentrations in the brain, however, no comparative studies of these two agents have been performed. Itraconazole does not enter the CSF; however, in animal studies it has been found to be superior to fluconazole. It is the preferred azole for follow-up therapy [8]. In patients with irreversible severe immunodeficiency, life-long maintenance therapy may be required. Persistent pleocytosis or the presence of *Histoplasma* antigen after 1 year of therapy would support continued treatement [6]. Focal cerebral or spinal cord lesions that are not associated with meningitis should be treated with amphotericin B induction, but itraconazole may be used for follow-up therapy [6].

The treatment of meningitis and encephalitis is mostly supportive, but specific interventions, such as anticonvulsant medication for seizures or CSF diversion or shunting for hydrocephalus may be necessary.

## *Prognosis*

Prognosis in cases of Histoplasma meningitis often depends on treatment of the underlying problem.

## References

1. Medoff G, Kobayashi GS, Painter A, Travis S. Morphogenesis and pathogenicity of *Histoplasma capsulatum*. *Infect Immun*. 1987; 55:1355–1358.
2. Leggiadro RJ, Barrett F, Hughes WT. Disseminated histoplasmosis of infancy. *Pedatr Infect Dis*. 1988; 7:799–805.
3. Odio CM, Navarrete M, Carrillo JM, Mora L, Carranza A. Disseminated histoplasmosis of infants. *Pediatr Infect Dis J*. 1999; 18:1065–1068.
4. Wheat LJ, Batteiger BE, Sathapatayavongs B. *Histoplasma capsulatum* infections of the central nervous system. A clinical review. *Medicine* (Baltimore) 1990; 69:244–260.
5. Ciulla TA, Piper HC, Wheat LJ. Presumed ocular histoplasmosis syndrome: update on epidemiology, pathogenesis, and photodynamic, antiangiogenic, and surgical therapies. *Curr Opin Ophthalmol*. 2001; 6:442–449.
6. Wheat LJ, Musial CE, Jenny-Avital E. Diagnosis and management of central nervous system histoplasmosis. *Clin Infect Dis*. 2005; 40:844–852.
7. Wheat LJ, Kohler RB, Tewari RP. Diagnosis of disseminated histoplasmosis by detection of *Histoplasma capsulatum* in serum and urine specimens. *N Engl J Med*. 1986; 314:83–88.
8. Wheat LJ, Freifeld AG, et al. Clinical practice guidelines for the management of patients with histoplasmosis: 2007 Update by the Infectious Diseases Society of America *Clin Infect Dis*. 2007; 45:807–825.

# Chapter 33
# *Coccidioides* Species

**Barbara Stechenberg, M.D.**

## Coccidioidomycosis

### *Introduction*

Coccidioidomycosis is an infection caused by the closely related dimorphic fungi, *Coccidioides immitis*, and the recently identified, *Coccidioides posadasii*. It is endemic in generally arid regions of the southwestern United States, Central America, and South America. Primary infection often goes unrecognized; extrapulmonary dissemination is rare. Coccidioidal meningitis is the most severe manifestation of dissemination.

### *Epidemiology*

The fungus grows best in damp, alkaline soil. Primary infection occurs most frequently in the summer and fall, after the rainy seasons that facilitate hyphal growth. The minute arthroconidia of the mycelial saprophytic phase are highly infectious; airborne, they are inhaled, or, rarely, enter the host through non-intact skin. In the infected host, they round up into spherules, which develop endospores that develop into new spherules. Variation in seasonal infection rates may be attributed to the occurrence of dust storms, earthquakes, or other events. Clustering has occurred after archaeologic digging or recreational activities. Filipinos, Hispanics, blacks, neonates, elderly, pregnant women, and immunocompromised persons, particularly those with human immunodeficiency virus (HIV) infection are at increased risk of dissemination. Person-to-person transmission does not occur. There are more than 100,000 cases per year in the United States; probably less than 0.1% are associated with meningitis.

L.L. Barton and N.R. Friedman (eds.), *The Neurological Manifestations of Pediatric Infectious Diseases and Immunodeficiency Syndromes.*

## Pathogenesis

Primary infection occurs in the lungs. Growth of the organism stimulates intense inflammation. This initial neutrophilic inflammatory response does not control infection, and granulomatous formation eventually predominates. Histologically, one finds pyogranulomatous inflammation containing spherules and endospores. Clinically apparent extrapulmonary disease occurs in approximately 1% of infected individuals by lymphohematogenous spread.

## Clinical Manifestations

The incubation period is typically 10 to 16 days, with a range from 1 week to 1 month. Primary infection, acquired by the respiratory route, is often asymptomatic or self-limited. Symptomatic disease, approximately 40% of infections, resembles influenza with malaise, fever, cough, chest pain, headache, fatigue, and myalgias. Transient rashes are frequent in children; early in the disease, they may be erythematous and maculopapular, whereas, later, one may see erythema multiforme or erythema nodosum. Arthralgias or arthritis may occur as a hypersensitivity manifestation. Pulmonary involvement is highly variable, but patchy, diffuse, or miliary pneumonic infiltrates with hilar adenopathy are common. Chronic pulmonary infiltrates are rare.

## Neurological Manifestations

Meningitis may be the sole manifestation of dissemination, particularly in Caucasians or it may occur with widespread dissemination including skin, lungs, bones, and joints; it usually develops within several months of the initial infection but may develop many months later. The most common symptoms are headache, lethargy, ataxia, and vomiting. Because signs of meningeal irritation are often absent, it may be hard to differentiate from the headache of primary disease. The headache associated with meningitis is usually more persistent and severe. Sometimes there are signs of focal neurological deficits. Tremulousness and intention tremor are common. Papilledema is very frequent in children [1]. Meningismus is seen in approximately half of cases. Hydrocephalus with signs and symptoms of intracranial hypertension may be the dominant finding on presentation [2].

## Neuropathology

The neuropathology is characterized by granulomatous and suppurative basilar meningitis, with frequent parenchymal involvement with granulomas and abscesses of the spinal cord and brain [3,4]. Vasculitis, observable pathologically, may be associated with the abrupt appearance of infarction and stroke-like focal findings [5].

## *Diagnosis*

The diagnosis of primary pulmonary coccidioidomycosis is based on serology and, less commonly, sputum culture. Eosinophilia is a frequent hematologic finding. Routine cerebrospinal fluid (CSF) analysis in patients with meningitis is not specific, but usually reveals moderate mononuclear pleocytosis. There may be an eosinophilic CSF pleocytosis, a finding not specific to this organism. The CSF glucose level is usually low and the protein level is elevated. Ventricular fluid abnormalities are often not as dramatic as those found in CSF from the lumbosacral space.

CSF culture for fungus is often negative, whereas CSF serology using complement-fixing (CF) antibody is often positive. The diagnosis is confirmed by culture, serology, or both. Occasionally, the diagnosis must be inferred from an abnormal CSF result, with positive serum serology (CF or immunodiffusion test) results, or culture from a nonmeningeal source.

Neuroimaging is an important adjunct to diagnosis. Magnetic resonance imaging (MRI) scan detected abnormalities in 76% of patients with coccidioidal meningitis, compared with 41.6% seen with computed tomographic scan in a recent study [6]. The most common abnormalities were hydrocephalus, basilar meningitis, and cerebral infarction. Significantly increased mortality was seen with hydrocephalus and with hydrocephalus with infarction [6].

The differential diagnosis of pulmonary coccidioidomycosis includes pneumonia caused by other fungi, numerous bacteria, and mycobacteria. Coccidioidal meningitis must, likewise, be differentiated from central nervous system infection by viruses, mycobacteria, and other fungi.

## *Treatment*

The therapy of primary pulmonary coccidioidomycosis is generally supportive. Patients with severe, progressive disease or in high-risk categories are candidates for antifungal therapy, generally oral azoles.

In contrast, coccidioidal meningitis was almost universally fatal before amphotericin B treatment. Death from this disease is rare now. Treatment guidelines for coccidioidal disease have been published by the Infectious Disease Society of America [7]. Treatment with fluconazole or itraconazole has supplanted amphotericin because of their efficacy and safety.

Therapy with fluconazole without concurrent amphotericin B has been associated with response rates of approximately 80% [8]. The dose of fluconazole in children is 12 mg/kg/d. Itraconazole has been reported to be comparably effective in adults [6].

Some physicians also initiate intrathecal amphotericin B in addition to an azole with the belief that response is more rapid with this approach. Recent reports of successful treatment of Coccidioidal meningitis with voriconazole in adults are intriguing and open further therapeutic possibilities [9,10]. Improvement is usually gradual, over months; because of a very high relapse rate, therapy is lifelong.

Attention to CSF flow dynamics is crucial because almost all children develop obstructive hydrocephalus requiring shunting [2,11]. Rarely, a second shunt is required to drain a "trapped" fourth ventricle. Follow-up MRI scan evaluations may be necessary because focal complications may emerge during treatment.

## References

1. Harrison HR, Galgiani JN, Reynolds AF Jr, Sprunger LW, Friedman AD. Amphotericin B and imidazole therapy for coccidioidal meningitis in children. *Pediatr Infect Dis.* 1983; 2:216–221.
2. Johnson RH, Einstein HE. Coccidioidal Meningitis. *Clin Infect Dis.* 2006; 42:103–107.
3. Erly WK, Bellon RJ, Seeger JF, Carmody RF. MR imaging of acute coccidioidal meningitis. *AJNR* 1999; 20:509–514.
4. Mischel PS, Vinters HV. Coccidioidomycosis of the central nervous system: neuropathological and vasculopathic manifestations and clinical correlates. *Clin Infect Dis.* 1995; 20:400–405.
5. Williams PL, Johnson R, Pappagianis D, et al. Vasculitic and encephalitic complications associated with *Coccidioides immitis* infection of the central nervous system in humans: report of 10 cases and review. *Clin Inf Dis.* 1992; 14:673–682.
6. Arsura EL, Johnson R, Penrose J, et al. Neuroimaging as a guide to predict outcomes for patients with coccidioidal meningitis. *Clin Infect Dis.* 2005; 40:624–627.
7. Galgiani JN, Ampel NM, Blair JE, et al. Coccidioidomycosis. *Clin Infect Dis.* 2005; 41:1217–1223.
8. Galgiani JN, Catanzaro A, Cloud GA, et al. Fluconazole therapy for coccidioidal meningitis. The NIAID-Mycoses Study Group. *Ann Intern Med.* 1993; 119:28–35.
9. Cortez KJ, Walsh TJ, Bennett JE. Successful treatment of coccidioidal meningitis with voriconazole. *Clin Infect Dis.* 2003; 36:1619–1622.
10. Proia LA, Tenorio AR. Successful use of voriconazole for treatment of *Coccidioides* meningitis. *Antimicrob Agents Chemother.* 2004; 48:2341.
11. Shehab ZM, Britton H, Dunn JH. Imidazole therapy of coccidioidal meningitis in children. *Pediatr Infect Dis J.* 1988; 7:40–44.

# Chapter 34
# Phaeohyphomycoses

**Barbara Stechenberg, M.D.**

## Cerebral Phaeohyphomycosis

### *Introduction and Epidemiology*

Dematiaceous fungi have melanin-like pigments in the cell walls and spores. They rarely cause a variety of infections in humans known as phaeohyphomycosis, the most severe of which is cerebral disease. The most common cause of cerebral phaeohyphomycosis is *Cladophialophora bantiana*, accounting for 48% in a large series [1,2]. The next most common was *Ramichloridium mackenzei* (13%), followed by *Ochroconis gallopavum* (5%) [1]. Many are found throughout the world in soil and decaying vegetation, although *R. mackenzei* has only been seen in the Middle East. They are most common in tropical and subtropical zones [3].

### *Pathogenesis*

Most cerebral infections were thought to arise from extension from adjacent paranasal sinuses; the spores were presumably inhaled and proliferated in the sinuses. Other infections result from penetrating trauma or contaminated wounds. However, in a recent review, most cases had no underlying cause or immunodeficiency [1]. The pathogenesis is, therefore, largely unknown. Melanin itself may act as a virulence factor and have a predilection for central nervous system localization.

### *Clinical and Neurological Manifestations*

Most cases present as brain abscess with focal neurological deficits or seizures. Symptomatic sinusitis, fever, and headache are uncommon. A small number of cases have presented as meningitis, encephalitis, or myelitis.

L.L. Barton and N.R. Friedman (eds.), *The Neurological Manifestations of Pediatric Infectious Diseases and Immunodeficiency Syndromes.*

## *Diagnosis*

Neuroimaging usually shows a single enhancing lesion in the frontal or parietal lobe. Cerebrospinal fluid examination reveals increased protein and decreased glucose levels and no visible organisms. Opening pressure may be normal or extremely elevated. Etiologic diagnosis is made by aspiration of the abscess or surgical resection. The fungal pigments cause the hyphae to appear golden brown when the fluid is examined microscopically. The fungi grow relatively quickly from clinical specimens, but identification may require the assistance of a reference laboratory.

## *Treatment*

Treatment requires both antifungal therapy and reduction of the abscess. Complete surgical evacuation is optimal. Most clinical strains have been susceptible to itraconazole and amphotericin B [4]. Combination therapy has been used initially with prolonged itraconazole treatment as follow-up. Other newer azoles, such as voriconazole and posaconazole, may be useful therapies [5]. Survival rates have improved, but are in the 50% range. Seizures are treated with anticonvulsant medications, often, long term.

## References

1. Revankar SG, Sutton DA, Rinaldi MG. Primary central nervous system phaeohyphomycosis: a review of 101 cases. *Clin Infect Dis*. 2004; 38:206–216.
2. Banerjee U, Mohapatra AK, Sarkar C, Chaudhery R. Cladosporiosis (cerebral phaeohyphomycosis) of brain—a case report. *Mycopathologia*. 1989; 105:163–166.
3. Palaoglu S, Sav A, Basak T, Yalcinlar Y, Scheithauer BW. Cerebral phaeohyphomycosis. *Neurosurgery*. 1993; 33:894–897.
4. Caligoirne RB, Resende MA, Melillo PH, Pelusco CP, Carmo FH, Azevedo V. In vitro susceptibility of chromoblastomycosis and phaeohyphomycosis agents to antifungal drugs. *Med Mycol*. 1999; 37:405–409.
5. Revankar SG. Phaeohyphomycosis. *Infect Dis Clin N Am*. 2006; 20:609–620.

# Section V
# Protozoa

# Chapter 35
# Protozoal Infections

Ana M. Alvarez, M.D. and Mobeen H. Rathore, M.D., C.P.E., F.A.A.P.

## Protozoal Infections

Protozoa cause a wide variety of clinical syndromes, from asymptomatic infections to severe and fatal illnesses. Some of these organisms predominantly affect the nervous system, whereas others only rarely do so. When parasitic infections are suspected, areas of endemicity, risk factors, and mode of acquisition must be considered and pertinent history and appropriate diagnostic workup should be performed.

## Toxoplasmosis

### *Introduction*

Infection with *Toxoplasma gondii*, although relatively common in humans, is usually asymptomatic. Clinically significant disease occurs only in a small percentage of cases. The disease may result from congenital infection ("congenital toxoplasmosis") or infection acquired after birth ("acquired toxoplasmosis").

### *Epidemiology*

Toxoplasmosis has a worldwide distribution. In the United States, the incidence of acquired infection ranges from 3 to 20% in different population groups [1] and of congenital toxoplasmosis from 1 in 1,000 to 1 in 10,000 live births [2]. Transplacental infection rates are 17% in the first trimester, 25% in the second trimester, and 65% in the third trimester [3]. However, there is an inverse correlation between the incidence of fetal infection and the severity of fetal damage at different stages of gestation. The toxoplasmosis seroprevalence among HIV-infected patients in the United States varies from 10 to 45% [4]. The incidence of toxoplasmic encephalitis (TE) among patients receiving antiretroviral therapy and prophylactic regimens has decreased

L.L. Barton and N.R. Friedman (eds.), *The Neurological Manifestations of Pediatric Infectious Diseases and Immunodeficiency Syndromes.*

markedly [4]. This presentation is rare in children and generally is a consequence of congenital infection. Most of the reported cases have occurred in children with underlying medical conditions such as bone marrow transplantation, neoplasms of the reticuloendothelial system, and acquired immunodeficiency syndrome (AIDS) [5].

## *Pathogenesis*

*Toxoplasma gondii* is an obligate intracellular protozoan of the class coccidia. It possesses two distinct life cycles. The sexual cycle occurs in cats, which are the definitive hosts. The asexual cycle occurs in other mammals, including humans, and in some birds. Human infection occurs mainly by ingestion of oocysts in soil, cat litter, or contaminated food, by consumption of under-cooked meat, which contains tissue cysts, and transplacentally. Most congenital infections occur after primary maternal infection during pregnancy. Women co-infected with human immunodeficiency virus (HIV) and toxoplasma may transmit toxoplasma transplacentally to their offspring at times of reactivated maternal parasitemia [6]. Infection has also occurred after solid organ and bone marrow transplantation [2].

## *Clinical Manifestations*

### Congenital Toxoplasmosis

Infections occurring in the first two trimesters of pregnancy are frequently associated with miscarriages, stillbirths, and severe disease. However, most infections occur in the last trimester, and most infants are asymptomatic at birth. When signs and symptoms are present in the neonatal period, they include hepatosplenomegaly, generalized lymphadenopathy, a maculopapular rash, jaundice, anemia, chorioretinitis, microcephaly or hydrocephalus, and seizures [3]. The most severely affected neonates may die within a few days of birth. A large percentage of the initially asymptomatic patients eventually develop symptoms months to years later. Chorioretinitis is the most common finding, usually bilateral in neonates and unilateral thereafter. Ocular lesions appear as ill-defined yellow areas that develop central scarring and hyperpigmentation near the macula [7]. Hypopituitarism, manifested as growth hormone deficiency, has been described as an additional complication of congenital toxoplasmosis [8]. Most children with untreated congenital infection have permanent ocular and/or neurological sequelae regardless of their age at presentation [9,10]. However, when infection is diagnosed and treated early, the overall prognosis is much better [11,12].

### Acquired Toxoplasmosis

It is estimated that only 10 to 20% of infected immunocompetent persons develop clinical signs and symptoms [4]. Lymphadenopathy is the most frequent presentation.

The cervical lymph nodes are most commonly affected. However, suboccipital, supraclavicular, axillary, and inguinal lymph nodes can be affected [13]. Patients are usually afebrile. In a few cases, patients present with a clinical picture similar to infectious mononucleosis (fever, malaise, fatigue, sore throat, and myalgias). Chorioretinitis seems to be a more common manifestation than previously recognized [14]. Myocarditis and polymyositis have also been reported, but they are rare in immunocompetent hosts [15].

Immunocompromised hosts are at higher risk for severe and potentially life-threatening toxoplasmosis. Encephalitis is the most common manifestation. Patients may also present with pneumonitis, myocarditis, and chorioretinitis [16,17].

## *Neurological Manifestations*

### Congenital Toxoplasmosis

Neonatal neurological manifestations include microcephaly, hydrocephalus, seizures, intracranial calcifications, and increased cerebrospinal fluid (CSF) protein and mononuclear cells. Diffuse cerebral calcifications are frequently demonstrable by cranial radiography, ultrasonography, or computed tomographic (CT) scan.

Neurological sequelae of congenital toxoplasmosis, which may occur after a symptomatic or an asymptomatic neonatal period, include mental retardation, seizures, spasticity, visual defects, and deafness [9,10]. Of 70 untreated, congenitally infected infants with symptomatic neurological disease followed for at least 4 years by Eichenwald, 89% had psychomotor retardation, 83% had seizures, 76% had spasticity, 69% had severe visual impairment, 44% had hydrocephalus or microcephaly, and 17% had deafness [3]. Similar sequelae were noted in the 31 infants who presented with systemic symptomatology (e.g., fever, jaundice, hepatosplenomegaly, and lymphadenopathy), but to a slightly lesser degree. Nine percent of the group with neurological disease on presentation and 16% of the group with systemic presenting abnormalities were healthy at 4 years of age. Follow-up studies of untreated infants with subclinical infection are sparse; the numbers comprising each study are small and duration of follow-up is generally short [3]. Of the four initially asymptomatic patients followed for 4 years by Eichenwald, two were mentally retarded and two had seizures. Others have noted chorioretinitis, often recurrent, in approximately 40 to 50% of untreated patients older than 5 years of age.

Early detection and treatment has a significant impact on the prognosis. In a French cohort of 327 congenitally infected children who received early treatment, only 24% had at least one retinochoroidal lesion, and 64% of these children had normal vision in both eyes [11]. In a cohort of 120 treated children in the United States, of the 24 without substantial systemic/neurological findings at birth, 100% had normal hearing, motor and cognitive function, and 85% had normal vision. Of the 96 children with moderate to severe systemic/neurological findings at birth, 100% had normal hearing, 80% had normal motor function, 73% had normal cognitive function, but only 15% had normal vision at subsequent follow up [12].

### Acquired Toxoplasmosis

TE is the most common neurological manifestation of acquired toxoplasmosis in immunocompromised patients, particularly in patients with AIDS [17]. Typically, the presentation is subacute, but it may be abrupt in a few patients. Headaches and neurological abnormalities, such as hemiparesis and abnormalities of speech, are common initial symptoms. Other clinical findings that may be present include cranial nerve palsies, altered mental status, seizures, weakness, cerebellar signs, and movement disorders. Neuropsychiatric manifestations, such as paranoid psychosis, dementia, anxiety, and agitation may be the predominant symptoms in some patients. A few patients present with signs and symptoms of a radiculomyelopathy. Other less common manifestations include panhypopituitarism, hyponatremia (either secondary to the syndrome of inappropriate antidiuretic hormone secretion or cerebral salt wasting) [18], and a diffuse form of encephalitis that occurs acutely and progresses rapidly to a fatal outcome [4,19]. Characteristic radiologic findings in HIV-infected patients with TE include multiple ring-enhancing lesions in brain CT and magnetic resonance imaging (MRI) scans. MRI scanning has superior sensitivity [20]. These characteristic radiologic findings may be absent in bone marrow transplant patients with TE. In these patients, the brain lesions are often initially hemorrhagic [21]. Permanent sequelae, such as seizure disorders and focal neurological deficits, may occur in these patients.

## *Neuropathology*

Histopathologic examination may reveal focal leptomeningitis with adjacent necrosis in the cerebral cortex, subcortical white matter, and basal ganglia; focal cerebral calcifications; and scattered glial nodules [7]. Parasites can be found within the intima of arterioles, venules, and capillaries [3].

## *Diagnosis*

The diagnosis of congenital toxoplasmosis can be made by visualization of tachyzoites in body fluids (CSF, blood, bone marrow aspirates) or in tissue biopsy (brain, placenta), by serology, or by polymerase chain reaction (PCR) [22–24]. Serologic diagnosis is based on IgM or IgA assays performed within the first 6 months of life or IgG beyond the first year of life. Specific IgA antibody seems to be more sensitive than IgM in the neonatal period [25]. These tests should be sent to a reference laboratory.

Serologic tests are the most common methods of diagnosis of acquired toxoplasmosis in immunocompetent hosts. However, serologic diagnosis in immunocompromised patients is often problematic. In a patient with characteristic clinical and radiological findings, improvement after an empiric therapeutic trial supports a presumptive diagnosis [4]. Demonstration of the organism by direct visualization or by PCR may be necessary to confirm the diagnosis [24].

## *Treatment*

### Congenital Toxoplasmosis

Treatment is recommended for all infected infants. Therapy during the first year of life has been shown to arrest signs of active disease, to improve cognitive and motor outcome, and to diminish the frequency of seizures and chorioretinitis [9,11,12]. Pyrimethamine and sulfadiazine with leucovorin (folic acid) should be administered for 1 year [26]. Corticosteroids are a consideration for patients with CSF protein equal to or more than 1 g/dl or with active vision-threatening chorioretinitis [1]. Seizures are managed with anticonvulsants. Hydrocephalus may necessitate ventriculoperitoneal shunt placement.

Treatment of primary infection in pregnant women with spiramycin is recommended because it may prevent transmission to the fetus. If there is confirmation of fetal infection after 17 weeks of gestation or if maternal infection occurs in the third trimester of pregnancy, maternal/fetal treatment with pyrimethamine/sulfadiazine should be instituted [26].

### Acquired Toxoplasmosis

Treatment of immunocompetent children is limited to those who have chorioretinitis or significant organ damage. However, all immunocompromised children with toxoplasmosis should receive treatment. Pyrimethamine and sulfadiazine supplemented with leucovorin are the agents of choice. Clindamycin is an acceptable alternative to sulfadiazine, when the latter agent is not available or not tolerated [2]. The recommended duration of therapy is 2 weeks beyond resolution of signs and symptoms in immunocompetent children, and 4 to 6 weeks beyond complete resolution of signs and symptoms in immunocompromised children [1]. Lifelong suppressive therapy is recommended for HIV-infected children with a history of toxoplasmosis. There is not enough data regarding the safety of discontinuing primary or secondary prophylaxis in HIV-infected children who are receiving highly active antiretroviral therapy (HAART) [2].

# Malaria

## *Introduction*

Malaria is a febrile illness that results from invasion of erythrocytes by protozoa of the genus *Plasmodium*. Although uncommon in the United States, malaria is one of the major causes of morbidity in tropical and semitropical regions of the world.

## Epidemiology

Worldwide, 300 to 500 million cases and 1.5 to 2.7 million deaths are reported annually [27]. Mortality has increased in recent years, most likely secondary to rising resistance to conventional antimalarial agents [28]. Children aged 6 months to 5 years are the most frequently affected. Congenital infection occurs in 0.3% and 7.4% of infants born to immune and nonimmune infected mothers, respectively. Approximately 1,000 cases are reported in the United States annually; most are imported [29]. However, locally acquired cases have been reported in several states, including recent cases in Florida [30,31]. Possible sources for these cases include international travelers and immigrant population [27,32]. Local transmission from imported infected mosquitoes to persons working or living near international airports has also been reported [33].

## Pathogenesis

The genus *Plasmodium* belongs to the class sporozoa. Four species of *Plasmodium* can infect humans: *P. vivax*, *P. falciparum*, *P. malariae*, and *P. ovale*. The two most common species worldwide are *P. vivax* and *P. falciparum*. The transmission principally occurs by the bite of an infected female Anopheles mosquito. Inside the human host, these parasites undergo an exoerythrocytic cycle of growth in the liver and an erythrocytic cycle within the red blood cells as part of their complex life cycle. Transmission can also occur congenitally and through transfusion, organ transplantation, and the use of contaminated needles or syringes [27].

## Clinical Manifestations

Clinical manifestations vary with the infecting species and the malaria-specific immune status of the host. Nonimmune individuals tend to have more severe disease [34]. The classic symptoms are periodic fever, chills, sweating, and headaches. Very young children may present only with a very high and continuous fever without the cyclic pattern observed in older children and adults [35]. Other symptoms include nausea, vomiting, diarrhea, cough, arthralgia, and abdominal and back pain. Hepatosplenomegaly is common [36,37].

*P. falciparum* malaria infections are associated with the highest morbidity and mortality. Severe anemia, hypoglycemia, metabolic acidosis, respiratory and renal failure, abnormal bleeding, shock, and cerebral malaria may occur [38]. *P. vivax* and *P. ovale* malaria may relapse for up to 3 to 5 years after the primary infection because of latent stages of the parasite in the liver. Malaria secondary to *P. malariae* has been associated with glomerulonephritis and chronic parasitemia, which may be asymptomatic [34].

Children with congenitally acquired malaria usually present at 2 to 8 weeks of age. Clinical manifestations may be similar to acquired malaria and include irritability, fever, chills, jaundice, and hepatosplenomegaly [35,39]. Seizures are indicative of central nervous system involvement and carry a poor prognosis [7].

## *Neurological Manifestations*

Seizures, often prolonged, are very common in children with severe malaria. They may be secondary to hyperpyrexia, hypoglycemia, or cerebral malaria. Differentiating between febrile seizures and cerebral malaria is often problematic.

Cerebral malaria is the most serious neurological complication of *P. falciparum* malaria. Typically, there is a 1- to 3-day history of fever, after which, the onset of neurological symptoms is abrupt; the transition from a normal sensorium to coma can be a matter of hours. Early symptoms include decreased oral intake, vomiting, cough, headache, confusion, and irritability. Seizures may occur before or after the onset of coma and may have subtle presentations (e.g., nystagmus, salivation, minor twitching of extremities or lips, or an irregular breathing pattern). Abnormalities on physical examination of patients with cerebral malaria include opisthotonos, pupillary changes, gaze abnormalities, abnormal corneal reflexes, retinal hemorrhages, papilledema, hypotonia, and Cheyne–Stokes or Kussmaul respirations. Nuchal rigidity is usually absent [34,40,41].

Cerebral malaria should be considered in a patient with malaria who remains unconscious for more than 1 hour after a convulsion. The depth of coma should be assessed using a coma scale. The Blantyre Coma Scale (BCS) (Table 35.1) is a modified and simplified Glasgow Coma scale, which has been used in a number of studies of cerebral malaria in children, especially in young, nonverbal children.

**Table 35.1** The Blantyre Coma Scale

| | | Score |
|---|---|---|
| Best motor response | Localizes painful stimulus[a] | 2 |
| | Withdraws limb from pain[b] | 1 |
| | Nonspecific or absent response | 0 |
| Verbal response | Appropriate cry | 2 |
| | Moan or inappropriate cry | 1 |
| | None | 0 |
| Eye movements | Directed (e.g., follows mother's face) | 1 |
| | Not directed | 0 |
| | Total | 0–5 |

[a]Rub knuckles on patient's sternum.
[b]Firm pressure on thumbnail bed with horizontal pencil.
A state of unarousable coma is reached at a score of less than 3.
This scale can be used repeatedly to assess improvement or deterioration.

A BCS score of 2 or less in children with *P. falciparum* parasitemia and no other identified cause of encephalopathy is considered indicative of cerebral malaria. This scale is also useful to assess subsequent improvement or deterioration [38,42]. Children with cerebral malaria often have increased intracranial pressure (ICP), which is not clinically apparent [43]. Lumbar puncture can exclude other causes of mental status changes.

Less than 10% of survivors of cerebral malaria may have long-term neurological sequelae such as motor impairment (hemiplegia, generalized spasticity, and cerebellar ataxia), speech disorders, cortical blindness, and behavioral and learning deficits [40,44]. Depth of coma on admission, multiple convulsions, and duration of unconsciousness have been identified as risk factors for these sequelae [45].

Neurological sequelae, such as cranial nerve dysfunction, polyneuropathy, and cerebellar ataxia, can also develop after severe malaria even in the absence of diagnosis of cerebral malaria [42]. A postmalaria neurological syndrome has been described in patients who recover from *P. falciparum* malaria. This syndrome is transient and can occur up to 2 months after the acute illness. Manifestations include acute confusional state or psychosis, one or more generalized seizures, and/or tremor. Patients recover completely without any permanent sequelae [46,47].

Some antimalarial drugs are potentially neurotoxic. The use of mefloquine and chloroquine has been associated with an acute self-limiting neuropsychiatric syndrome. Tremor has been reported to occur before or after treatment with chloroquine, quinine, mefloquine, and artemether [48,49].

The mortality of cerebral malaria is high, ranging from 6 to 50%, with an average of 18.6% in African children [42,50]. Risk factors that have been associated with higher mortality are respiratory distress, impairment of consciousness, hypoglycemia, jaundice, intractable seizures, lactic acidosis, and papilledema [51].

## Neuropathology

The pathogenesis of cerebral malaria is controversial. It may be the result of sequestration of parasitized erythrocytes in the microvasculature of the brain leading to localized ischemia, release of inflammatory cytokines and mediators such as tumor necrosis factor and nitric oxide, and subsequent tissue injury [42,52]. The classic histopathological findings in malignant cerebral malaria are brain vessels plugged with parasitized red cells, accompanied by ring hemorrhages and small focal inflammatory reactions (called malarial or Durck granulomas) [52,53].

## Diagnosis

Diagnosis is made by identification of the parasite on stained thick and thin blood films. Confirmation and species identification are crucial in guiding therapy. Other diagnostic modalities include detection of parasite DNA by PCR and antigen detection tests (known as rapid diagnostic tests [RDT]), but they are considered experimental in the United States [27].

CSF parameters are usually normal, but mild pleocytosis (<20 white blood cells/ml) and slightly elevated protein levels (<40 mg/dl) can be present. The electroencephalogram (EEG) is diffusely abnormal [54]. Abnormalities found on CT scans of the head include loss of sulci and loss of spaces around the cisterns [55]. MRI scans of the brain may show nonenhancing high-density signal foci suggestive of capillary occlusion [56]. However, these neuroradiological findings are nonspecific.

## *Treatment*

The treatment of choice of malaria is a blood schizontocide, such as chloroquine, quinine, quinidine, mefloquine, halofantrine, and artemisinin and its derivatives. These drugs act rapidly, inducing remission of symptoms. The choice of antimalarial treatment depends on the species, possibility (or probability) of drug resistance, and the severity of the illness. Resistance to all classes of antimalarials, except, to date, to the artemisinin derivatives, has been reported [28]. Chloroquine resistance is widespread, limiting its use in certain geographic locations. Malaria acquired in Africa is most commonly secondary to chloroquine-resistant *P. falciparum* [27].

Patients with severe malaria and cerebral malaria in the United States should be treated with intravenous quinidine. This drug has potential cardiac toxicity and should be administered with continuous cardiac monitoring. As soon as patients are conscious and able to swallow, treatment should be changed to oral quinine. The total duration of therapy (intravenous and oral) is 5 to 7 days [28,35,42]. Artemisinin derivatives are active against multidrug-resistant *P. falciparum* and have been shown effective for severe malaria, including cerebral malaria [28,57,58]. Artemisinin-based combinations (ACTs) are currently recommended by the World Health Organization to treat malaria in all countries experiencing resistance problems [59]. Intravenous artesunate is now available in the United States.

Treatment for uncomplicated *P. falciparum* malaria depends on the susceptibility to chloroquine. If susceptible, patients can be treated with chloroquine orally for 48 hours. For chloroquine-resistant malaria, the recommendation is to use oral quinine in combination with doxycycline, tetracycline, or clindamycin for 7 days, or atovaquone–proguanil for 3 days [60].

*P. vivax* malaria and *P. ovale* malaria should be treated with a 14-day course of chloroquine followed by a 3-day course of primaquine. Primaquine is an effective tissue schizontocide and is the drug of choice to eradicate the dormant stages of *P. vivax* and *P. ovale* in the liver [28,35].

Supportive measures include antipyretics, rehydration, seizure control, and close monitoring. Patients with severe or cerebral malaria should be admitted to an intensive care unit for monitoring and management of potential complications (respiratory failure, renal failure, hypoglycemia, hypovolemia, and lactic acidosis) [38,42]. When parasitemia exceeds 15%, or when it is between 5% and 15% in a patient with other signs of poor prognosis, exchange transfusion should be considered [61]. The use of phenobarbital to prevent seizures in children with cerebral malaria has been associated with an increased mortality and is, therefore, not recommended [62,63].

# Amebiasis

## *Epidemiology*

Amebiasis is the disease caused by the pathogenic protozoa *Entamoeba histolytica*. It is a major cause of infectious diarrhea in the developing countries of the world.

It is estimated that worldwide approximately 500 million people are carriers, 50 million people have active disease, and 50,000 to 100,000 people die of amebiasis per year [64]. Areas of high prevalence include Africa, the Indian subcontinent, the Far East, and Central and South America. Although the prevalence rate in the United States is only approximately 4%, travel to endemic areas with a prolonged stay (>1 month) predisposes individuals to amebic infections [65]. Amebiasis can occur in all age groups. However, the incidence peaks in the very young (<3 years of age) and in people older than 40 years [64].

## *Pathogenesis*

*E. histolytica* is responsible for a wide variety of symptomatic diseases. In contrast, morphologically identical *E. dispar* has only been associated with an asymptomatic carrier state. The two species exist as cysts and trophozoites. Human are the natural host and reservoir. Transmission occurs via the fecal–oral route.

## *Clinical Manifestations*

When clinically apparent, amebiasis may present as intestinal or extraintestinal disease. Intestinal disease varies from mild diarrhea to severe illness with fever, chills, abdominal pain, and bloody diarrhea (amebic dysentery). Complications include perforation with peritonitis, intussusception and necrotizing enterocolitis, and amebomas (large intestinal masses of trophozoites) [64,66].

Extraintestinal manifestations include liver abscesses and metastatic amebiasis (pleuropulmonary, pericardial, and cerebral abscesses). Liver abscesses are the most common extraintestinal presentation and occur in 1 to 7% of children with invasive amebiasis [66]. Symptoms in children include high fever, abdominal distention, irritability, tachypnea, and hepatomegaly. Diarrhea is uncommon. Mortality rate is high in young children, primarily because of delayed diagnosis [64].

Metastatic disease is thought to be secondary to direct extension from liver abscesses and less often from the intestine. Thoracic amebiasis (pleuropulmonary abscess, empyema, and bronchohepatic fistulae) is the most common type of metastatic disease, occurring in approximately 10% of patients with liver abscess. Pericardial amebiasis occurs in approximately 3% of patients with liver abscess, whereas cerebral amebiasis has been reported in 0.7 to 4.7% of patients with liver abscess [64,66,67].

## *Neurological Manifestations*

Patients with cerebral amebiasis present abruptly with altered consciousness and focal neurological deficits. Headaches are common. Seizures can occur. The disease may progress rapidly to death within 12 to 72 hours. Other sites are usually affected and non-neurological symptoms (abdominal pain and distention, cough, chest pain, and dyspnea) may predominate and be present for weeks or months before neurological symptoms [68].

The mortality rate is extremely high (>90%) although most reported cases are diagnosed postmortem. However, there are several reported survivors and the disease is no longer considered invariably fatal [69–72].

## *Neuropathology*

Amebic brain abscesses are thought to result from hematogenous spread from hepatic or pulmonary lesions. Their size varies from a centimeter in diameter to massive lesions that can occupy almost an entire lobe [68]. Histologically, the walls are composed of a thin connective tissue capsule containing amebic trophozoites. The fluid itself does not usually contain the amebas or inflammatory cells [66].

## *Diagnosis*

The diagnosis of intestinal amebiasis is made by identification of trophozoites or cysts in stool specimens. Serologic tests are used for the diagnosis of extraintestinal amebiasis [73]. CT scans may show single or multiple ring-like lesions [68,74] or irregular lesions without a surrounding capsule or enhancement [65,71]. MRI scans may offer better structural differentiation [74]. Brain biopsy demonstrates the trophozoites [68].

## *Treatment*

Treatment of amebiasis encompasses the elimination of organisms in the intestinal lumen (with a luminal agent) as well as eradication of tissue-invading trophozoites.

Asymptomatic carriers of *E. histolytica* should be treated with luminal agents such as iodoquinol, paromomycin, or diloxanide furoate. Patients with symptomatic intestinal or with extraintestinal disease should receive a 10-day course of metronidazole (or tinidazole) followed by a luminal agent [73].

Patients with invasive disease who fail the initial treatment should be treated with dehydroemetine followed by a luminal agent. Patients with liver abscess may also be treated with chloroquine phosphate and dehydroemetine followed by metronidazole or tinidazole [73]. Additionally, percutaneous or surgical aspiration may be beneficial for patients with large liver abscesses [75].

Cerebral amebiasis should be treated as other extraintestinal disease. Metronidazole has been used effectively in treating some cases. Surgical drainage in addition to medical treatment may be of benefit in selected cases [69–72,76].

## Amebic Meningoencephalitis

### *Introduction*

Infections of the central nervous system with free-living amebae were first described in 1965 [77]. Although rare, they have been reported worldwide and are associated with extremely high mortality. Amebic meningoencephalitis can be divided into two separate clinical entities: primary amebic meningoencephalitis (PAM) and granulomatous amebic encephalitis (GAE).

### *Epidemiology*

PAM is caused by *Naegleria fowleri* and occurs mostly in healthy children and young adults [78]. GAE secondary to *Acanthamoeba* occurs in immunocompromised and chronically ill patients [79,80]. GAE secondary to *Balamuthia* has been described in healthy and immunodeficient children and adults [81–83].

### *Pathogenesis*

The free-living amebae that have been linked to disease in humans are *N. fowleri*, *Acanthamoeba* species, and *Balamuthia mandrillaris*. *N. fowleri* is found in moist soil and in warm fresh water. It exists in three forms: trophozoites, flagellate forms, and cysts. *Acanthamoeba* are found as trophozoites and cysts in soil, fresh water, hot tubs, and sewage. Several species have been implicated in human disease. *Balamuthia mandrillaris*, formerly known as the leptomyxid ameba, is found in stagnant water [84].

## *Clinical Manifestations*

*N. fowleri* produces PAM, a fulminant and almost always fatal disease that resembles acute bacterial meningitis. It is a consequence of trophozoitic invasion of the brain through the cribriform plate via the olfactory nerves. Most infections occur during the spring and summer months and have been associated with swimming, diving, bathing, or playing in warm fresh water. However, cases without a history of contact with water have been reported [78,85].

Both *Acanthamoeba* and *Balamuthia* cause GAE, which has a subacute or chronic clinical course. Central nervous system infection with *Acanthamoeba* results from hematogenous spread from primary inoculation sites in the lungs or skin [7]. The pathogenesis and route of infection with *Balamuthia* are unclear, but probably similar [81]. Besides GAE, *Acanthamoeba* can also produce osteomyelitis, lung and sinus infection, skin infections, and keratitis [84]. This latter manifestation has been described in healthy individuals who wear contact lenses [86].

## *Neurological Manifestations*

### Primary Amebic Meningoencephalitis

After an incubation period of several days to 1 week, patients with PAM develop headaches, fever, and alterations in taste or smell. The disease progresses rapidly to vomiting, lethargy, altered mental status, nuchal rigidity, and seizures. Cerebellar ataxia and third, fourth, and sixth cranial nerve palsies are common. Increased ICP, cerebral herniation, and death occur within 3 to 7 days after the onset of symptoms [78,84].

More than 95% of patients with PAM succumb to the disease. Interestingly, long-term sequelae in survivors have been minimal [78].

### Granulomatous Amebic Encephalitis

The clinical manifestations of GAE are more indolent than those of PAM. Signs and symptoms are usually subacute or chronic and may include headache, fever, nausea and vomiting, somnolence, seizures, nuchal rigidity, behavioral changes, and focal neurological findings (ataxia, diplopia or other visual field disturbances, anisocoria, nystagmus, paresthesias, and hemiparesis) [87]. Signs and symptoms resembling a tumor or space-occupying lesion of the brain have been described in a few cases [7]. A vesicular, pustular, or nodular skin lesion may be present. The incubation period is unknown.

## Neuropathology

Histologic findings in PAM include diffuse cerebral edema; fibrinopurulent exudates along the leptomeninges of the cerebral hemispheres, brainstem, cerebellum, and upper portions of the spinal cord; and superficial hemorrhagic necrosis of the gray matter and olfactory bulbs. Abundant amebic trophozoites can be detected in the perivascular space, and in small numbers in the exudates [7,78].

The histological findings in GAE consist of brain edema and multifocal, subacute hemorrhagic parenchymal lesions, with focal chronic leptomeningitis in the adjacent areas. Amebic trophozoites and cysts are seen within the perivascular spaces and within the parenchymal lesions [88].

## Diagnosis

CSF findings in PAM include pleocytosis with neutrophil predominance, markedly elevated protein (frequently >500 mg/dl), and normal or decreased glucose level. Results of Gram stain and bacterial cultures are negative, but trophozoites may be identified on examination of fresh, warm CSF [7]. Neuroimaging (CT or MRI scan) findings vary from normal at the beginning of the illness to signs of increased ICP and meningeal enhancement later on [89,90]. Areas of cerebral infarction have been reported. Severe cerebral edema is indicative of a poor outcome.

CSF analysis in GAE usually reveals less inflammation than that seen in PAM, with low to moderate pleocytosis with mononuclear predominance, and normal or slightly abnormal protein and glucose levels. Typically, no trophozoites are visualized in the CSF, but cysts can be detected in brain biopsy specimens [7]. Free-living amoeba can be isolated in culture [91,92]. Determination of the species can be performed by immunofluorescent tests through the Centers for Disease Control and Prevention (CDC) [83,85,87]. Molecular techniques, such as PCR and DNA probes, have been reported to be useful in the diagnosis and differentiation of the free-living amebas [93–95]. Serology can also be diagnostic [87]. CT and MRI scans commonly reveal multifocal enhancing lesions. Mass effect and small areas of necrosis are common [89,90,96].

## Treatment

A 10-day course of amphotericin B either alone or in combination with rifampin, doxycycline, or miconazole, is the treatment of choice for PAM [85]. Azithromycin has also shown promising in vitro and in vivo activity against *N. fowleri* [97].

Effective treatment of GAE is not established. Reported successful regimens for *Acanthamoeba* infections include prolonged courses (months) of different combinations of pentamidine, ketoconazole, fluconazole, itraconazole, sulfadiazine, flucytosine, rifampin, and trimethoprim–sulfamethoxazole [98]. There are two reported survivors of *B. mandrillaris* meningoencephalitis [83,88,96]. These patients were treated with a combination of pentamidine, a macrolide (clarithromycin or azithromycin), fluconazole, sulfadiazine, and flucytosine. Phenothiazine compounds have in vitro efficacy against *Balamuthia*, and were also used in these two patients [83]. In vitro susceptibilities have shown pentamidine to be the most effective, followed by fluconazole and ketoconazole [92].

# Trypanosomiasis

## *Introduction*

There are two distinct forms of human trypanosomiasis: African trypanosomiasis or sleeping sickness and American Trypanosomiasis or Chagas disease. They occur in separate continents and are caused by different organisms.

## *African Trypanosomiasis*

African trypanosomiasis is a febrile illness with initial blood and lymphatic system, and subsequent central nervous system infection. It is also known as "sleeping sickness."

### Epidemiology

Historically, African trypanosomiasis has been a major obstacle to the social and economic development of Central and East Africa, with an estimated 200,000 to 300,000 people infected each year [99]. In the United States, 31 imported cases have been reported, most of which have been the Rhodesian form [100]. Children are infected less frequently than adults, but symptomatology is similar in all age groups [7].

### Pathogenesis

African trypanosomiasis is caused by two variants of *Trypanosoma brucei*: *T. brucei gambiense* and *T. brucei rhodesiense*. Both are extracellular hemoflagellate protozoans that infect humans mainly through the bite of the tsetse fly (*Glossina* species). Humans are the only important reservoir of *T. brucei gambiense*; wild game animals are the reservoir of *T. brucei rhodesiense*. Other modes of transmission include blood transfusion and transplacental transmission [7,99].

### Clinical Manifestations

The East African or Rhodesian form of the disease is acute and more severe than the West African or Gambian variety. Clinical manifestations occur in three stages. A cutaneous chancre may develop at the inoculation site within days after the bite. Fever, malaise, myalgia, headache, urticarial rash, and generalized lymphadenopathy characterize the second or hemolymphatic stage. The meningoencephalitic or late stage occurs within weeks to a month in the East African form, but may appear only after months to years in the West African type [101].

### Neurological Manifestations

Signs and symptoms of central nervous system involvement include persistent headaches, daytime somnolence with nighttime insomnia, backache, nuchal rigidity, tremors, ataxia, cranial nerve palsies, hemiplegia, incontinence, mood swings, psychotic behavior, anorexia, wasting syndrome, decreased proprioceptive reflexes, stupor, and coma [7] Seizures are frequent in children, but rare in adults [100]. Without treatment, the disease is typically fatal. Treatment during the first two stages is successful in most patients. Cure rates are also high (95%) with treatment during the meningoencephalitic stage. However, toxicity of antiparasitic therapy can complicate the outcome. As many as 10% of melarsoprol-treated patients develop an encephalopathy manifested by seizures, psychosis, coma, and death within days of initiation of therapy. This complication is more common in severely debilitated patients [102,103].

Central nervous system relapses are common and are characterized by the return of neurological symptoms and reappearance of parasitemia or CSF pleocytosis. Periodic assessments of the CSF (every 3–6 months for 1–2 years after initial treatment) are recommended to detect relapses [99,100].

### Diagnosis

The diagnosis is established by identification of trypomastigotes in clinical specimens (blood, skin lesions, lymph node, and CSF). This is very difficult in the Gambian variety, in which serologic diagnosis is preferred [104]. Analysis of CSF shows increased protein secondary to hypergammaglobulinemia and pleocytosis with mononuclear predominance. Trypomastigotes may be found in the CSF using double centrifugation. The detection of specific IgM and trypanosome DNA by PCR in CSF appear to be more sensitive than parasitologic techniques [105]. Neuroimaging studies show cerebral edema (CT scan) and nonspecific, diffuse white matter enhancement (MRI scan) [106].

### Treatment

For early stages of infection, pentamidine or suramin are the drugs of choice. Melarsoprol (for the Rhodesian variety) or eflornithine (for the Gambian variety) are indicated for CNS disease [60,102,103,107]. These drugs are available through the World Health Organization and the CDC. The concomitant use of corticosteroids may prevent melarsoprol-induced encephalopathy [108].

## *American Trypanosomiasis*

### Epidemiology

Chagas disease occurs exclusively in the Western Hemisphere in endemic areas of Mexico and Central and South America. An estimated 16 to 18 million people are infected [109]. Although rare in the United States, with increased immigration, transmission by blood transfusion has become more important [110]. Additionally, reactivation of disease in immunocompromised patients is being increasingly recognized.

### Pathogenesis

American trypanosomiasis is caused by *T. cruzi*, a protozoan hemoflagellate, which is transmitted to humans through the feces of reduviid insects or "kissing bugs." These insects defecate while ingesting human blood. Bitten individuals inoculate themselves by rubbing the insect's feces into the site of the bite, abraded skin, or mucous membranes of the eyes, nose, or mouth. Humans, cats, and dogs are the most important reservoirs. Other modes of transmission include blood transfusion, organ transplantation, laboratory accident, and transplacental transmission [99,101,110,111].

### Clinical Manifestations

The clinical manifestations of acquired Chagas disease are divided into three stages: acute, latent or undifferentiated, and chronic. Up to one third of infected individuals develop acute symptoms; most of these are young or immunocompromised patients. A nodular lesion (chagoma) at the site of inoculation occurs first. In children, it is also common to find unilateral palpebral edema (Romaña's sign). Other signs and symptoms include intermittent fever, headache, anorexia, generalized lymphadenopathy, mild to moderate hepatosplenomegaly, vomiting, and diarrhea. Myocarditis is frequent and meningoencephalitis occurs occasionally. A latent stage of 10 to 40 years may ensue. The most common manifestation of chronic disease is chagasic cardiomyopathy, followed by gastrointestinal tract disorders (megaesophagus and megacolon). Autonomic, central, and peripheral nervous system abnormalities have also been noted. Immunodeficient patients may have reactivation of acute disease with neurological involvement [99,1018].

Congenital Chagas disease is often asymptomatic [112], but it may resemble the acute stage of acquired disease or it may be indistinguishable from other more familiar congenital infections (toxoplasmosis, syphilis, rubella, and cytomegalovirus) [7,99]. Infants co-infected with HIV have a more severe disease [112].

## Neurological Manifestations

Acute chagasic meningoencephalitis is primarily seen in infants and young children. Manifestations include headache, irritability, mental status changes, focal or generalized seizures, and coma. Early onset of seizures carries a poor prognosis, with death occurring within 48 hours.

Neonates with congenital Chagas disease may present with meningoencephalitis with or without associated cardiac manifestations. Signs and symptoms include hypotonia, weak suck, and seizures. Approximately one half of these patients die within 4 months secondary to either neurological or cardiac complications.

Reactivation of Chagas disease has been reported in patients with AIDS, hematologic malignancies, and after transplantation [113–117]. Although these patients may have myocarditis, neurological manifestations (acute multifocal meningoencephalitis or a brain mass) predominate. Typical symptoms include fever, headache, signs and symptoms of increased ICP, and focal neurological deficits.

Reported mortality rates for children with acute chagasic meningoencephalitis are between 25 and 50% [50,99]. Neurological sequelae in survivors include choreoathetosis, deviant behavior and poor communication skills apparent initially, and minimal cerebral dysfunction detected subsequently (7–13 years of age) [50].

In older individuals with chronic Chagas disease, chronic headaches, focal epilepsy, and hypothalamic dysfunction have been reported as sequelae. Some investigators have suggested that these sequelae are secondary to cerebral ischemia and infarction caused by heart failure and embolic phenomena, rather then direct brain parasitic invasion [50,118].

## Neuropathology

Pathological findings include perivascular lymphocytic infiltrates, nodules of microglial cells, hemorrhage, and intracellular amastigote forms of *T. cruzi* in the meninges and gray matter. These findings are observed in patients with congenital infection [7] (with or without clinical neurological abnormalities), as well as in patients with acquired menigoencephalitis [50]. Histological findings in chronic chagasic encephalopathy are nonspecific, and may reflect ischemia and infarction. In immunocompromised hosts, large necrotic or granulomatous mass lesions have been described [114].

## Diagnosis

The diagnosis of Chagas disease is established by visualization of the parasite (Giemsa staining or wet mount) or PCR during the acute phase, and by xenodiagnosis, special cultures, serology, and/or PCR during the chronic phase [101,117,119]. Hematologic examination during acute Chagas disease also demonstrates trypomastigote forms, lymphocytosis, hypergammaglobulinemia, and elevated erythrocyte sedimentation rate.

Analysis of CSF in acute Chagasic meningoencephalitis may show mononuclear pleocytosis and/or mild elevation of protein levels, but, more frequently, CSF results are within normal limits. Organisms are rarely seen in the CSF. Results of head CT scans are usually normal [50].

However, head CT findings are remarkably different in reactivated Chagas disease, with single or multiple hypodense lesions, with or without ring enhancement. Occasionally, hyperdense lesions in the subcortical areas are found [115,116]. These radiological findings may be indistinguishable from central nervous system toxoplasmosis [101].

### Treatment

Specific treatment for Chagas disease is effective during the acute phase and, to a lesser extent, during reactivation in immunosuppressed patients. Treatment is also recommended for congenital Chagas disease. The drugs of choice are nifurtimox (available through the CDC) or benznidazole. Therapy during the latent and chronic stages improves parasite-related outcomes. Its efficacy in improving clinical outcomes seems promising, but needs further evaluation [120,121]. Trypanosomal DNA PCR seems to be better than serology to monitor success of treatment during and after therapy [122,123]. Other modes of therapy, such as interferon gamma, allopurinol, and antifungal treatments, remain largely investigational.

## References

1. Boyer KM, McLeod RL. *Toxoplasma gondii* (Toxoplasmosis) In: Long SS, Pickering LK, Prober CG, eds. *Principles and Practice of Pediatric Infectious Diseases*. 2nd ed. New York, NY: Churchill Livingstone; 2003; 1303–1322.
2. American Academy of Pediatrics. *Toxoplasma gondii* infections. In: Pickering LK, Baker CJ, Long SS, McMillan JA, ed. *Red Book: 2006 Report of the Committee on Infectious Diseases*. 27th ed. Elk Grove Village, IL: American Academy of Pediatrics; 2006; 666–671.
3. Remington JS, McLeod R, Thulliez P, Desmonts G. Toxoplasmosis. In: Remington JS, Klein JO, Wilson CB, Baker CJ, eds. *Infectious Diseases of the Fetus and Newborn Infant*. 6th ed. Philadelphia, PA: Elsevier Saunders; 2006; 947–1091.
4. Montoya JG, Kovacs JA, Remington JS. *Toxoplasma gondii*. In: Mandell GL, Bennett JE, Dolin R, eds. *Principles and Practice of Infectious Diseases*. 6th ed. Philadelphia, PA: Churchill Livingstone; 2005; 3170–3193.
5. Khan EA, Correa AG. Toxoplasmosis of the central nervous system in non-human immunodeficiency virus-infected children: case report and review of the literature. *Pediatr Infect Dis J*. 1997; 16:611–618.
6. Mitchell CD, Erlich SS, Mastrucci MT, Hutto, SC, Parks WP, Scott GB. Congenital toxoplasmosis occurring in infants perinatally infected with human immunodeficiency virus 1. *Pediatr Infect Dis J*. 1990; 9:512–518.

7. Lowichik A, Siegel JD. Parasitic infections of the central nervous system in children. Part I: congenital infections and meningoencephalitis. *J Child Neurol.* 1995; 10:4–17.
8. Massa G, Vanderschueren-Lodeweyckx M, Van Vliet G, Craen M, de Zegher F, Eggermont E. Hypothalamo-pituitary dysfunction in congenital toxoplasmosis. *Eur J Pediatr.* 1989; 148:742–744.
9. McAuley J, Boyer KM, Patel D. et al. Early and longitudinal evaluations of treated infants and children and untreated historical patients with congenital toxoplasmosis: the Chicago Collaborative Treatment Trial. *Clin Infect Dis.* 1994; 18:38–72.
10. Wilson CB, Remington JS, Stagno S, Reynolds DW. Development of adverse sequelae in children born with subclinical congenital *Toxoplasma* infection. *Pediatrics.* 1980; 66:767–774.
11. Wallon M, Kodjikian L, Binquet C, et al. Long-term ocular prognosis in 327 children with congenital toxoplasmosis. *Pediatrics.* 2004; 113:1567–1572.
12. McLeod R, Boyer K, Karrison T, et al. Outcome of treatment for congenital toxoplasmosis, 1981–2004: the National Collaborative Chicago-Based, Congenital Toxoplasmosis Study. *Clin Infect Dis.* 2006; 42:1383–1394.
13. McCabe RE, Brook RG, Dorfman RF, Remington JS. Clinical spectrum in 107 cases of toxoplasmic lymphadenopathy. *Rev Infect Dis.* 1987; 9:754–774.
14. Montoya JG, Remington JS. Toxoplasmic chorioretinitis on the setting of acute acquired toxoplasmosis. *Clin Infect Dis.* 1996; 23:277–282.
15. Montoya JG, Jordan R, Lingamneni S, Berry GJ, Remington JS. Toxoplasmic myocarditis and polymyositis in patients with acute acquired toxoplasmosis diagnosed during life. *Clin Infect Dis.* 1997; 24:676–683.
16. Israelski DM, Remington JS. Toxoplasmosis in the non-AIDS immunocompromised host. *Curr Clin Top Infect Dis.* 1993; 13:322–356.
17. Luft BJ, Remington JS. Toxoplasmic encephalitis in AIDS. *Clin Infect Dis.* 1992; 15:211–222.
18. Duzovali O, Choroszy MS, Chan KW. Hyponatremia as the presenting feature of cerebral toxoplasmosis. *Bone Marrow Transplantation.* 2005; 35:1221–1222.
19. Gray F, Gherardi R, Wingate E, et al. Diffuse "encephalitic" cerebral toxoplasmosis in AIDS. Report of four cases. *J Neurol.* 1989; 236:273–277.
20. Levy RM, Mills CM, Posin JP, Moore SG, Rosenblum ML, Bredesen DE. The efficacy and clinical impact of brain imaging in neurologically symptomatic AIDS patients: a prospective CT/MRI study. *J Acquir Immune Defic Syndr.* 1990; 3:461–471.
21. Mueller-Mang C, Mang TG, Kalhs P, Thurnher MM. Imaging characteristics of toxoplasmosis encephalitis after bone marrow transplantation: report of two cases and review of literature. *Neuroradiology.* 2006; 48:84–89.
22. Willis MS, Southern P, Latimer MJ. *Toxoplasma* infections: making the best use of laboratory tests. *Infect Med.* 2002; 19:522–532.
23. Boyer KM. Diagnostic testing for congenital toxoplasmosis. *Pediatr Infect Dis J.* 2001; 20:59–60.
24. Montoya JG. Laboratory diagnosis of *Toxoplasma gondii* infection and toxoplasmosis. *J Infect Dis.* 2002; 185 (Suppl 1):S73–82.
25. Naessens A, Jenum PA, Pollak A, et al. Diagnosis of congenital toxoplasmosis in the neonatal period: a multicenter evaluation. *J Pediatr.* 1999; 135:714–719.
26. Boyer KM. Congenital toxoplasmosis: current status of diagnosis, treatment, and prevention. *Semin Pediatr Infect Dis.* 2000; 11:165–171.
27. American Academy of Pediatrics. Malaria. In: Pickering LK, Baker CJ, Long SS, McMillan JA, eds. *Red Book: 2006 Report of the Committee on Infectious Diseases.* 27th ed. Elk Grove Village, IL: American Academy of Pediatrics; 2006; 435–441.
28. WHO. Guidelines for the Treatment of Malaria. Geneva, Switzerland: World Health Organization; 2006.
29. Gubler DJ. Resurgent vector-borne diseases as a global health problem. *Emerg Infect Dis.* 1998; 4:442–450.

30. Centers for Disease Control and Prevention (CDC). Local transmission of *Plasmodium vivax* malaria—Palm Beach County, Florida, 2003. *MMWR.* 2003; 52:908–911.
31. Centers for Disease Control and Prevention (CDC). Multifocal autochthonous transmission of malaria—Florida, 2003. *MMWR.* 2004; 53:412–413.
32. Zucker JR. Changing patterns of autochthonous malaria transmission in the United States: a review of recent outbreaks. *Emerg Infect Dis.* 1996; 2:37–43.
33. Isaacson M. Airport malaria: a review. *Bull World Health Organ.* 1989; 67:737–743.
34. Wilson CM. *Plasmodium* Species (Malaria). In: Long SS, Pickering LK, Prober CG, eds. *Principles and Practice of Pediatric Infectious Diseases.* 2nd ed. New York, NY: Churchill Livingstone; 2003; 1295–1301.
35. Mehta PN. Malaria. *eMedicine* [serial online]. February 2006.
36. Viani RM, Bromberg K. Pediatric imported malaria in New York: delayed diagnosis. *Clin Pediatr (Phila).* 1999; 38:333–337.
37. Winters RA, Murray HW. Malaria—the mime revisited: fifteen more years of experience at a New York City teaching hospital. *Am J Med.* 1992; 93:243–246.
38. WHO. *Management of Severe Malaria: A practical handbook.* 2nd ed. Geneva, Switzerland: World Health Organization; 2000.
39. Hulbert TV. Congenital malaria in the United States. Report of a case and review. *Clin Infect Dis.* 1992; 14:922–926.
40. Sowunmi A. Clinical study of cerebral malaria in African children. *Afr J Med Sci.* 1997; 26:9–11.
41. Olumese PE, Gbadegesin RA, Adeyemo AA, Brown B, Walker A. Neurological features of cerebral malaria in Nigerian children. *Ann Trop Pediatr.* 1999; 19:321–325.
42. John CC, Idro RI. Cerebral malaria in children. *Infect Med.* 2003; 20:53–58.
43. Newton CR, Crawley J, Sowumni A, et al. Intracranial hypertension in Africans with cerebral malaria. *Arch Dis Child.* 1997; 76:219–226.
44. Brewster DR, Kwiatkowski D, White NJ. Neurological sequelae of cerebral malaria in children. *Lancet.* 1990; 336:1039–1043.
45. van Hensbroek MB, Palmer A, Jaffar S, Schneider G, Kwiatkowski D. Residual neurologic sequelae after childhood cerebral malaria. *J Pediatr.* 1997; 131:125–129.
46. Nguyen TH, Day NP, Ly VC, et al. Post-malaria neurological syndrome. *Lancet.* 1996; 348:917–921.
47. Senanayake N, de Silva HJ. Delayed cerebellar ataxia complicating falciparum malaria: a clinical study of 74 patients. *J Neurol.* 1994; 241:456–459.
48. White NJ. Neurological dysfunction following malaria: disease- or drug-related? *Clin Inf Dis.* 2000; 30:836.
49. Elias Z, Bonnet E, Marchou B, Massip P. Neurotoxicity of artemisinin: possible counseling and treatment of side effects. *Clin Infect Dis.* 1999; 28:1330–1331.
50. Lowichik A, Ruff AJ. Parasitic infections of the central nervous system in children. Part II: Disseminated infections. *J Child Neurol.* 1995; 10:77–87.
51. Marsh K, Forster D, Waruiru C, et al. Indicators of life-threatening malaria in African children. *N Engl J Med.* 1995; 332:1399–1404.
52. Fairhurst RM, Wellems TE. Plasmodium species (Malaria). In: Mandell GL, Bennett JE, Dolin R, eds. *Principles and Practice of Infectious Diseases.* 6th ed. Philadelphia, PA: Churchill Livingstone; 2005; 3121–3144.
53. McAdam AJ, Sharpe AH. Infectious Diseases. In: Kumar V, Abbas AK, Fausto N, eds. *Robbins & Cotran: Pathologic Basis of Disease.* 7th ed. Philadelphia, PA: Elsevier Saunders; 2005; 343–414.
54. Crawley J, Smith S, Muthinji P, Marsh K, Kirkham F. Electroencephalographic and clinical features of cerebral malaria. *Arch Dis Child.* 2001; 84:247–253.
55. Newton CR, Peshu N, Kendall B, et al. Brain swelling and ischaemia in Kenyans with cerebral malaria. *Arch Dis Child.* 1994; 70:281–287.
56. Looareesuwan S, Wilairatana P, Krishna S, et al. Magnetic resonance imaging of the brain in patients with cerebral malaria. *Clin Infect Dis.* 1995; 21:300–309.

57. Karunajeewa HA, Kemiki A, Alpers MP, et al. Safety and therapeutic efficacy of artesunate suppositories for treatment of malaria in children in Papua New Guinea. *Pediatr Infect Dis J*. 2003; 22:251–255.
58. McIntosh HM, Olliaro P. Artemisinin derivatives for treating severe malaria. *Cochrane Database Syst Rev*. 2000; 2:CD000527.
59. WHO. Facts on ACTS (Artemisinin-based Combination Therapies). January 2006 Update, World Health Organization, Geneva.
60. American Academy of Pediatrics. Drugs for Parasitic Infections. In: Pickering LK, Baker CJ, Long SS, McMillan JA, eds. *Red Book: 2006 Report of the Committee on Infectious Diseases*. 27th ed. Elk Grove Village, IL: American Academy of Pediatrics; 2006; 790–817.
61. White NJ. The treatment of malaria. *N Engl J Med*. 1996; 335:800–806.
62. Crawley J, Waruiru C, Mithwani S, et al. Effect of phenobarbital on seizure frequency and mortality in childhood cerebral malaria: a randomised, controlled intervention. *Lancet*. 2000; 355:701–706.
63. Meremikwu M, Marson AG. Routine anticonvulsants for treating cerebral malaria. *Cochrane Database Syst Rev*. 2006; 2:CD002152.
64. Yost J. Amebiasis. *Pediatr Rev*. 2002; 23:293–294.
65. Horga MA, Naparst TR, Dhawan VK. Amebiasis. *eMedicine* [serial online]. March 2006.
66. Hotez PJ, Strickland AD. Amebiasis. In: Feigin RD, Cherry JD, eds. *Textbook of Pediatric Infectious Diseases*. 5th ed. Philadelphia , PA: WB Saunders; 2004; 2660–2668.
67. Hughes FB, Faehnle ST, Simon JL. Multiple cerebral abscesses complicating hepatopulmonary amebiasis. *J Pediatr*. 1979; 86:95–96.
68. Lowichik A, Ruff AJ. Parasitic infections of the central nervous system in children. Part III: space-occupying lesions. *J Child Neurol*. 1995; 10:177–190.
69. Shah AA, Shaikh H, Karim M. Amoebic brain abscess: a rare but serious complication of *Entamoeba histolytica* infection. *J Neurol Neurosurg Psychiatry*. 1994; 57:240–241.
70. Schmutzhard E, Mayr U, Rumpl E, Prugger M, Pohl P. Secondary cerebral amebiasis due to infection with *Entamoeba histolytica*. A case report with computer tomographic findings. *Eur Neurol*. 1986; 25:161–165.
71. Becker GL, Knep S, Lance KP, Kaufman L. Amebic abscess of the brain. *Neurosurgery*. 1980; 6:192–194.
72. Kchouk M, Ghedas K, Bouhaouala MH, et al. [Amebic brain abscess. Apropos of a case.] *Ann Radiol* (Paris). 1993; 36:332–335.
73. American Academy of Pediatrics. Amebiasis. In: Pickering LK, Baker CJ, Long SS, McMillan JA, eds. *Red Book: 2006 Report of the Committee on Infectious Diseases*. 27th ed. Elk Grove Village, IL: American Academy of Pediatrics; 2006; 204–206.
74. Dietz R, Schanen G, Kramann B, Erpelding J. Intracranial amebic abscesses: CT and MR findings. *J Comput Assist Tomogr*. 1991; 15:168–170.
75. van Sonnenberg E, Mueller PR, Schiffman HR, et al. Intrahepatic amebic abscess: indications for and results of percutaneous catheter drainage. *Radiology*. 1985; 156:631–635.
76. Ohnishi K, Murata M, Kojima H, Takemura N, Tsuchida T, Tachibana H. Brain abscess due to infection with *Entamoeba histolytica*. *Am J Trop Med Hyg*. 1994; 51:180–182.
77. Fowler M, Carter RF. Acute pyogenic meningitis probably due to *Acanthamoeba sp*: a preliminary report. *Br Med J*. 1965; 2:740–742.
78. Barnett ND, Kaplan AM, Hopkin RJ, Saubolle MA, Rudinsky MF. Primary amoebic meningoencephalitis with *Naegleria fowleri*: clinical review. *Pediatr Neurol*. 1996; 15:230–234.
79. Bottone EJ. Free-living amebas of the genera *Acanthamoeba* and *Naegleria*: an overview and basic microbiology correlates. *Mt Sinai J Med*. 1993; 60:260–270.
80. Martinez AJ. Free-living amebas: infection of the central nervous system. *Mt Sinai J Med*. 1993; 60:271–278.
81. Denney CF, Iragui VJ, Uber-Zak LD, et al. Amebic meningoencephalitis by *Balamuthia mandrillaris*: case report and review. *Clin Infect Dis*. 1997; 25:1354–1358.
82. Griesemer DA, Barton LL, Reese CM, et al. Amebic meningoencephalitis caused by *Balamuthia mandrillaris*. *Pediatr Neurol*. 1994; 10:249–254.

83. Deetz TR, Sawyer MH, Billman G, et al. Successful treatment of *Balamuthia* amoebic encephalitis: presentation of 2 cases. *Clin Infect Dis*. 2003; 37:1304–1312.
84. Seidel JS. *Naegleria, Acanthamoeba*, and Balamuthia. In: Feigin RD, Cherry JD, eds. *Textbook of Pediatric Infectious Diseases*. 5th ed. Philadelphia, PA: WB Saunders; 2004; 2748–2755.
85. American Academy of Pediatrics. Amebic meningoencephalitis and keratitis. In: Pickering LK, Baker CJ, Long SS, McMillan JA, eds. *Red Book: 2006 Report of the Committee on Infectious Diseases*. 27th ed. Elk Grove Village, IL: American Academy of Pediatrics; 2006; 206–208.
86. Asbell PA. *Acanthamoeba* keratitis: there and back again. *Mt Sinai Med J.*, 1993; 60:279–282.
87. Schuster FL, Honarmand S, Visvesvara GS, Glaser CA. Detection of antibodies against free-living amoebae *Balamuthia mandrillaris* and *Acanthamoeba* species in a population of patients with encephalitis. *Clin Infect Dis*. 2006; 42:1260–1265.
88. Martinez AJ, Visvesvara GS. *Balamuthia mandrillaris* infection. *J Med Microbiol*. 2001; 50:205–207.
89. Schumacher DJ, Tien RD, Lane K. Neuroimaging findings in rare amebic infections of the central nervous system. *Am J Neuroradiol*. 1995; 16:930–935.
90. Kidney DD, Kim SH. CNS infections with free-living amebas: neuroimaging findings. *Am J Roentgenol*. 1998; 171:809–812.
91. Schuster FL. Cultivation of pathogenic and opportunistic free-living amebas. *Clin Microbiol Rev*. 2002; 15:342–354.
92. Schuster FL, Visvesvara GS. Axenic growth and sensitivity studies of *Balamuthia mandrillaris*, an agent of amebic meningoencephalitis in humans and other animals. *J Clin Microbiol*. 1996; 34:385–388.
93. Sparagano O, Drouet E, Denoyel G, Pernin P, Ruchard-Sparagano MH. Differentiation of *Naegleria fowleri* from other species of *Naegleria* using monoclonal antibodies and the polymerase chain reaction. *Trans R Soc Trop Med Hyg*. 1994; 88:119–120.
94. Reveiller FL, Cabanes PA, Marciano-Cabral F. Development of a nested PCR assay to detect the pathogenic free-living amoeba *Naegleria fowleri*. *Parasitol Res*. 2002; 88:443–450.
95. Lai S, Asgari M, Henney HR. Non-radioactive DNA probe and polymerase chain reaction procedures for the specific detection of *Acanthamoeba*. *Mol Cell Probes*. 1994; 8:81–89.
96. Healy JF. *Balamuthia* amebic encephalitis: radiographic and pathologic findings. *Am J Neuroradiol*. 2002; 23:486–489.
97. Goswick SM, Brenner GM. Activities of azithromycin and amphotericin B against *Naegleria fowleri* in vitro and in a mouse model of primary amebic meningoencephalitis. *Antimicrob Agents Chemother*. 2003; 47:524–528.
98. Singhal T, Bajpai A, Kalra V, et al. Successful treatment of *Acanthamoeba* meningitis with combination oral antimicrobials. *Pediatr Infect Dis J*. 2001; 20:623–627.
99. Ortega-Barria E. Trypanosoma species. In: Long SS, Pickering LK, Prober CG, eds. *Principles and Practice of Pediatric Infectious Diseases*. 2nd ed. New York, NY: Churchill Livingston; 2003; 1324–1330.
100. Kiminyo KK, Lucey DR. African Trypanosomiasis (Sleeping Sickness). *eMedicine Journal* 2002.
101. Wittner M, Tanowitz HB. Trypanosomiasis. In: Feigin RD, Cherry JD, eds. *Textbook of Pediatric Infectious Diseases*. 5th ed. Philadelphia, PA: WB Saunders; 2004; 2739–2748.
102. Truc P, Lejon V, Magnus E, et al. Evaluation of the micro-CATT, CATT/*Trypanosoma brucei gambiense*, and LATEX/T.b. gambiense methods for serodiagnosis and surveillance of human African trypanosomiasis in West and Central Africa. *Bull World Health Organ*. 2002; 80:882–886.
103. Jamonneau V, Solano P, Garcia A, et al. Stage determination and therapeutic decision in human African trypanosomiasis: value of polymerase chain reaction and immunoglobulin M quantification on the cerebrospinal fluid of sleeping sickness patients in Cote d' Ivoire. *Trop Med Int Health*. 2003; 8:589–594.

104. Gill DS, Chatha DS, del Carpio-O'Donovan R. MR imaging findings in African trypanosomiasis. *Am J Neuroradiol.* 2003; 24:1383–1385.
105. Legros D, Ollivier G, Gastellu-Etchegorry M, et al. Treatment of human African trypanosomiasis: present situation and needs for research and development. *Lancet Infect Dis.* 2002; 2:437–440.
106. Burri C, Nkunku S, Merolle A, Smith T, Blum J, Brun R. Efficacy of new, concise schedule for melarsoprol in treatment of sleeping sickness caused by *Trypanosoma brucei gambiense*: a randomised trial. *Lancet.* 2000; 355:1419–1425.
107. Burri C, Brun R. Eflornithine for the treatment of human African trypanosomiasis. *Parasitol Res.* 2003; 90:S49–52.
108. Pepin J, Milord F, Guern C, Mpia B, Ethier L, Mansinsa D. Trial of prednisolone for prevention of melarsoprol-induced encephalopathy in gambiense sleeping sickness. *Lancet.* 1989; 1:1246–1250.
109. Prata A. Clinical and epidemiological aspects of Chagas disease. *Lancet Infect Dis.* 2001; 1:92–100.
110. Centers for Disease Control and Prevention (CDC). Chagas disease after organ transplantation—Los Angeles, California, 2006. *MMWR.* 2006; 55:798–800.
111. Centers for Disease Control and Prevention (CDC). Chagas disease after organ transplantation—United States, 2001. *MMWR.* 2002; 51:210–212.
112. Freilij H, Altcheh J. Congenital Chagas disease: diagnostic and clinical aspects. *Clin Infect Dis.* 1995; 21:551–555.
113. Del Castillo M, Mendoza G, Oviedo J, Perez Bianco RP, Anselmo AE, Silva M. AIDS and Chagas disease with central nervous system tumor-like lesion. *Am J Med.* 1990; 88:693–694.
114. Ferreira MS, Nishioka Sde A, Silvestre MT, Borges AS, Nunes-Araujo FR, Rocha A. Reactivation of Chagas' disease in patients with AIDS: report of three new cases and review of the literature. *Clin Infect Dis.* 1997; 25:1397–1400.
115. Di Lorenzo GA, Pagano MA, Taratuto AL, Garau ML, Meli FJ, Pomsztein, MD. Chagasic granulomatous encephalitis in immunosuppressed patients. Computed tomography and magnetic resonance imaging findings. *J Neuroimaging.* 1996; 6:94–97.
116. Goldani LZ. A 32-year-old Brazilian woman with severe headache and fever. *Clin Infect Dis.* 2002; 35:1549–1550.
117. Walker M, Zunt JR. Parasitic central nervous system infections in immunocompromised hosts. *Clin Infect Dis.* 2005; 40:1005–1015.
118. Silva AA, Roffe E, Marino AP, et al. Chagas' disease encephalitis: intense CD8+ lymphocytic infiltrate is restricted to the acute phase, but is not related to the presence of *Trypanosoma cruzi* antigens. *Clin Immunol.* 1999; 92:56–66.
119. Wincker P, Telleria J, Bosseno MF, et al. PCR-based diagnosis for Chagas' disease in Bolivian children living in an active transmission area: comparison with conventional serological and parasitological diagnosis. *Parasitology.* 1997; 114:367–373.
120. Villar JC, Marin-Neto JA, Ebrahim S, Yusuf S. Trypanocidal drugs for chronic asymptomatic *Trypanosoma cruzi* infection. *Cochrane Database Syst Rev.* 2002; 1:CD003463.
121. Reyes PA, Vallejo M. Trypanocidal drugs for late stage, symptomatic Chagas disease (*Trypanosoma cruzi* infection). *Cochrane Database Syst Rev.* 2005; 4:CD004102.
122. Solari A, Ortiz S, Soto A, et al. Treatment of *Trypanosoma cruzi*-infected children with nifurtimox: a 3 year follow-up by PCR. *J Antimicrob Chemother.* 2001; 48:515–519.
123. Galvao LM, Chiari E, Macedo AM, Laguetti AO, Silva SA, Andrade AL. PCR assay for monitoring *Trypanosoma cruzi* parasitemia in childhood after specific chemotherapy. *J Clin Microbiol.* 2003; 41:5066–5070.

# Chapter 36
# *Babesia* Species

**Abeer Khayat, M.D. and Mobeen H. Rathore, M.D., C.P.E., F.A.A.P.**

## Babesiosis

### *Introduction*

Babesiosis is a zoonotic disease caused by intraerythrocytic protozoa of the genus *Babesia* [1,2]. This malaria-like illness affects a variety of wild and domestic animals, and only occasionally humans [3]. Since the first recognized human case in 1957, babesiosis has been reported with increasing frequency in humans.

### *Epidemiology*

In the United States, babesiosis occurs in clusters, and clinically apparent disease is seen primarily in patients with underlying risk factors (*vide infra*); most reported cases have occurred in patients with intact spleens [4,5]. In contrast, babesiosis in Europe has been described as a sporadic disease that occurs almost exclusively in asplenic patients, with a clinical course that has almost always been fatal [4–6]. The disease occurs mainly in coastal areas in the northeastern United States and in the Midwest during the spring and summer months [4,7]. Although most cases have been reported in adults, serologic surveys in epidemic areas suggest that babesial infections occur in children as commonly as in adults.

### *Pathogenesis*

More than 100 species of *Babesia* have been identified, but only a few are associated with human infection [4,8]. *Babesia microti* prevails in the United States and *Babesia divergens* in Europe. In addition, a similar but distinct *Babesia* species designated WA-1 has been identified in cases from the western United States and MO-1 from

L.L. Barton and N.R. Friedman (eds.), *The Neurological Manifestations of Pediatric Infectious Diseases and Immunodeficiency Syndromes.*

Missouri [1,2]. *Babesia divergens* is transmitted by the nymph stage of the tick, *Ixodes ricinus*, in Europe and *Ixodes scapularis* in the United States. Concurrent Lyme disease has been reported in approximately 20% of cases of babesiosis. Rarely, babesiosis is transmitted transplacentally or through blood transfusion [1,2,6,9].

After the sporozoites are introduced into the host's bloodstream by tick saliva, *Babesiae* gain entry into red blood cells. The parasite subsequently buds asexually to produce two or four daughter cells that appear as the characteristic "Maltese cross" in Giemsa-stained blood smears. Newly formed trophozoites are released, infecting other erythrocytes. Most of the clinical manifestations of babesiosis are caused by hemolysis and the systemic inflammatory response to the parasites [1,2,10].

## *Clinical Manifestations*

Babesial infections are usually asymptomatic or mild and self-limited [8]. They can be severe, however, particularly in asplenic persons, the elderly, or the immunocompromised [5–7,9,11]. After an incubation period of 1 to 4 weeks (up to 9 weeks in transfusion-associated babesiosis) symptoms occur, with the gradual onset of fever (up to 40°C), chills, diaphoresis, headache, myalgia, arthralgia, and fatigue. Patients may later develop jaundice and dark urine, hepatomegaly, and splenomegaly. Gastrointestinal and upper respiratory symptoms include abdominal pain, anorexia, nausea, vomiting, conjunctival injection, pharyngeal erythema, and nonproductive cough. Pulmonary edema and adult respiratory distress syndrome as well as heart failure, renal failure, and disseminated intravascular coagulation may occur with fulminant babesiosis [1,2,4,10,12]. Children generally develop a milder disease than adults [2]. The illness can last for a few weeks to several months, with a recovery period as long as 18 months. Untreated patients may remain parasitemic for months or years, with subsequent recrudescence of disease [6].

## *Neurological Manifestations*

Headache is one of the most common symptoms and has been reported in approximately 80% of patients. Although uncommon, other neurological manifestations may occur, including photophobia, neck and back stiffness, altered sensorium, hyperesthesia, incoordination, emotional liability, and depression [2,6,13].

## *Diagnosis*

Babesiosis should be suspected in any febrile patient living or traveling in an endemic area, irrespective of history of exposure to ticks or tick bites. Specific diagnosis of babesiosis can be achieved by microscopic examination of Wright- or Giemsa-stained peripheral blood smears. Typically, *Babesia* organisms appear as intraerythrocytic ring forms [8,11]. Tetrads of merozoites are visible [1,3,6,7,9]. Both IgM and IgG immunofluorescent antibodies are markedly elevated during acute illness and decline within 12 months [2,8,13]. Polymerase chain reaction (PCR) is a more sensitive technique than microscopic examination of thin blood smear and has comparable specificity [2]. However, PCR is expensive, time consuming, and requires specialized laboratories. Syrian hamster inoculation has been used for parasite detection, but this technique is less sensitive than PCR and is generally available only in research laboratories.

Other laboratory abnormalities that are characteristic of babesiosis are related to hemolysis. These include anemia, reticulocytosis, hemoglobinuria, decreased haptoglobin, and elevated liver enzymes, lactate dehydrogenase, and unconjugated bilirubin. Thrombocytopenia is common. The white blood cell count may be normal or decreased. Proteinuria and elevated blood urea nitrogen and creatinine levels also may occur [2,3,6].

## *Treatment*

The recommended treatment for babesiosis consists of the combination of clindamycin and oral quinine for 7 days or atovaquone and azithromycin for 7 to 10 days [1,2,5,8,10,14]. Therapy is generally reserved for patients who have been splenectomized or who are immunosuppressed, elderly, or significantly symptomatic [1,3]. The dosage of clindamycin for children is 20 to 40 mg/kg/d administered in three oral doses. The dosage of quinine is 25 mg/kg/d administered in three doses. Exchange transfusion in combination with clindamycin and quinine therapy should be considered for severely ill patients with life-threatening babesiosis [2,5,6,8,10].

## *Prevention*

The prevention of babesiosis is best accomplished by avoidance of tick-infested areas and deer and mice habitats, especially from May through September. Tick bites may be prevented by use of clothing that covers all exposed areas and by the use of insect repellents on exposed skin as well as clothing. After venturing in areas where ticks, deer, and mice thrive, a complete and thorough examination of the skin for the presence of ticks and their removal using a tweezer, if promptly performed, is a very effective preventive tool [15].

## References

1. Krause PJ. Babesiosis. *Med Clin N Am*. 2002; 86:361–373.
2. Lantos PM, Krause PJ. Babesiosis: similar to malaria but different. *Pediatr Ann*. 2002; 31:192–197.

3. Alonso GO. In: Ferri FF, ed. *Ferri's Clinical Advisor: Diagnosis and Treatment*. 2005 ed. Philadelphia, PA: Mosby, Inc; 2005; 111–112.
4. Pruthi RK, Marshall WF, Wiltsie J, Persing DH. Human Babesiosis. *Mayo Clin Proc*. 1995; 70:853–862.
5. Spach DH, Liles WC, Campbell GL, Quick RE, Anderson DE Jr, Fritsche TR. Tick-borne diseases in the United States. *N Engl J Med*. 1993; 329:936–947.
6. Mylonakis E. When to suspect and how to monitor babesiosis. *Am Fam Physician*. 2001; 63:1969–1974.
7. Gelfand JA. Vannier. Babesia species. In: Mandell GL, Bennett JE, Dolin R, eds. *Principles and Practice of Infectious Diseases*. 6th ed. Philadelphia, PA: Churchill Livingstone; 2004; 3209–3214.
8. Ortega-Barria E. Babesia species (Babesiosis). In: Long SS, Pickering LK, Prober CG, eds. *Principles and Practice of Pediatric Infectious Diseases*. 2nd ed. Philadelphia, PA: Churchill Livingstone; 2003; 1261–1264.
9. Pearson RD. Other protozoan diseases. In: Goldman L, Ausiello D, eds. *Cecil Textbook of Medicine*. 22nd ed. Philadelphia, PA: Saunders; 2004; 1973–1974.
10. Boustani MR, Gelfand JA. Babesiosis. *Clin Infect Dis*. 1996; 22:611–615.
11. Roos KL. Nonviral Infections. In: Goetz CG, Pappert EJ, ed. *Textbook of Clinical Neurology*. 2nd ed. Philadelphia, PA: Saunders; 2003; 936.
12. Kumar V, Abbas AK, Fausto N, eds. *Robbins & Cotran Pathologic Basis of Disease*. 7th ed. Philadelphia, PA: Saunders; 2005; 403.
13. Krause PJ, McKay K, Thompson CA, et al. Disease-specific diagnosis of coinfecting tick-borne zoonoses: babesiosis, human granulocytic ehrlichiosis, and Lyme disease. *Clin Infect Dis*. 2002; 34:1184–1191.
14. American Academy of Pediatrics. Babesios. In: Pickering LK, Baker CJ, Long SS, McMillan JA, eds. *Red Book: 2006 Report of the Committee on Infectious Diseases*. 27th ed. American Academy of Pediatrics. Elk Grove Village, IL: American Academy of Pediatrics; 2006; 223–224.
15. Wormser GP, Dattwyler RJ, Shapiro ED, et al. The clinical assessment, treatment and prevention of Lyme disease, human granulocytic anaplasmosis, and babesiosis: clinical practice guidelines by the Infectious Diseases Society of America. *Clin Infect Dis*. 2006; 43:1089–1134.

# Section VI
# Helminths

# Chapter 37
# Helminth Infections

Patrick J. Gavin, M.B., M.R.C.P.I.D.(A.B.M.M.)

## Introduction

Helminth (worm) infections are among the most prevalent of parasitic infections in the world. Approximately 2 billion people, or one third of the world's population, are affected, half are school-aged children [1]. Although helminth infections of the central nervous system (CNS) are unusual, because of the associated mortality and potential for neurological devastation, it is important that they not be overlooked. In addition, involvement of the CNS is undoubtedly underdiagnosed in endemic areas, because of a lack of confirmatory diagnostic testing, and unrecognized in the developed world, because of a lack of familiarity. As international travel and immigration increase, helminth parasites normally only seen in tropical and subtropical regions are likely to present with increasing frequency in non-endemic areas. Recognition of the possibility of a helminthic etiology for select neurological presentations is an important first step in diagnosis. This chapter focuses on those members of the three classes of helminths, cestodes (flatworms), nematodes (roundworms), and trematodes (flukes), most commonly associated with CNS infection (Table 37.1)

## General Considerations

Unfortunately, helminth infections of the CNS are not easy to diagnose. In the majority of cases, presentation is nonspecific, with seizures, or symptoms and signs of a space-occupying lesion, stroke, meningitis, encephalitis, focal deficit, or paraplegia. However, a detailed history may provide vital clues regarding potential exposures. Specific inquiry should be made regarding travel to or immigration from endemic areas, consumption of local foods (especially freshwater crustacean, fish, or snails), rash and swellings (especially if migratory), or exposure to freshwater. It is also important to remember that lack of a travel history should not exclude the diagnosis. Local transmission of helminths in non-endemic

L.L. Barton and N.R. Friedman (eds.), *The Neurological Manifestations of Pediatric Infectious Diseases and Immunodeficiency Syndromes.*

**Table 37.1** Helminth infections of the central nervous system

| Disease | Helminth parasite | Definitive host | Intermediate host | Exposure risk |
|---|---|---|---|---|
| Cestodes | | | | |
| Neurocysticercosis | *Taenia solium*[a] | Humans | Pigs | Ingestion of infective eggs in feces of human tapeworm carriers |
| Coenurosis | *Taenia serialis and multiceps*[a] | Dogs | Herbivores | Ingestion of infective eggs in dog feces |
| Hydatid disease | *Echinococcus* sp. | Dogs and canids | Herbivores | Ingestion of infective eggs in dog feces |
| Sparganosis | *Spirometra* sp. | Cats and dogs | Crustaceans, frogs, and snakes | Ingestion of larvae in freshwater, and raw or undercooked frogs, fish, and snakes |
| Nematodes | | | | |
| Angiostrongyliasis | *Angiostrongylus cantonensis*[a] | Rats | Freshwater snails, crustaceans, and frogs | Ingestion of larvae in snails, crustaceans, and frogs |
| Toxocariasis | *Toxocara* sp. | Dogs and cats | | Ingestion of infective eggs in dog feces |
| Baylisascariasis | *Baylisascaris procyonis* | Raccoons | Small mammals and birds | Ingestion of infective eggs in raccoon feces or soil |
| Trichinosis | *Trichinella* sp. | Rats | Pigs | Ingestion of larvae in raw or undercooked pork |
| Strongyloidiasis | *Strongyloides stercoralis* | Humans | | Penetration of intact skin by infective larvae in soil |
| Gnathostomiasis | *Gnathostoma spinigerum*[a] | Cats and dogs | Freshwater crustaceans, fish, and fowl | Ingestion of larvae in raw or undercooked crustaceans, fish, and fowl |
| Trematodes | | | | |
| Schistosomiasis | *Schistosoma* sp. | Humans | Freshwater snails | Penetration of intact skin by larvae in infested freshwater |
| Paragonimiasis | *Paragonimus westermani* | Humans | Freshwater crustaceans | Ingestion of larvae in raw or undercooked crustaceans |

[a]Larvae demonstrate neurotropism.

regions is well documented. Infection with larva of *Taenia solium*, the pork tapeworm, is described in individuals who have never left the United States, and whose religion proscribes the consumption of pork [2–4]. Here infection is attributed to contamination of food by family members or domestic employees who are tapeworm carriers.

Although most routine laboratory tests are neither sensitive nor specific for helminth infections of the CNS, the presence of eosinophilia, particularly eosinophilic meningitis, should alert the physician to the possibility of a parasitic etiology [5–7]. Eosinophils are not normally present in cerebrospinal fluid (CSF) and should never be ignored. Eosinophilic meningitis is associated with relatively few conditions, particularly helminth infections or inflammatory diseases (Table 37.2); its presence narrows the differential diagnosis of CNS disease and may provide an early or the only etiologic clue. Eosinophils and their cytotoxic granular contents in the CSF also contribute to the neurological damage and adverse sequelae associated with many of these conditions [6–8]. The nematode parasites, *Angiostrongylus*, *Baylisascaris*, and *Gnathostoma*, are most consistently associated with eosinophilic meningitis. Although the presence of eosinophils in the CSF provides strong supportive evidence for helminth infection of the CNS, their absence does not exclude the diagnosis. Eosinophils are easily missed in unstained or Gram-stained CSF, and are best detected by Wright's or Giemsa stain of cytocentrifuged specimens. Thus, if helminth infection is suspected, the clinician should request that the laboratory stain the CSF specifically for eosinophils.

**Table 37.2** Causes of eosinophilic meningitis

| Infectious | | Noninfectious |
|---|---|---|
| Helminths | Non-helminths | |
| Nematodes | Fungi | Ventriculoperitoneal shunts[a] |
| *Angiostrongylus cantonensis*[a] | *Coccidioides immitis*[a] | CNS leukemia/lymphoma |
| *Baylisascaris procyonis*[a] | *Cryptococcus* | Drugs |
| *Gnathostoma spinigerum*[a] | Viruses | Antimicrobials (intraventricular) |
| *Toxocara* sp. | Coxsackie | Nonsteroidal anti-inflammatories |
| *Trichinella* sp. | Lymphocytic choriomeningitis | Myelography contrast |
| Cestodes | Bacteria | Hypereosinophilia syndrome |
| *Taenia solium* (cysticercosis) | Myiasis | Sarcoidosis |
| Trematodes | | |
| *Paragonimus westermani* | | |
| *Schistosoma* sp. | | |

[a]Common causes.

# Cestodes

## *Neurocysticercosis*

### Epidemiology

Neurocysticercosis, the most common parasitic infection of the CNS, is caused by infection with the larval form (cysterci) of *Taenia solium*, the pork tapeworm [9,10]. Neurocysticercosis has a worldwide distribution and is endemic in areas where pigs are raised in unsanitary conditions. It is especially prevalent in Central and South America (notably, Mexico), sub-Saharan Africa, India, Southeast Asia, and China, and seems to be on the rise in the United States [11–16]. In Latin America alone, an estimated 400,000 people have symptomatic disease [17]. In the United States, it is widely distributed and highly prevalent in certain populations (e.g., Hispanics, immigrants and travelers returned from endemic areas) and regions (e.g., the Southwest) [12–15,18].

### Pathogenesis

Humans can act as both definitive and intermediate host for *T. solium*. In taeniasis, humans act as the definitive host for the adult tapeworm. Pigs are the source of human infection. Humans ingest cysticerci larvae, in undercooked infested ("measly") pork, which develop into adult cestodes in the human gut. The head (scolex) of the adult worm attaches to the human jejunum via suckers and hooklets. The scolex is connected by an actively growing neck region to a long chain of hermaphroditic egg-producing segments (proglottids). Both eggs and gravid proglottids are shed in human feces. In the natural life cycle, pigs ingest human feces containing infective *Taenia* eggs, which hatch, penetrate the gut wall, and migrate to the pig's tissues where they encyst.

Unfortunately, humans may also act as intermediate hosts for larvae of *T. solium*, giving rise to cysticercosis. Cysticercosis is acquired by ingesting food contaminated with *Taenia* eggs shed in the feces of a human tapeworm carrier. Ingested eggs hatch and larvae penetrate the human gut and migrate to tissues, where they encyst. *Taenia* larvae have a predilection to encyst in brain, skeletal muscle, and the eye. Thus, taeniasis is caused by ingestion of larva in infested pork, while cysticercosis is a fecal–oral infection caused by ingestion of eggs in the feces of a human tapeworm carrier.

In neurocysticercosis, the CNS is affected by the presence of the parasite and the resulting inflammatory response, fibrosis, and residual calcification [19]. Symptoms depend on the number, location, and developmental stage of the cysts, and the inflammatory response [9,10]. Most children with neurocysticercosis have only a single parenchymal cyst, but massive infestation can occur [19,20]. Cysticerci are typically less than 1 cm across and, when not actively growing or degenerating, do not elicit an inflammatory immune response [11]. The majority of patients remain asymptomatic until, after a variable number of years (2–5 years in adults), the cysticercus begins to degenerate and loses its ability to modulate the host immune response [9,10]. Neurological symptoms appear as the inflammatory response develops. The final stage of infection involves granuloma formation, calcification, and death of the larva. Residual calcification and scarring act as foci for ongoing seizures [21].

## Clinical and Neurological Manifestations

Typically, neurocysticercosis presents with seizures (in 50–90% of cases) or signs of increased intracranial pressure (headache, nausea, and vomiting) [10,16,18,20]. Neurocysticercosis is the most common cause of late-onset epilepsy in adults from endemic areas and is a prominent cause of seizures in children [22]. Seizures are more commonly focal motor or complex partial in nature, rather than primary generalized tonic-clonic, and are characteristically afebrile [12,13,16,18]. Less common neurological manifestations include encephalitis and intracranial hypertension from multiple parenchymal cysts, obstructive hydrocephalus secondary to blockage of CSF flow from intraventricular cysts, or a slowly progressive paraplegia from involvement of the spinal cord. A minority of patients present with psychosis or visual disturbances. Cases of racemose cysticercosis in which grape-like clusters of cysticerci grow in the ventricles or basilar meninges, are locally invasive, and lead to hydrocephalus have also been reported [15]. Cerebrovascular accidents related to angiitis-induced infarctions are another rare manifestation of neurocysticercosis [2].

## Diagnosis

Clinical diagnosis of neurocysticercosis is difficult. No signs or symptoms are pathognomonic, and laboratory studies are neither sensitive for nor predictive of the diagnosis [16]. Patients are generally afebrile and signs of meningeal irritation are absent [18]. CSF is normal or shows mild, nonspecific pleocytosis or elevated protein levels [10,11,16]. Diagnosis is usually by neuroimaging and serology in a patient with appropriate risk of exposure (Fig. 37.1) [10]. A combination of computed tomographic (CT) and magnetic resonance imaging (MRI) scans provides the best diagnostic workup [10,16,20]. MRI scanning is most sensitive for detection of acute inflammatory changes, and, particularly, posterior fossa, intraventricular, or subarachnoid lesions, whereas CT scanning is best for demonstrating calcified granulomata. Cysts are classically thin walled with an eccentric hyperintensity corresponding to the scolex. As cysts die, they appear as dense granulomas with surrounding edema, and may be indistinguishable from CNS tumors. Definitive diagnosis of such solitary lesions commonly requires histological examination. Newer serologic tests for detection of antibodies to the cysticercus of *T. solium* are highly sensitive and specific, even with solitary parenchymal cysts and in areas in which *Taenia* and other helminths are highly endemic [10,11,20,23,24]. Nevertheless, as many as 30% of

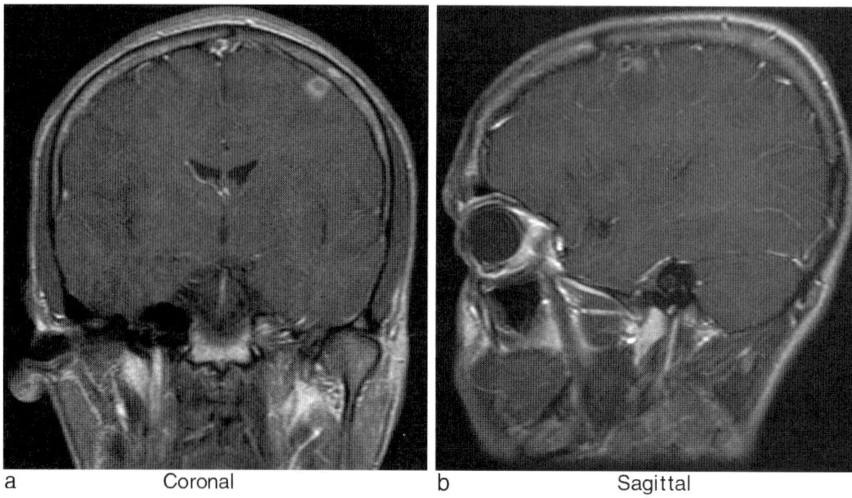


**Fig. 37.1** Neurocysticercosis in a 17-year-old boy who presented with afebrile seizures. **a** Coronal and **b** sagittal T1-weighted post-gadolinium MRI scans demonstrate left frontal cortical ring-enhancing lesions surrounded by mild vasogenic edema.

patients with a single CNS lesion may have negative test results [25]. To aid diagnosis, a set of criteria has been proposed that includes results of histology, imaging, and serology, with clinical features, response to treatment, and epidemiology [26].

## Treatment

The decision to treat neurocysticercosis is complex and should be made on an individual case basis [10]. Use of anthelminthics is controversial and largely depends on cyst number, viability, and activity [18,20]. Consensus treatment guidelines have recently been published [20,27]. In addition, recent double-blind placebo-controlled trials of albendazole in adults with multiple non-enhancing (viable) cysticerci and children with solitary enhancing (dying) cysticerci on neuroimaging demonstrated significant reductions in late-onset seizures, and more rapid resolution of brain cysts among the albendazole-treated groups [28,29]. Although both anthelminthics are highly effective in CNS disease, albendazole is considered superior to praziquantel [10,17,20]. In general, anthelminthic therapy is well tolerated and the long-term prognosis for treated patients is excellent. In contrast, extraparenchymal and racemose cysticercosis are associated with a poor prognosis [15]. Cysts outside the brain parenchyma grow irregularly and trigger a more intense inflammatory response [10]. Corticosteroids are usually used as adjunctive therapy to control any inflammatory reaction induced by destruction of the cyst and increased intracranial pressure, and are the mainstay of treatment of encephalitis, angiitis, and chronic meningitis, and particularly for extraparenchymal disease [10,20,27].

### Prevention

In areas of high endemicity, efforts to control cysticercosis focus on inspection of pork, removal of infected carcasses from the food chain, and public health initiatives to ensure sanitary disposal of human feces. In non-endemic areas, efforts focus on detection and treatment of tapeworm carriers to prevent additional cases [14]. In an effort to identify the source of infection and prevent further transmission, it is recommended that stools from pediatric cases and their family members are examined for presence of *Taenia* eggs [20].

## *Coenurosis*

### Epidemiology

Coenurosis is a zoonosis caused by larva of *Taenia* species of dog tapeworms: *T. serialis*, in Africa, Europe, and South America; and *T. multiceps* in North America [11,12,30].

### Pathogenesis

The pathogenesis is similar to that of cysticercosis, except that dogs rather than humans are the definitive hosts for the adult cestode. In the natural life cycle, herbivores and small mammals act as intermediate hosts. Human infection is more commonly seen in patients from rural areas, particularly in those who raise sheep.

Coenurosis is a rare but potentially serious disease. Neurotropism of the larva ensures that the CNS is preferentially involved [12,30]. Untreated, it progresses and the outcome is poor. Humans become accidental intermediate hosts by ingestion of eggs contained in dog feces. All North American cases have had significant previous exposure to dogs [30]. The eggs hatch and larvae exit the intestine and migrate to the CNS, where they develop into a fluid-filled cyst, the "coenurus," which often involves the ventricles, subarachnoid space, and spinal cord.

### Clinical and Neurological Manifestations

Coenurosis is more commonly diagnosed in adults, but a few cases have been described in young children, all of whom had CNS disease [30]. Clinical presentation is usually indolent with symptoms and signs of an intracranial mass lesion.

Occipital headache, vomiting, cranial nerve palsy, and seizures are common secondary to basal arachnoiditis and obstructing hydrocephalus.

### Diagnosis

Findings on neuroimaging are nonspecific and definitive diagnosis requires histological examination.

### Treatment

Surgical removal has been curative and is the only recognized treatment [11,12].

## *Hydatid Disease (Echinococcosis)*

### Epidemiology

Hydatid disease is caused by cestodes of the genus *Echinococcus*, common parasites of dogs and wild canids. It is a zoonosis of worldwide importance [31,32]. The two major species of medical and public health importance are *E. granulosus*, the cause of cystic hydatid disease, and *E. multilocularis*, the cause of alveolar hydatid disease. Both cause serious and severe diseases and are regarded as emerging or reemerging pathogens [31,32].

Cystic hydatid disease is problematic in Mediterranean regions, the Middle East, East Africa, South and Central America, China, and Australia, predominantly in rural areas where dogs and herbivores, the definitive and intermediate hosts, respectively, are found [31,32]. The small adult tapeworm lives in the intestine of dogs and sheds gravid proglottids or eggs in dog feces. Sheep and cattle or humans act as intermediate hosts by ingestion of dog feces containing infective larvae. In the intermediate host, larvae penetrate the gut wall and travel via lymphatics or blood vessels to the liver, lungs, or other organs. In tissue, *E. granulosus* larvae develop into slowly enlarging fluid-filled hydatid cysts. The natural life cycle is completed when dogs eat uncooked sheep carcasses or viscera that contain hydatid cysts. Humans are dead-end hosts.

### Pathogenesis

In humans, hydatid cysts are most commonly found in the liver (50–70%) or lungs (20–30%) [31]. Intracranial involvement occurs in 1 to 2% of infections [31–33]. Fifty to 75% of intracranial disease is seen in young children, especially boys [34,35]. Hydatid cysts in the CNS are usually solitary, parenchymal (commonly in the distribution of the middle cerebral artery), and slow growing, often to a very large size [36]. Hydatid cysts are filled with increasing numbers of protoscoleces (embryonic tapeworms) and daughter cysts.

## Clinical and Neurological Manifestations

Most patients remain asymptomatic for months to years, only developing symptoms if the cyst ruptures or exerts mass effect [32,33]. Rupture of the fragile cysts can lead to aseptic meningitis, anaphylaxis, and development of metastatic cysts with subsequent recurrence of disease. The majority of patients present with symptoms of raised intracranial pressure or focal signs [33,35]. The focal signs are typically secondary to pressure effects, and the specific neurological manifestation depends on the location of the cyst. In contrast to neurocysticercosis, hydatid disease of the CNS is rarely associated with seizures. Hydatid disease of the CNS should be in the differential diagnosis of any patient with a CNS mass lesion who has lived in an endemic area [12,37].

## Diagnosis

Diagnosis is most frequently made by neuroimaging. CT scans most commonly reveal a single large cystic lesion with signs of mass effect, but without the associated edema or enhancement characteristic of abscesses or tumors. The presence of additional cysts, in the liver or lung, supports the diagnosis. Serology for antibodies to *E. granulosus* are useful in diagnosis and follow-up of liver and lung disease, but are relatively insensitive in CNS disease [32]. Peripheral blood eosinophilia is present in a minority of cases.

## Treatment

Surgical excision remains the treatment of choice for CNS disease. Preoperative diagnosis is important to ensure that precautions are taken to minimize risk of cyst rupture at surgery, which can convert a curable disease to an incurable chronic one that is potentially fatal. In large series, mortality of CNS disease has approached 20% [33–35]. Postoperative seizure rates of 14% have been reported [35].

Experience and data regarding the efficacy of anthelminthic therapy are limited. However, mebendazole, albendazole, and praziquantel shrink and sterilize cysts, and are used as preoperative and postoperative adjuncts or if surgery is contraindicated [32].

## Prevention

Preventive strategies aim to decrease prevalence of infection in dogs and intermediate hosts by control of stray dogs, slaughter of livestock, and disposal of viscera.

## Other

*E. multilocularis* is a parasite of wild carnivores that infects humans living in Alaska, Arctic regions, central Europe, Russia, the Asian Republics, China, and Japan [32]. The cyst of *E. multilocularis* is a tumor-like, infiltrating structure composed of multiple small vesicles that are locally invasive. If diagnosed late or managed incorrectly, mortality and morbidity rates are high [31]. Fortunately, intracranial involvement by alveolar hydatid disease is very unusual.

## Sparganosis

### Epidemiology

Sparganosis is an uncommon disease caused by infection with larva of the genus *Spirometra,* cestodes of cats and dogs. The majority of cases occur in China, Korea, South East Asia, Japan, and Australia, although cases caused by *S. mansonoides* have occurred in the United States [12,38]. Disease is caused by aberrant migration of larvae, most frequently through subcutaneous tissue and muscle. Cerebral sparganosis is exceedingly rare in children, with only a handful of case reports [39,40].

### Pathogenesis

The life cycle of *Spirometra* is complex, involving a definitive host (a cat or dog) and two intermediate hosts (crustaceans and frogs or snakes). In endemic areas, adult *Spirometra* live in the intestines of cats or dogs and shed eggs in their feces. If eggs reach fresh water, they are ingested by a minute fresh water crustacean, *Cyclops*, and develop into larva. *Cyclops* are, in turn, ingested by frogs or snakes, and a further larval stage occurs. The natural life cycle is completed when cats or dogs ingest larvae, in tissues of infected frogs or snakes, which then develop into adult intestinal tapeworms. Humans serve as accidental intermediate hosts by ingesting larvae in untreated fresh water, raw or undercooked frogs, fish, and snakes, and directly through skin and conjunctivae with use of local, traditional raw snake or frog poultices [39,40].

### Clinical and Neurological Manifestations

Sparganosis presents most frequently as a superficial ocular or subcutaneous swelling [40]. CNS disease is uncommon; 5 (15%) of 34 reported cases in Thailand [40]. Patients with CNS involvement present with headache, generalized seizures, and focal signs, specifically hemiparesis and migratory cranial nerve palsies [39].

### Diagnosis

Neuroimaging is not specific, although change in position of cerebral lesions on serial imaging, caused by continued larva migration, is suggestive of the diagnosis. A serologic test with high reported sensitivity and specificity exists but is not readily available [39]. Definitive diagnosis requires histological identification of the worm.

### Treatment

Surgical excision is the only effective treatment. Albendazole has been used as additional treatment in deep visceral infection.

# Nematodes

## *Angiostrongyliasis*

### Epidemiology

The rat lungworm, *Angiostrongylus cantonensis*, is the most common infectious cause of eosinophilic meningitis in humans [7]. Most cases occur in Southeast Asia, the Pacific Basin, and Australia, where it is endemic, but recent outbreaks have been reported in North America and the Caribbean [7,38,41].

### Pathogenesis

In the rat, eggs laid in the pulmonary arteries by the adult worm, *A. cantonensis*, migrate to the intestine and are subsequently shed in feces. Humans are infected by ingestion of larvae in intermediate hosts, particularly fresh water snails and slugs that feed on rat feces; or transport hosts, such as prawns, crabs, and frogs; or fresh produce, such as lettuce, contaminated with infected snails or their slime [41,42]. Children are at high risk of infection and severe disease because they ingest higher inocula of larva [38,43].

Larvae of *A. cantonensis* are actively neurotropic in both rats and humans. Although humans are dead-end hosts for larvae, before they die, larval migration produces small (<0.1 mm) tracks and vascular thromboses in the brain and spinal cord [12]. Symptoms usually develop after an incubation period of up to 2 weeks (range, 2–45 days) [44]. Spinal fluid eosinophilia appears in response to the dying larvae, 2 to 4 weeks later, waxes and wanes, reappears at 6 to 8 weeks, and disappears after 12 weeks [44,45].

### Clinical and Neurological Manifestations

Typically, *A. cantonensis* infection presents as eosinophilic meningitis, with persistent severe headache, neck stiffness, vomiting, and paresthesiae [46]. In young children, presentation with persistent fever and encephalitis is common [47]. Although systemic infection is rare, presentation with acute abdominal distention, mimicking appendicitis has been reported [43,48]. As it progresses, development of hyperesthesia of the trunk or a limb is relatively common [45]. Angiostrongyliasis is usually short-lived and the prognosis favorable. Infection is generally self-limiting, with resolution within approximately 4 weeks of onset. The case fatality rate is generally low: 1 of 484 cases in Thailand [45]. However, long-term sequelae, adverse neurological outcome, and fatalities are reported, particularly in children [38,43,49]. Meningoencephalitis, cranial nerve palsy, coma, and residual neurological deficit have been described in association with ingestion of large inocula of larvae, particularly after the ingestion of raw snails, a delicacy in Vietnam and Thailand [12,42].

### Diagnosis

Definitive diagnosis is difficult. Among travelers at risk, the clinical diagnosis is suggested by headache, elevated opening pressure on lumbar puncture, and CSF pleocytosis with eosinophilia, particularly if accompanied by paresthesiae or hyperesthesiae [41]. Absence of eosinophilia (peripheral or in the CSF) is well described in the acute stages, and does not exclude the diagnosis [41,43,45,47,50,51]. When present, neuroimaging reveals nonspecific generalized edema and meningeal enhancement. Results of CT and MRI scans may be normal or reveal increased signal intensity in the basal ganglia, meningeal enhancement, and small hemorrhages [52]. Sensitive and specific tests for anti-*A. cantonensis* antibodies in serum or CSF are available in endemic areas [53,54].

### Treatment

Treatment is directed at reducing symptoms of meningitis and intracranial hypertension with analgesics, serial lumbar punctures, and corticosteroids [41]. Anthelminthic therapy has not changed the clinical outcome.

## *Toxocariasis*

### Epidemiology

Toxocariasis is caused by human infection with larvae of *Toxocara canis* or *Toxocara catis*, common roundworm parasites of dogs and cats, respectively. *Toxocara* has a worldwide distribution in dogs, with more than 90% of puppies infected soon after birth [12,55].

## Pathogenesis

Dogs defecate indiscriminately, and outdoor parks and children's play areas are generally heavily contaminated with feces containing *Toxocara* eggs. Eggs can remain infective in soil for years. Humans are infected by ingestion of soil contaminated with infective eggs. After the eggs hatch, larvae penetrate the intestine and migrate throughout the body. Larva migrans refers to the prolonged migration or persistence of helminth larvae in organs and tissues of animals or humans. *Toxocara canis* is the most common cause of visceral and ocular larva migrans in humans and animals worldwide [55]. This is a result of large numbers of infected dogs and cats, widespread environmental contamination with their feces, and the level of human contact with both. Infected dogs and cats shed enormous numbers of eggs in their feces daily [55].

## Clinical and Neurological Manifestations

Most *Toxocara* infections are considered to be asymptomatic, but subtle clinical features, which, in isolation, are nonspecific, are increasingly recognized [56]. Visceral larva migrans is seen in young children with heavy infestation, particularly those with pica. Visceral migration leads to tissue damage and an eosinophilic inflammatory reaction, and typically presents with fever, hepatomegaly, hypergammaglobulinemia, and peripheral eosinophilia [57]. Infection slowly resolves over months to years, although fatalities are occasionally reported.

Ocular larva migrans is associated with visual impairment and blindness. Although *Toxocara* sp. are a common cause of visceral larva migrans, they are a most unusual cause of neural larva migrans [55,57,58]. Rare cases of CNS infection, reported more commonly in adults than children, have presented with seizures, eosinophilic meningitis, or meningoencephalitis [59]. In contrast, the related raccoon nematode, *Baylisascaris*, invariably causes CNS disease.

## Diagnosis

Diagnosis is usually by serology in patients with a compatible history and clinical findings [55]. Humans, as dead-end hosts, do not pass *Toxocara* eggs or larvae in their feces.

## Treatment

Albendazole is considered the anthelminthic of choice for toxocariasis [58,59]. Corticosteroids are administered as adjunctive therapy for severe disease and, in particular, for ocular involvement.

## Prevention

Efforts to prevent infection have focused on treatment of puppies, control of the spread of dog feces, and protection of children's play areas.

## *Baylisascariasis*

### Epidemiology

Larvae of *Baylisascaris procyonis*, the common roundworm of raccoons (*Procyon lotor*), are the most common and widespread cause of clinical larva migrans in animals in the United States [60]. More recently, the zoonotic potential of *B. procyonis* has also become apparent [61,62]. To date, 13 confirmed human cases of CNS disease have been documented in the United States [63,64]. In humans, *B. procyonis* neural larva migrans, is a neurologically devastating and potentially fatal encephalitis. Contact with infected raccoons or their feces and geophagic pica are the most important risk factors for infection [60,63].

### Pathogenesis

Adult *B. procyonis* live in the raccoon small intestine. Infected raccoons contaminate the domestic environment by shedding millions of *B. procyonis* eggs daily in their feces. Raccoons defecate in latrines found at the bases of trees or on raised flat surfaces such as logs, tree-stumps, wooden decks, and rooftops [60]. Similar to *Toxocara* eggs, *B. procyonis* eggs are extremely resistant to degradation and decontamination and remain viable in moist soil for years. In the natural life cycle, fatal neural larva migrans develops in small mammals and birds after ingestion of infective eggs. The cycle is completed when raccoons ingest larvae in tissues of these animals. Humans are infected by ingestion of infective eggs in soil or other materials (e.g., bark/wood chips) contaminated with raccoon feces. Infants and young children, especially those with pica or geophagia, are at greatest risk of infection when exposed to contaminated environments. After ingestion, eggs hatch and larvae migrate aggressively and invade the CNS, where they continue to grow and incite a vigorous eosinophilic inflammatory response [60,63].

### Clinical and Neurological Manifestations

The clinical spectrum depends on the numbers of *B. procyonis* larvae entering the CNS, the extent of larval migration, and the severity of the inflammatory reaction. In addition to mechanical damage, the combination of larval products and the eosinophilic inflammatory response is markedly neurotoxic [8]. In animal and human infection, the brain is the most severely affected organ. Fatal human cases demonstrate massive larval invasion of the CNS [61]. Clinical presentation is one of rapidly progressive eosinophilic meningoencephalitis and is almost exclusively restricted to young infants and toddlers [63]. In contrast, in adults, *B. procyonis* causes retinitis rather than encephalitis, presumably reflecting smaller inocula of eggs and a larger adult brain.

## Diagnosis

In the absence of specific symptoms or signs, clinical diagnosis is difficult. Neuroimaging is nonspecific, lags behind the clinical signs, and has not led to early diagnosis (Fig. 37.2) [65]. Diagnosis is most frequently by serology for antibodies in CSF and serum in the setting of a compatible clinical and exposure history. Unfortunately, by the time serology is performed, severe CNS damage has already occurred. In North America or Europe, baylisascariasis should be considered strongly in any person with encephalitis, CSF and peripheral eosinophilia, with or without retinitis. A history of exposure to raccoons or their feces should be sought.

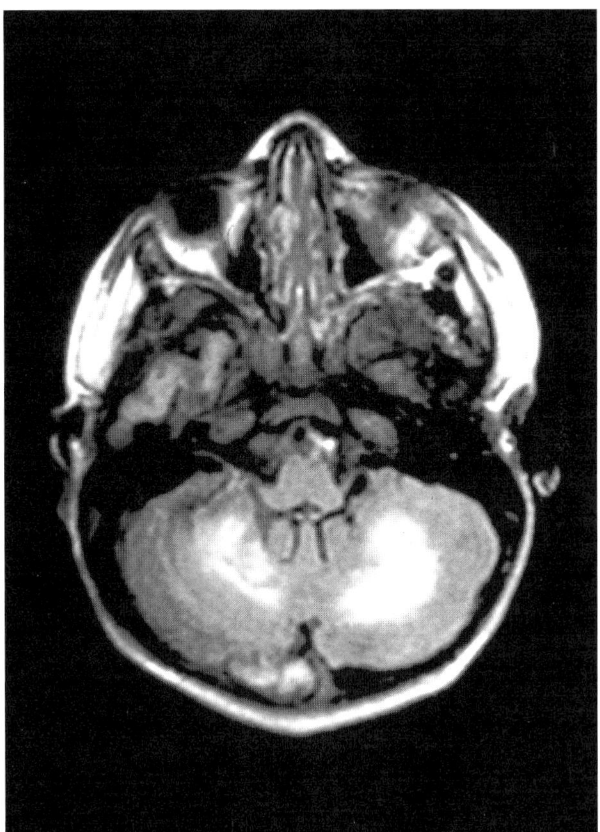

**Fig. 37.2** *Baylisascaris procyonis* neural larva migrans in a 2.5-year-old boy who presented with acute fulminant eosinophilic meningoencephalitis. Axial fluid-attenuated inversion recovery MRI scan at the level of the posterior fossa demonstrates an abnormal hyperintense signal of cerebellar white matter.

### Treatment

The current prognosis for *B. procyonis* neural larva migrans is grave, with or without treatment. Empiric anthelmintic therapy has failed to prevent unfavorable outcomes. Although several recent cases have not been fatal, there are no documented neurologically intact survivors [63]. For therapy to be effective, it should be started before larvae enter the CNS. However, at this early stage, the diagnosis is rarely apparent. Of the anthelminthic drugs available for *B. procyonis* infection, albendazole and diethylcarbamazine are considered to have the best CSF penetrance and larvicidal activity [60,63]. Because the larvicidal effect of anthelminthics may induce further inflammation and neurological damage, adjunctive corticosteroids are given.

### Prevention

In the absence of early diagnosis and effective therapy, prevention remains the best strategy. Public health education is crucial to minimize risk of exposure to raccoons or their feces. In many parts of the United States, widespread contamination of the domestic environment by infected raccoons suggests that the risk of human infection is substantial and likely to increase [66].

## *Trichinosis*

### Epidemiology

Trichinosis is a zoonosis, with worldwide distribution, caused by the nematode *Trichinella spiralis*.

### Pathogenesis

Humans are not the normal host. Infection is usually acquired by eating undercooked pork containing trichinella cysts. *Trichinella spiralis* exists in two forms: adult and cystic [67]. The adult worm lives in the mammalian intestine, where its eggs hatch and its larvae emerge. Motile larvae migrate via lymphatics and the circulation to encyst in striated muscle, where they can remain dormant for many years.

### Clinical and Neurological Manifestations

Trichinosis is usually self-limited. Intestinal infection is normally silent but may be associated with gastrointestinal upset. Larval migration is commonly associated with fever (90%), severe myalgia (86%), headaches (56%), periorbital edema, and eosinophilia [12,68]. Involvement of the CNS is seen in 10 to 20% of infections, usually in heavy infestation, when sufficient numbers of larvae reach the CNS. Although trichinella larvae only encyst in striated muscle, larval migration through the CNS and heart and the ensuing inflammatory response may have severe and potentially fatal complications [12,67]. Infection of the CNS presents as meningitis, meningoencephalitis, seizures, or focal deficits (plegias and cranial nerve palsy).

### Diagnosis

Diagnosis is serologic, by antigen detection, or by demonstration of larvae in tissue. Peripheral eosinophilia, caused by tissue invasion, is characteristic, and muscle enzyme elevation is found in approximately half of cases. Larvae may occasionally be identified in the CSF.

### Treatment

Therapy is directed at encysted larvae (mebendazole) and the inflammatory reaction they evoke (corticosteroids) [12,67].

### Prevention

Trichinosis can be prevented by thorough cooking or adequate refrigeration of pork and changes in animal husbandry that prevent pigs from eating contaminated garbage [12,67].

## *Strongyloidiasis*

### Epidemiology

Strongyloidiasis is caused by a small intestinal nematode, *Strongyloides stercoralis*, that infects an estimated 10 million people worldwide [69]. Although most infections are asymptomatic, CNS involvement and a fulminant fatal hyperinfection syndrome may develop in infected patients in the setting of compromised cell-mediated immunity. *Strongyloides stercoralis* is prevalent in tropical and subtropical regions worldwide, but endemic foci are found in the United States [69,70].

### Pathogenesis

The life cycle is unusual in having free living (moist soil), parasitic (intestinal), and endogenous (autoinfective) phases. Humans are usually infected transcutaneously by filariform (infective) larvae in soil. After skin penetration, rapid larval migration may cause a rapidly creeping urticarial rash, which is followed by migration to the lungs and small intestine. In the small intestine, adult female worms can persist and lay eggs for decades. Eggs hatch into rhabditidiform (free-living) larvae, which are shed in feces. In moist soil, rhabditidiform larvae develop into infective (filariform) larvae and wait to penetrate the intact skin of a passing host. Less commonly, in the endogenous cycle, rhabditidiform larvae develop into infective filariform larvae in the intestine, where they can penetrate the bowel wall or perianal skin and disseminate widely to tissues, including the CNS.

The ability of *S. stercoralis* to complete its life cycle in one host sets it apart from other helminth parasites. Hyperinfection describes the uncommon syndrome of accelerated "autoinfection." It is classically described in military veterans or immigrants who become immunocompromised and become symptomatic many years after returning from an endemic area [71]. Recipients of corticosteroids, cytotoxic chemotherapy, or organ transplants are most vulnerable [69,72]. Rare case of hyperinfection are reported in children with asymptomatic infection and compromised cell-mediated immunity [72].

### Clinical and Neurological Manifestations

Strongyloidiasis of the CNS classically presents as Gram-negative bacterial meningitis [68,69,72]. Meningitis occurs when enteric bacteria are carried in the wake of *Strongyloides* larvae migrating from the intestine to the CNS or by meningeal seeding during episodes of recurrent enteric bacteremia. Eosinophilic meningitis is not described.

### Diagnosis

Disseminated strongyloidiasis should be considered in any immunocompromised patient with unexplained enteric bacterial meningitis. A history of geographic exposure, creeping urticarial skin eruptions, gastrointestinal complaints, and peripheral eosinophilia should also arouse suspicion [71,72]. Diagnosis is by microscopy of stool or duodenal aspirates for the presence of characteristic larvae. After 1 or 2 days at room temperature, culture of stool on blood agar demonstrates serpiginous tracts of bacterial growth along the paths of motile larvae. Serologic testing is widely available, is sensitive but not specific, and does not distinguish between past or present infection [69,73]. Abnormalities on neuroimaging are non-specific, but include prominent atrophy, abscess, and mycotic aneurysm.

### Treatment

Anthelminthic therapy with ivermectin, albendazole, or thiabendazole is effective, particularly in chronic disease, but individualized and prolonged or repeated courses may be required [69,71,72]. Even with optimal therapy, the mortality rate in CNS disease is high.

Disseminated infection may be prevented by screening patients from endemic areas to identify and eradicate asymptomatic carriage before they undergo corticosteroid or cytotoxic chemotherapy [68,69]. Patients with *Strongyloides* hyperinfection should be nursed in contact isolation.

## *Gnathostomiasis*

### Epidemiology

Gnathostomiasis is caused by ingestion of raw or partially cooked foods infected with larva or cysts of *Gnathostoma spinigerum*, a nematode parasite of cats and dogs. *Gnathostoma* species are endemic in China, Southeast Asia, and, more recently, Central and South America (notably Mexico) [74,75]. Increased travel and immigration has led to an increasing number of cases in non-endemic areas [76].

### Pathogenesis

Eggs passed in the feces of cats and dogs hatch in fresh water and larvae infect a range of intermediate hosts, which include fish, crab, shrimp, crayfish, and fowl. Human infection follows ingestion of larvae in raw or inadequately cooked food [74,75].

It is postulated that *Gnathostoma* larvae enter the CNS by migrating directly through spinal or cranial nerve roots. Symptoms are caused by mechanical injury to neural tissue, nerves, and blood vessels caused by migrating larvae, the toxins they produce, and the resultant host inflammatory response [75]. In contrast to the microscopic migratory tracts of *Angiostrongylosis* larvae, in the CNS, migratory tracts of *Gnathostoma* larvae are much larger and visible to the naked eye [74].

### Clinical and Neurological Manifestations

Gnathostomiasis most often presents as recurrent migratory red, itchy, subcutaneous swellings with marked peripheral eosinophilia [75]. Invasion of the CNS is well described [74,75]. The highly motile larva cannot mature in humans but its migration, the resulting tissue destruction, and host inflammatory reaction produces clinical symptoms. Pain, specifically radicular pain, is the hallmark of neurological involvement in gnathostomiasis [74]. With rapid and widespread larval migration, radiculomyelitis, encephalomyelitis, hemiplegia, subarachnoid hemorrhage, eosinophilic meningitis, or multiple cranial nerve palsies may ensue. Initially, peripheral nervous system involvement is suggested by the sudden onset of agonizing radicular pain followed (1–5 days later) by paralysis or weakness of one or more limbs, and

CNS involvement including eosinophilic meningitis and occasionally subarachnoid hemorrhage [74]. In a series from Thailand, 16% of subarachnoid hemorrhages in infants and children were caused by gnathostomiasis [77]. In comparison with aneurysmal hemorrhage, bleeding caused by gnathostomiasis occurs in atypical locations and is associated with eosinophils in the CSF [77]. Mortality rates for *Gnathostoma* infection of the CNS range from 10 to 25% [74]. Death is usually caused by brainstem involvement, massive hemorrhage, or secondary bacterial infection. One third of survivors have neurological sequelae.

### Diagnosis

Definitive diagnosis requires isolation of the worm. Clinical diagnosis is most often made in patients with a compatible exposure history (residence or travel in an endemic area and consumption of implicated food) and supportive serologic tests. Eosinophilic meningitis and xanthochromia are characteristic of *Gnathostoma* infection of the CNS, but are not absolute requirements for the diagnosis [74]. Neuroimaging has been helpful in assessing extent and severity of disease. MRI scan of the spine has demonstrated enlargement of the cervical cord with diffuse, ill defined, high signal intensity on T2-weighted images, especially involving the central grey matter [78]. In a patient with cauda equina syndrome, MRI scan of the lumbosacral spine showed slight enlargement of the conus medullaris, with gadolinium enhancement of the cauda equina nerve roots [79]. MRI scan of the brain has shown scattered deep intracerebral hemorrhages and hemorrhagic tracts, as well as diffuse T2-weighted hyperintensities involving the periventricular white matter, with small nodular enhancing lesions [78].

### Treatment

Surgical removal is the only effective therapy for CNS disease, providing the worm can be located in an accessible area. Blind surgical exploration is not recommended [75]. Gnathostomiasis can be effectively prevented by proper cooking of food that might contain infective larvae or cysts.

# Trematodes

## *Schistosomiasis*

### Epidemiology

Schistosomiasis is caused by infection with parasitic mammalian blood flukes, whose adults live and mate within the human vasculature. Three species cause the majority of human disease: *S. hematobium*, *S. mansoni*, and *S. japonicum*. Schistosomiasis is one of the most widespread of all parasitic diseases, and ranks second only to malaria in terms of socioeconomic and public health importance [1]. It is endemic in 76 countries worldwide: *S. hematobium* in the Middle East and Africa; *S. mansoni* in Africa (particularly, the Nile valley, Egypt, and the Sudan) and South America (particularly Brazil); and *S. japonicum* in China, Indonesia, and the Philippines [80]. In endemic areas, children have the highest prevalence of infection [81]. In 1977, it was estimated that there were 400,000 imported cases of schistosomiasis in the United States [82]. In a CDC investigation, prompted by cases of schistosomiasis in returning Peace Corps volunteers, one third of expatriates residing in Malawi were found to be infected [83].

## Pathogenesis

The *Schistosoma* life cycle is complex, involving a definitive human host, intermediate freshwater snail hosts, and repeated human exposures to freshwater contaminated with human excreta. In humans, pairs of adult *S. hematobium* preferentially inhabit venules in the bladder wall and pelvic venous plexus, whereas those of *S. mansoni* and S. *japonicum* inhabit the inferior and superior mesenteric venules, respectively. For the duration of their 3- to 8-year life span, adult female worms lay eggs in the vasculature [80]. Some eggs pass through the vessel wall into the lumen of the bladder (*S. hematobium*) or bowel (*S. mansoni* and *S. japonicum*) and are shed in urine or feces. Many other eggs embolize from the vasculature to reach the liver, lung, or other sites, including the CNS. The burden of schistosomal disease results from ectopic deposition of the eggs and the granulomatous inflammatory immune response they provoke.

Eggs, shed in human excreta, reach fresh water and hatch into motile larvae, which infect specific aquatic snails. After further development and incubation, actively swimming microscopic infective forms (cercariae) emerge from snails. Humans are infected by cercariae that penetrate intact skin or mucosa during exposure to infested fresh water.

## Clinical and Neurological Manifestations

School-aged children are most heavily infected by cercariae because of more intense water exposure, lack of partial immunity, and relatively poor hygiene. Skin penetration may be associated with acute cercarial dermatitis ("swimmer's itch") and a delayed serum sickness-like illness, with rash, fever, and swelling, and intense eosinophilia, termed "Katayama fever." Occasionally, in young Caucasians from non-endemic areas, self-limiting neurological symptoms may accompany Katayama fever [84]. In human tissues, cercariae become shistosomulae, which migrate to the venules, where they develop into adults, mate, and lay eggs. Adult worms in human vasculature cause little pathology and evade the immune system for decades. In contrast, eggs deposited in tissues provoke the intense granulomatous inflammation and fibrosis responsible for symptoms and signs of chronic infection. *Schistosoma hematobium* is associated with bladder fibrosis, chronic painless hematuria, and bladder cancer, whereas *S. mansoni* and *S. japonicum* cause colonic polyposis, chronic diarrhea, hepatic cirrhosis, and portal hypertension.

Neuroschistosomiasis manifests as cerebral or spinal cord disease. Eggs of the three *Schistosoma* species have been found in brain and spinal cord. *Schistosoma* eggs are thought to reach the CNS via Batson's valveless intervertebral venous plexus, by arterial embolism, or by local production by ectopic adult worms. Although cerebral involvement is more often associated with *S. japonicum* and *S. haematobium*, myelopathy is most commonly caused by *S. mansoni* [68,84]. It is postulated that the smaller eggs of *S. japonicum* are more likely to reach the brain, whereas the larger eggs of *S. mansoni*, with their lateral spine, lodge in the lower cord.

Most cases of cerebral egg deposition are asymptomatic. When symptomatic, acute cerebral schistosomiasis presents with meningoencephalitis. Chronic CNS involvement presents with seizures (generalized, focal motor or temporal lobe), signs of a space-occupying lesion, or stroke [68,80]. In contrast, spinal cord disease is rarely asymptomatic and frequently presents with areflexic flaccid paraplegia, sphincter dysfunction, and altered sensation [84–86]. The majority of schistosomal myelopathy is caused by intramedullary granulomas in the conus medullaris. Most patients develop paraplegia within a week of the onset of symptoms [84]. Although schistosomal myelopathy is prevalent in endemic areas, because of the worm's longevity, disease may present in the developed world many years after initial infection.

## Diagnosis

Definitive diagnosis is by visualization of eggs in stool, urine, tissue biopsies, or rectal snips. CSF analysis often reveals mild lymphocytic pleocytosis, and elevated protein and normal glucose levels [84,86]. Peripheral and CSF eosinophilia are characteristic, but their absence does not exclude the diagnosis [84,86]. Positive serologic tests suggest infection and support a compatible clinical presentation [80,81]. Because acutely infected travelers from endemic areas may have relatively low numbers of eggs in their excreta and seroconversion can take up to 12 weeks, repeated examinations may be required to make the diagnosis [38]. Neuroimaging may demonstrate a cerebral space-occupying lesion or cord abnormality.

## Treatment

Anthelminthic therapy with praziquantel is effective, cheap, and well tolerated [68]. Cure rates for urinary and intestinal disease approach 80%, but are more variable in neuroschistosomiasis. In one review, 54% of patients recovered, 34% remained paraplegic, and 11% died [84]. Early empiric therapy of suspected schistosomal myelopathy and laminectomy improve the prognosis [80,84]. Adjunctive use of corticosteroid remains controversial.

### Prevention

In Africa, where 85% of infected people live, World Health Organization control strategies aim to decrease morbidity by reducing the worm burden in infected people with regular population-based anthelminthic therapy. Strategies to prevent infection focus on health education and improved sanitation and water supplies.

## *Paragonimiasis*

### Epidemiology

Paragonimiasis is primarily a pulmonary disease caused by species of adult lung flukes of the genus *Paragonimus*. Infection is prevalent in Southeast Asia, West Africa, and South and Central America [86]. *Paragonimus westermani*, the Oriental lung fluke, is the most common etiologic agent in Asia and worldwide.

### Pathogenesis

Humans are infected by the ingestion of raw, pickled, or undercooked fresh water crabs and crayfish containing *Paragonimus* larvae. Larvae penetrate the gut wall and migrate from the peritoneal cavity, through the diaphragm, and into the lungs, where they mature into adult worms. In the lung, the adults create a cystic space, where they may survive for up to 20 years, and begin to lay eggs, which are either expectorated in sputum or passed in feces. The eggs hatch in fresh water, and pass through an intermediate snail host before encysting in the tissues of a crustacean.

### Clinical and Neurological Manifestations

Typically, paragonimiasis manifests as a chronic cough with production of purulent, bloodstained or rusty brown sputum and parasite eggs. Involvement of the CNS by *Paragonimus* is a consequence of aberrant larval migration into the CNS through the skull foramina. The posterior region of the CNS is affected most frequently [87]. Involvement of the CNS is most common in young children [87,88]. In a large South Korean series, 75% of patients with CNS paragonimiasis were younger than 20 years old [88]. In two thirds of patients, the onset of disease was insidious. Half of the cases had pulmonary disease, which frequently preceded involvement of the CNS. Cerebral paragonimiasis presents as focal seizures (40–60%), visual impairment (50%), headache, meningitis, space-occupying lesion, or hemiplegia. Spinal lesions may present as spastic paraplegia.

### Diagnosis

The clinical diagnosis of *Paragonimus* infection of the CNS is suggested by a compatible clinical picture, dietary history, or residence in an endemic area, and chronic hemoptysis. Definitive diagnosis is by demonstration of eggs in sputum, feces, or cerebral tissue. CSF findings may mimic tuberculosis, with a mononuclear pleocytosis and elevated protein level, or xanthochromia. Eosinophilic meningitis is unusual. Neuroimaging, typically, shows grape-like clusters of ring-enhancing lesions followed by "soap-bubble" calcifications. Results of chest radiography are also frequently abnormal [88].

### Treatment

Praziquantel is the anthelminthic of choice and is highly effective in pulmonary disease, although caution is advisable in CNS disease [87].

### Prevention

Prevention of disease depends on public health education to change cultural food preparation and consumption practices, and on early identification of pulmonary disease, particularly in children.

## References

1. World Health Organization. The World Health Report 1999. Geneva, 1999.
2. Stamos JK, Rowley AH, Hahn YS, Chadwick EG, Schantz PM, Wilson M. Neurocysticercosis: report of unusual pediatric cases. *Pediatrics* 1996; 98:974–977.
3. Schantz PM, Moore AC, Munoz JL, Hartman BJ, Schaefer JA, Aron AM, Persaud D, Sarti E, Wilson M, Flisser A. Neurocysticercosis in an Orthodox Jewish community in New York city. *N Engl J Med* 1992; 327:692–695.
4. Kruskal BA, Moths L, Teele DW. Neurocysticercosis in a child with no history of travel outside the continental United States. *Clin Infect Dis* 1992; 16:290–292.
5. Rothenberg ME. Eosinophilia. *N Engl J Med* 1998; 338:1592–1600.
6. Weller PF. Eosinophilic meningitis. *Am J Med* 1993; 95:250–253.
7. Re VL, Gluckman SJ. Eosinophilic meningitis. *Am J Med* 2003; 114:217–223.
8. Moertel CL, Kazacos KR, Butterfield JH, Kita H, Watterson J, Gleich GJ. Eosinophil-associated inflammation and elaboration of eosinophil-derived proteins in two children with raccoon roundworm (*Baylisascaris procyonis*) encephalitis. *Pediatrics* (http://www.pediatrics.org/cgi/content/full/108/5/e93). 2001; 108.

9. White AC. Neurocysticercosis: a major cause of neurological disease worldwide. *Clin Infect Dis* 1997; 24:101–115.
10. Garcia HH, Del Bruto OH, for the Cysticercosis Working Group in Peru. Neurocysticercosis: updated concepts about an old disease. *Lancet Neurol* 2005; 5:653–661.
11. Baily GC. Other Cestode Infections. In: Cook GC, Zumla AI, eds. *Manson's Tropical Diseases*. 21st ed Philadelphia: WB Saunders, 2003; 1583–1597.
12. Cameron ML, Durack DT. Helminthic Infections of the Central Nervous System. In: Scheld W, Whitley R, Durack D, eds. *Infections of the Central Nervous System*. New York: Raven Press, 1997; 825–858.
13. Ong S, Talan DA, Moran GJ, Mower W, Newdow M, Tsang VC, Pinner RW. Neurocysticercosis in radiographically imaged seizure patients in U.S. emergency departments. *Emerg Infect Dis* 2002; 8:608–613.
14. Townes JM, Hoffmann CJ, Kohn MA. Neurocysticercosis in Oregon, 1995–2000. *Emerg Infect Dis* 2004; 10:508–510.
15. Sorvillo FJ, Portigal L, DeGiorgio C, Smith L, Waterman SH, Berlin GW, Ash LR. Cysticercosis-related deaths, California. *Emerg Infect Dis* 2004; 10:465–469.
16. Rosenfeld EA, Byrd SE, Shulman ST. Neurocysticercosis among children in Chicago. *Clin Infect Dis* 1996; 23:262–268.
17. Bern C, Garcia HH, Evans C, Gonzalez AE, Verastegui M, Tsang VC, Gilman RH. Magnitude of the disease burden from neurocysticercosis in a developing country. *Clin Infect Dis* 1999; 29:1203–1209.
18. Sotelo J, Guerrero V, Rubio F. Neurocysticercosis: a new classification based on active and inactive forms. *Arch Intern Med* 1985; 145:442–445.
19. Mitchell WG, Crawford TO. Intraparenchymal cerebral cysticercosis in children: diagnosis and treatment. *Pediatrics* 1988; 82:76–82.
20. St. Geme JW, Maldonado Y, Enzmann D, Hotez PJ, Overturf GD, Schantz PM. Consensus: diagnosis and management of neurocysticercosis in children. *Pediatr Infect Dis J* 1993; 12:455–461.
21. Del Brutto OH. Prognostic factors for seizure recurrence after withdrawal of antiepileptic drugs in patients with neurocysticercosis. *Neurology* 1994; 44:1706–1709.
22. Garcia HH, Brutto OHD. *Taenia solium* cysticercosis. *Infect Dis Clin North Am* 2000; 14:97–119.
23. Sloan L, Schneider S, Rosenblatt J. Evaluation of enzyme-linked immunoassay for serological diagnosis of cysticercosis. *J Clin Microbiol* 1995; 33:3124–3128.
24. Tsang VCW, Brand JA, Boyer AE. An enzyme-linked immunoelectrotransfer blot assay and glycoprotein antigens for diagnosing human cysticercosis (*Taenia solium*). *J Infect Dis* 1989; 159:50–59.
25. Wilson M, Bryan RT, Fried JA, Ware DA, Schantz PM, Pilcher JB, Tsang VC. Clinical evaluation of the cysticercosis enzyme-linked immunoelectrotransfer blot in patients with neurocysticercosis. *J Infect Dis* 1991; 164:1007–1009.
26. Del Brutto OH, Rajshekhar V, White AC Jr., Tsang VCW, Nash TE, Takayanagui OM, Schantz PM, Evans, CAW, Flisser A,Correa D, Botero D, Allan JC, Sarti E, Gonzalez AE, Gilman RH, García HH. Proposed diagnostic criteria for neurocysticercosis. *Neurology* 2001; 57:747–783.
27. Garcia HH, Evans CAW, Nash TE, Takayanagui OM, White AC, Botero D, Rajshekhar V, Tsang VCW, Schantz PM, Allan JC, Flisser A, Correa D, Sarti E, Friedland JS, Martinez MM, Gonzalez AE, Gilman RH, Del Bruto OH. Current consensus guidelines for treatment of neurocysticercosis. *Clin Microbiol Rev* 2002; 15:747–756.
28. Garcia HH, Pretell EJ, Gilman RH, Martinez SM, Moulton LH, Del Brutto OH, Herrera G, Evans CAW, Gonzalez AE. A trial of antiparasitic treatment to reduce the rate of seizures due to neurocysticercosis. *N Engl J Med* 2004; 350:249–258.
29. Baranwal AK, Singhi PD, Khandelwal N, Singhi SC. Albendazole therapy in children with focal seizures and single small enhancing computerized tomographic lesions: a randomized, placebo-controlled, double blind trial. *Pediatr Infect Dis J.* 1998; 17:696–700.

30. Ing MB, Schantz PM, Turner JA. Human Coenurosis in North America: Case reports and review. *Clin Infect Dis* 1998; 27:519–523.
31. Eckert J, Deplazes P. Biological, epidemiological, and clinical aspects of echinococcosis, a zoonosis of increasing concern. *Clin Microbiol Rev* 2004; 17:107–135.
32. McManus DP, Zhang W, Li J, Bartley PB. Echinococcosis. *Lancet* 2003; 362:1295–1304.
33. Gottstein B, Reichen J. Echinococcosis/Hydatidosis. In: Cook GC, Zumla AI, eds. *Manson's Tropical Diseases*. 21st ed. Philadelphia: WB Saunders, 2003; 1561–1582.
34. Ersahin Y, Mutluer S, Guzelbag E. Intracranial hydatid cysts in children. *Neurosurgery* 1993; 33:219–225.
35. Onal C, Unal F, Barlas O, Izgi N, Hepgul K, Turantan MI, Canbolat A, Turker K, Bayindir C, Gokay HK, Kaya U. Long-term follow-up and results of thirty pediatric intracranial hydatid cysts: Half a century of experience in the department of neurosurgery of the School of Medicine at University of Istanbul (1952–2001). *Pediatr Neurosurg* 2001; 35:72–81.
36. Onal C, Barlas O, Orakdofen M, Hepgul K, Izgi N, Unal F. Three unusual cases of intracranial hydatid cyst disease in the pediatric age group. *Pediatr Neurosurg* 1997; 26:208–213.
37. Pearl M, Kotsilimbos DG, Lehrer HZ, Hanumanth A, Fink H, Zaiman H. Cerebral *Echinococcus*, a pediatric disease: report of two cases with one successful five-year follow-up. *Pediatrics* 1978; 61:915–920.
38. Hughes A, Biggs B. Parasitic worms of the central nervous system: an Australian perspective. *Intern Med J* 2002; 32:541–553.
39. Kim C, Cho B, Kim I, Hwang Y, Wang K. Cerebral sparganosis in a child. *Pediatr Neurosurg* 1997; 26:103–106.
40. Wiwanitkit, V. A review of human sparganosis in Thailand. *Intern J Infect Dis* 2005; 9:312–316.
41. Slom TL, Cortese MM, Gerber SI, Jones RC, Holtz TH, Lopez AS, Zambrano CH, Sufit RL, Sakolvaree Y, Chaicumpa W, Herwaldt BL, Johnson S. An outbreak of eosinophilic meningitis caused by *Angiostrongylus cantonensis* in travelers returning from the Caribbean. *N Engl J Med* 2002; 346:668–675.
42. Chau T, Thwaites G, Chuong L, Sinh D, Farrar J. Headache and confusion: the dangers of a raw snail supper. *Lancet* 2003; 361:1866.
43. Lindo JF, Escoffery CT, Reid B, Codrington G, Cunningham-Myrie C, Eberhard M. Fatal autochthonous eosinophilic meningitis in a Jamaican child caused by *Angiostrongylus cantonensis. Am J Trop Med Hygiene* 2004; 70:425–428.
44. Hwang K, Chen E. Clinical studies on *Angiostrongylus cantonensis* among children in Taiwan. *Asian J Trop Med Public Health* 1991; 22:194–199.
45. Punyagupta S, Bunnag T, Juttijudata P, Rosen L. Eosinophilic meningitis in Thailand: epidemiologic studies of 484 typical cases and the etiologic role of *Angiostrongylus cantonensis. Am J Trop Med Hygiene* 1970; 19:950–958.
46. Kuberski T, Wallace G. Clinical manifestations of eosinophilic meningitis due to *Angiostrongylus cantonensis. Neurology* 1079; 29:1566–1570.
47. Shih S, Hsu C, Huang F, Shen E, Lin J. Fatal *Angiostrongylus* infection in a Jamaican child. *Am J Trop Med Hygiene* 1992; 70:425–428.
48. Hulbert TV, Larsen RA, Chandrasoma PT. Abdominal Angiostrongyliasis mimicking acute appendicitis and Meckel's diverticulum: report of a case in the United States and review. *Clin Infect Dis* 1992; 14:836–840.
49. Cooke-Yarborough CM, Kornberg AJ, Hogg GG, Spratt DM, Forsyth JR. A fatal case of Angiostrongyliasis in an 11-month-old infant. *Med J Aust* 1999; 170:541–543.
50. Shia SL, Hsu CH, Huang FY, Shen EY, Lin JC. *Angiostrongylus cantonensis* infection in infants and young children. *Pediatr Infect Dis J* 1992; 11:1064–1066.
51. Tsai HC, Liu YC, Kunin CM, Lee SS, Chen YS, Lin HH, Tsai TH, Lin WR, Huang CK, Yen MY, Yen CM. Eosinophilic meningitis caused by *Angiostrongylus cantonensis*: report of 17 cases. *Am J Med* 2001; 111:109–114.
52. Tsai HC, Liu YC, Kunin CM, Lai PH, Lee SS, Chen YS, Wann SR, Lin WR, Huang CK, Ger LP, Lin HH, Yen MY. Eosinophilic meningitis caused by *Angiostrongylus cantonensis* associated

with eating raw snails: correlation of brain magnetic resonance imaging scans with clinical findings. *Am J Trop Med Hygiene* 2003; 68:281–285.
53. Chye SM, Yen CM, Chen ER. Detection of circulating antigen by monoclonal antibodies for immunodiagnosis of angiostrongyliasis. *Am J Trop Med Hygiene* 1997; 56:408–412.
54. Ellis-Pegler R, Parry G. Eosinophilic meningitis due to Angiostrongylus cantonensis. *Clin Infect Dis* 2002; 35:777–778.
55. Kazacos KR. Protecting children from helminthic zoonoses. *Contemporary Pediatrics* 2000; 17(Suppl): 1–24.
56. Taylor MR, Keane C, O'Connor P, Mulvihill E, Holland C. The expanded spectrum of toxocaral disease. *Lancet* 1988; 1(8587):692–694.
57. Despommier D. Toxocariasis: Clinical aspects, epidemiology, medical ecology, and molecular aspects. *Clin Microbiol Reviews* 2003; 16:265–272.
58. Schantz PM. Toxocara Larva Migrans Now. *Am J Trop Med Hygiene* 1989; 41 Suppl:21–34.
59. Vidal JE, Sztajnbok J, Seguro AC. Eosinophilic meningoencephalitis due to *Toxocara canis*: Case report and review of the literature. *Am J Trop Med Hygiene* 2003; 69:341–343.
60. Kazacos KR. *Baylisascaris procyonis* and related species. In: Samuels WM, Pybus MJ, Kocan AA, eds. *Parasitic Diseases of Wild Mammals*. 2nd ed. Ames Iowa. Iowa State University Press, 2001; 301–341.
61. Fox AS, Kazakos KK, Gould NS, Heydemann PT, Thomas C, Boyer KM. Fatal eosinophilic meningoencephalitis and visceral larva migrans caused by the raccoon ascarid *Baylisascaris procyonis. N Engl J Med* 1985; 312:1619–1623.
62. Gavin PJ, Kazacos KR, Tan TQ, Brinkman WB, Byrd SE, Davis AT, Mets MB, Shulman. ST. Neural larval migrans caused by the raccoon roundworm *Baylisascaris procyonis. Pediatr Infect Dis J* 2002; 21:971–975.
63. Gavin PJ, Kazacos KR, Shulman ST. Baylisascariasis. *Clin Microbiol Rev* 2005; 18:703–718.
64. Murray WJ, Kazacos KR. Raccoon roundworm encephalitis. *Clin Infect Dis* 2004; 39:1484–1492.
65. Rowley HA, Uht RM, Kazakos KR, Sakanari J, Wheaton WV, Barkovich AJ, Bollen AW. Radiologic-pathologic findings in raccoon roundworm (*Baylisascaris procyonis*) encephalitis. *Am J Neuroradiol* 2000; 21:415–420.
66. Snyder DE, Fitzgerald PR. The relationship of *Baylisascaris procyonis* to Illinois raccoons (*Procyon lotor*). *J Parasitol* 1985; 71:596–598.
67. Giles HM. Trichinosis. In: Cook GC, Zumla AI, eds. *Manson's Tropical Diseases*. 21st ed. Philadelphia: WB Saunders, 2003; 1553–1560.
68. Bia FJ, Barry M. Parasitic infections of the central nervous system. *Neurol Clin* 1986; 4:171–206.
69. Keiser PB, Nutman TB. *Strongyloides stercoralis* in the immunocompromised population. *Clin Microbiol Rev* 2004; 17:208–217.
70. Berk SL, Verghese A, Alvarez S, Hall K, Smith B. Clinical and epidemiologic features of strongyloidiasis. A prospective study in rural Tennessee. *Arch Intern Med* 1987; 147:1257–1261.
71. Pelletier LL, Gabre-Kidan T. Chronic strongyloidiasis in Vietnam veterans. *Am J Med* 1985; 78:139–140.
72. Scowden EB, Schaffner W, Stone WJ. Overwhelming strongyloidiasis. *Medicine* 1978; 57:527–544.
73. Walker MD, Zunt JR. Neuroparasitic infections: nematodes. *Seminars Neurol* 2005; 25:252–261.
74. Boongird P, Phuapradit P, Siridej N, Chirachariyavej Y, Chuahirun S, Vejjajiva A. Neurological manifestations of gnathostomiasis. *J Neurol Sci* 1977; 31:279–291.
75. Rusnak JM, Lucey DR. Clinical gnathostomiasis: case report and review of the English language literature. *Clin Infect Dis* 1992; 16:33–50.
76. Moore DA, McCroddan J, Dekumyoy P, Chiodini PL. Gnathostomiasis: an emerging imported disease. *Emerg Infect Dis* 2003; 9:647–650.

77. Visudhiphan P, Chiemchanya S, Somburanasin R, Dheandhanoo D. Causes of spontaneous subarachnoid hemorrhage in Thai infants and children. *J Neurosurg* 1980; 53:185–187.
78. Sawanyawisuth K, Tiamkao S, Kanpittaya J, Dekumyoy P, Jitpimolmard S. MR imaging findings in cerebrospinal gnathostomiasis. *Am J Neuroradiol* 2004; 25:446–449.
79. Sawanyawisuth K, Tiamkao S, Nitinavakarn B, Dekumyoy P, Jitpimolmard S. MR imaging findings in cauda equina gnathostomiasis. *Am J Neuroradiol* 2005; 26:39–42.
80. Davis A. Schistosomiasis. In: Cook GC, Zumla AI, eds. *Manson's Tropical Diseases*. 21st ed. Philadelphia: WB Saunders, 2003; 1431–1469.
81. Doehring E. Schistosomiasis in childhood. *Eur J Pediatr* 1988; 147:2–9.
82. Mahmoud AA. Schistosomiasis: current concepts. *N Engl J Med* 1977; 297:1329–1331.
83. CDC. Schistosomiasis in U.S. Peace Corps volunteers—Malawi, 1992. *MMWR* 1993;Jul 30; 42:565–570.
84. Scrimgeour EM, Gajdusek DC. Involvement of the central nervous system in *Schistosoma mansoni* and *haematobium* infection. *Brain* 1985; 108:1023–1038.
85. Selwa L, Brunberg J, Mandell S, Garofalo E. Spinal cord schistosomiasis: a pediatric case mimicking intrinsic cord neoplasm. *Neurology* 1991; 41:755–777.
86. Nascimento-Carvalho C, Moreno-Carvalho O. Clinical and cerebrospinal fluid findings in patients less than 20 years old with a presumptive diagnosis of neuroschistosomiasis. *J Trop Pediatr* 2004; 50:98–100.
87. Haswell-Elkins M, Levri E. Food-borne Trematodes. In: Cook GC, Zumla AI, eds. *Manson's Tropical Diseases*. 21st ed. Philadelphia: WB Saunders, 2003; 1481–1486.
88. Oh SJ. Cerebral paragonimiasis. *Trans Am Neurol Assoc* 1967; 92:275–277.

# Section VII
# Primary Immunodeficiencies

# Chapter 38
# Neurological Disease and Primary Immunodeficiency

**Megan Connick, M.D.**

## Primary Immunodeficiencies

### *Introduction*

The primary immunodeficiencies are heritable disorders of the immune system. Neurological disease, either degenerative or developmental, is a feature of some of these disorders. Children with ataxia–telangiectasia suffer from relentless loss of cerebellar function [1] and those with Nijmegen breakage syndrome are microcephalic at birth or become so postnatally [2]. Distinctive neurological sequelae of immune system dysfunction also complicate some of the primary immunodeficiencies. Patients with X-linked agammaglobulinemia are vulnerable to chronic enteroviral meningoencephalitis [3], whereas children with Wiskott–Aldrich [4] or X-linked lymphoproliferative syndrome [5] develop hematologic malignancies with central nervous system involvement. Lymphohistiocytic infiltration of cranial nerves and brain occurs during the accelerated phase of Chédiak–Higashi syndrome [6]. Neurological manifestations of selected primary immunodeficiencies are listed in Table 38.1 [1–16].

### *Ataxia–Telangiectasia Syndrome*

#### Introduction

Ataxia–telangiectasia (AT) syndrome is an autosomal recessive disorder characterized by progressive cerebellar ataxia, oculocutaneous telangiectasia, frequent infection, radiosensitivity, and predisposition to malignancy [1].

L.L. Barton and N.R. Friedman (eds.), *The Neurological Manifestations of Pediatric Infectious Diseases and Immunodeficiency Syndromes.*

**Table 38.1** Neurological features of selected primary immunodeficiencies

| Disorder | Site of immune defect | Non-neurological features | Neurological features |
|---|---|---|---|
| C1q deficiency [7] | Complement cascade | Early-onset SLE-like syndrome | Autoimmune disease of CNS |
| | | Invasive bacterial infection | Bacterial meningitis |
| C5, C6, C7, C8, C9 deficiency [8] | Complement cascade | | Meningococcal meningitis |
| Chronic granulomatous disease [9,10] | Phagocyte | Abscess formation | Chorioretinopathy |
| | | Obstruction of hollow viscera | Intracranial infection (rare) |
| Chédiak–Higashi syndrome [6,11] | NK cell, T-cell | Oculocutaneous albinism | Variable (see text) with accelerated phase |
| | | Severe bacterial infections | Cerebellar ataxia (adults) |
| | | Uncontrolled lymphoproliferation | |
| Griscelli syndrome [12,13] | NK cell, T cell | See Chédiak–Higashi syndrome | Variable (see text) with accelerated phase |
| X-linked agammaglobulinemia [3] | B cell | Severe bacterial infections | Chronic enteroviral meningoencephalitis |
| X-linked lymphoproliferative syndrome [5] | NK, B, and T cell | Fatal EBV-associated mononucleosis | CNS involvement in mononucleosis |
| | | Predisposition to malignancy | Malignancy commonly involves CNS |
| Wiskott–Aldrich syndrome [4] | B and T cell | Eczema; bleeding tendency | Malignancy commonly involves CNS |
| | | Severe bacterial and viral infections | |
| | | Predisposition to malignancy | |
| Ataxia–telangiectasia [1] | B and T cell | Telangiectasia | Cerebellar degeneration |
| | | Sinopulmonary infections | Choreoathetosis |
| | | Predisposition to malignancy | Peripheral neuropathy (late in course) |
| Nijmegen breakage syndrome [2] | B and T cell | Dysmorphic facies | Microcephaly |
| | | Sinopulmonary infections | Borderline–mild mental retardation |
| | | Predisposition to malignancy | |

(continued)

**Table 38.1** Neurological features of selected primary immunodeficiencies (continued)

| Disorder | Site of immune defect | Non-neurological features | Neurological features |
|---|---|---|---|
| PNP deficiency [14] | B and T cell | Autoimmune hemolytic anemia | Limb spasticity |
| | | Severe bacterial and viral infections | Developmental delay |
| DiGeorge syndrome [15] | T cell | Congenital heart disease | Developmental delay |
| | | Hypoparathyroidism | Hypotonia |
| Hyperimmunoglobulin E syndrome [16] | Unknown | Dysmorphic facies, retained teeth, and osteopenia | Focal white matter lesions |
| | | Abscess formation | Chiari type I malformations |

SLE, systemic lupus erythematosus; CNS, central nervous system; NK, natural killer; EBV, Epstein-Barr virus; PNP, purine nucleoside phosphorylase.

## Epidemiology

The incidence of AT is 1 per 40,000 to 300,000 births. No specific racial predilection has been identified. The rate of heterozygous carriage among whites in the United States has been estimated at 1 to 2% [1,17,18].

## Pathogenesis

The gene mutated in AT, ATM, has been localized to 11q22–23 [19]. ATM encodes a kinase that participates in the cellular response to double-stranded DNA breaks [20]. Cultured lymphocytes from affected individuals develop abnormally high numbers of spontaneous and radiation-induced chromosomal breaks and rearrangements [21,22]. Immunoglobulin subclasses, particularly IgA and IgE, are often low, and defective T-cell function may be demonstrated in many patients [1,17]. How mutations in ATM result in neurodegeneration remains to be defined [20].

## Clinical Manifestations

Children with AT typically develop truncal ataxia by 3 years of age, and often during the first year of life [1,23]. Subsequently, characteristic telangiectasia appears on the interpalpebral bulbar conjunctivae (Fig. 38.1), [24] external ears, and occasionally elsewhere. The majority of patients also suffer from frequent bacterial infections, particularly otitis media, sinusitis, and pneumonia [1,23]. Lower respiratory tract infections become more frequent with age [17]. Bronchiectasis and pulmonary fibrosis may develop [1,23]. Malignancies, usually hematologic, occur at all ages; prognosis is generally poor, but long-term survival does occur [25–27]. Radiation therapy has had catastrophic results in some instances [28–30].

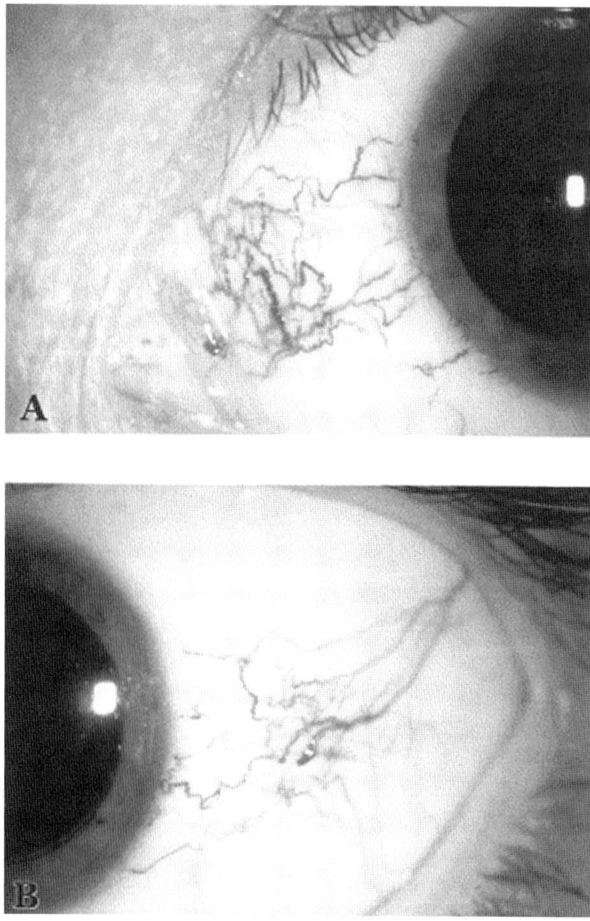


**Fig. 38.1** Telangiectasia of the nasal (**A**) and temporal (**B**) interpalpebral conjunctiva of a child with AT. Reprinted from reference 24, with permission from Elsevier [24].

Other reported manifestations of AT include eczema, hirsutism (in girls), graying of the hair, freckling, and warts. Actinic keratosis, basal cell carcinoma, and "hidebound" skin in sun-exposed areas may develop in older adolescents and young adults [23,31]. Endocrinopathy may include gonadal dysgenesis, diabetes mellitus, and adrenal cortical hypoplasia [1]. Short stature with a low weight-to-height ratio is the rule in AT, and the severity of growth failure correlates with the degree of neurological impairment [23,32]. Thymic dysplasia is always present [1].

Historically, death has occurred most commonly during the first or second decade of life, usually from chronic lung disease or malignancy [1]. However, life expectancy may be improving [17,23]. Furthermore, the phenotype of AT is very variable [1,23], probably because of residual production of functional protein associated with some mutations in the ATM gene [33]. Ataxia may start after age 4 years [1,23] or even in adulthood [34]; telangiectases may be sparse or absent; infections may be mild; and survival into the fourth and fifth decade has been described [1,17,23].

## Neurological Manifestations

The early clinical course of AT is usually dominated by progressive cerebellar dysfunction. Swaying of the head and trunk while sitting or standing occurs. Children may require assistance with balance in order to walk, although strength is preserved. Apparent improvement in cerebellar function may be noted in young children as motor skills develop, but, eventually, maturational gains are negated by further neurodegeneration. Basal ganglia dysfunction becomes apparent at a mean age of 5 years, but choreoathetosis is the initial neurological manifestation of AT in some children [1,23].

Over time, limb ataxia, generalized hypotonia, difficulty initiating voluntary movements, and intention tremor develop. Deep tendon reflexes may be diminished or lost, and the Babinski sign or equivocal plantar responses may be present [1]. Dystonia may also occur, and some patients have episodes of distressing, involuntary shaking of one limb [23]. The majority of patients are wheelchair-bound by age 10 years, but some remain ambulatory into their teenage years [1,23].

Abnormalities of ocular motility are usual in AT. Initiation of voluntary but not involuntary saccades is delayed, and attempts at smooth pursuit are characterized by step-like eye movements. Head thrusts are used to achieve fixation. Convergence and accommodation are deficient. Strabismus, nystagmus, and horizontal gaze apraxia may also be present [23,24].

Facial hypotonia results in a flat affect, which disappears when the patient is engaged [1]. Speech is slurred from the time the child starts talking or becomes so by the age of 10 years. Initiation of sounds may be delayed and speech may have a forced, whining quality. Speech may be clearer when the patient makes a conscious effort to swallow frequently [23]. Difficulty swallowing leads to drooling. Both silent and apparent aspiration become problematic as children get older [32].

In the third decade of life, peripheral neuropathy becomes apparent. Strength is lost, and muscle atrophy and contractures may occur. Lower limbs are affected more than upper limbs. Eventually, distal proprioception is impaired [1,23].

Cognitive development in early childhood is normal, but slows over time, such that intelligence quotient decreases somewhat with age. Nevertheless, adults with AT may have high levels of intellectual function [1,23]. A characteristic "affable personality" has also been described [1].

Magnetic resonance imaging of the head of patients with AT shows progressive cerebellar atrophy, with the lateral aspects of the hemispheres and the superior vermis showing the earliest changes [35]. Electromyography and nerve conduction studies are abnormal before the development of overt peripheral neuropathy, and findings are consistent with a nondemyelinating axonopathy of sensory and motor nerves [36]. Visual evoked potentials may be diminished in amplitude [37,38], whereas auditory brainstem responses [38] and electroencephalogram [1] are usually normal.

## Neuropathology

Histopathology in young children reveals a striking loss of Purkinje cells and, less dramatically, of granular cells in the cerebellum. Vermal degeneration is more prominent than that of the hemispheres. In older children and adults, pathologic abnormalities are found throughout the neuroaxis, spinal ganglia, peripheral nerves, and muscle [1]. Sural nerve biopsies are, for the most part, consistent with loss of large fibers, without evidence of primary demyelination [39]. Oddly, little degeneration of the basal ganglia is found until adulthood, despite the appearance of choreoathetosis in childhood [1].

## Diagnosis

The diagnosis of AT is based on the history and clinical examination, and is supported by an elevated serum alpha-fetoprotein level [40]. The latter finding is less specific in early infancy when serum fetal protein levels of healthy infants tend to be high [41]. Rarely, a patient with AT will have a normal serum alpha-fetoprotein level [1,23]. Genetic testing [42] and testing for radiosensitivity [43] are possible. Early diagnosis may avert unnecessary diagnostic and therapeutic exposure of patients to ionizing radiation or radiomimetic drugs [1,30]. Knowledge of the diagnosis also may permit identification of affected siblings and heterozygote relatives, and aid in family planning. Prenatal testing is available [44].

The differential diagnosis of AT is vast when the affected child comes to medical attention before the onset of telangiectasia, before the progressive nature of the ataxia is appreciated, and without a clear history of frequent infections. Tumor, infection, intoxication, congenital malformation, and metabolic or heredodegenerative disease may be considered. Patients with AT often receive an erroneous initial diagnosis of spastic cerebral palsy [1,23,45], and it has been suggested that serum alpha-fetoprotein should be measured in all young children with chronic or progressive ataxia of undetermined cause [45]. Friedreich's ataxia may be distinguished from AT by its later age of onset, and associated skeletal deformities, spinal signs, and normal alpha-fetoprotein level [1].

## Treatment

Treatment of patients with AT is directed toward amelioration of ongoing functional losses. Patients should receive therapy to optimize mobility, speech, feeding, and ability to perform activities of daily living. Corrective lenses that address exotropia and facilitate accommodation may benefit some patients [24]. Efforts to minimize chronic lung disease should include regular pulmonary toilet and prompt antibiotic therapy of bacterial sinopulmonary infections [1]. Intravenous immunoglobulin (IVIG) should be administered to patients who are unable to generate specific antibody responses [46].

Malignancies in AT are treated with the same agents and modalities that are used in immunocompetent patients. Although some oncologists use reduced dosages of radiomimetic drugs and avoid radiation therapy, this approach to therapy is controversial [26].

### Prevention

Preventive measures should include avoidance of non-essential radiological studies [1] and excessive sun exposure. Until the risk of malignancy in heterozygotes is better defined, [47,48] AT carriers also should avoid unnecessary exposure to ionizing radiation.

## *Nijmegen Breakage Syndrome*

### Introduction

Nijmegen breakage syndrome (NBS) is a rare, autosomal recessive disease associated with microcephaly, frequent infection, chromosomal instability, and predisposition to malignancy [2].

The gene mutated in NBS, NBS1, is located on chromosome 8q21 and encodes the protein nibrin. Nibrin is linked to the cellular response to breaks in DNA [49,50]. Thymic dysplasia or aplasia is usual. Most patients have mild-to-moderate lymphopenia, and abnormal T-cell function [2]. Dysgammaglobulinemia with poor generation of specific antibody is also common [51].

### Epidemiology

The majority of patients with NBS reported to date are of Slavic origin. A carrier frequency as high as 1 in 177 has been reported in some populations [52].

### Clinical Manifestations

Microcephaly is present in 75% of neonates with NBS, whereas birth weight and length are usually normal [2]. Children who are not microcephalic at birth become so during early infancy. Retardation of linear growth in proportion to weight, and bone age delay also occur after birth [53]. Dysmorphic facies, more evident in older children, include receding forehead, prominent midface with a long nose and philtrum, receding mandible, upward slanting palpebral fissures, and large ears with dysplastic helices. Dermatologic findings may include sparse hair, freckling on the cheeks and nose, café-au-lait spots, hypopigmented patches, subtle scleral telangiectasia, and pigment deposits in the ocular fundus. Syndactyly or clinomegaly is found in 50% of patients. A striking diversity of additional congenital malformations have been reported in NBS patients, including ovarian dysgenesis, anal atresia or stenosis, renal anomalies, hip dysplasia, and cerebral malformations [54].

Immunodeficiency is manifested by frequent episodes of otitis media, sinusitis, mastoiditis, pneumonia, and bronchitis. Bronchiectasis and death from respiratory failure may occur. Some patients have recurrent urinary tract infections. Viral infections are generally well tolerated [51,54].

Malignancy, particularly lymphoma, occurs in more than 40% of NBS patients. Prognosis is poor, but long-term survival after malignancy has been reported [2,27]. Fatal toxicity after radiation and chemotherapy has been reported in a patient with unrecognized NBS [55].

## Neurological Manifestations

Despite severe microcephaly, most patients with NBS have grossly normal psychomotor development. Feeding problems may occur in infancy, but are probably caused by mandibular hypoplasia. Developmental milestones usually are reached normally in the first year of life. Mental development is normal in 40% of patients, whereas 50% have borderline to mild retardation and 10% are moderately retarded. Hyperactivity is common [2]. Cranial magnetic resonance imaging scanning shows small frontal lobes with narrow anterior horns, and dilated lateral horns. Partial agenesis of the corpus callosum is sometimes seen, and focal white matter lesions, predominantly in the frontal lobes, may be present [56]. A simplified gyral pattern, most conspicuous in the frontal lobes, has been found at necropsy [57].

## Diagnosis

Diagnosis of NBS is made on the basis of clinical appearance. Genotyping may be performed in research laboratories [2].

## Treatment

At present, there is no curative treatment for NBS. Bacterial infections should be treated aggressively, and prophylactic antibiotics may be appropriate. IVIG may benefit patients unable to generate specific antibody [46]. Bone marrow transplantation may be considered.

## Prevention

Non-essential exposure to ionizing radiation and radiomimetic drugs should be avoided.

## *X-Linked Agammaglobulinemia*

### Introduction

X-linked agammaglobulinemia (XLA) is a rare disorder of B-cell maturation that results in frequent, often severe, bacterial infections and susceptibility to chronic enteroviral infection. B-cell development is blocked in the bone marrow at the pre-B-cell stage, and XLA is distinguished from other forms of hypogammaglobulinemia by the absence of B cells in the peripheral circulation and lymphoid tissue. Serum IgM, IgA, and IgG levels are low or undetectable [3,58].

### Clinical Manifestations

Maternal antibody protects infants with XLA from bacterial infection in the first months of life. The majority of patients become symptomatic with recurrent infection within the first year, most often with encapsulated bacteria. Sinopulmonary disease is common, and chronic lung disease may develop. Frequent skin infections, diarrhea, meningitis, sepsis, septic arthritis, and osteomyelitis also occur. Viral infections are generally well tolerated, with the exception of those caused by enteroviruses [3,58].

### Neurological Manifestations

Patients with XLA are vulnerable to chronic enteroviral meningoencephalitis and myelitis. Disease usually begins with slowly progressive loss of neurological function. Headache, sensorineural hearing loss, weakness, seizures, and altered mental status are common. Ataxia, paresthesias, hemiparesis, spastic paraplegia, cranial nerve palsies, aphasia, loss of cognitive skills, or altered personality may also occur. A waxing and waning course during several years followed by death is common, but there are long-term survivors. Occasionally, onset of disease is fulminant with fever, headache, and seizures. Edema, rash, and myositis or hepatitis accompanies central nervous system disease in some cases. Dermatomyositis-like symptoms may be present for months or years before central nervous system involvement becomes apparent [59,60].

Vaccine-associated paralytic polio is another well-recognized enteroviral complication of XLA, and differs from the disease in non-hypogammaglobulinemic patients. The incubation period may be prolonged and reversion to wild-type virus does not take place. Meningoencephalitis may develop in addition to myelitis. Mortality is high, and death often follows protracted illness [61]. The exclusive use of inactivated polio vaccine in the United States eliminates the risk of acquiring vaccine-associated polio in this country.

### Diagnosis

Diagnosis of chronic enteroviral infection is made by culture of virus [60] or amplification of viral nucleic acid [62,63] from the cerebrospinal fluid of patients in the appropriate clinical setting. Lumbar puncture may reveal elevated intracranial pressure, mild-to-moderate increases in cerebrospinal fluid protein level, leukocytosis, and hypoglycorrhachia [60]. Results of magnetic resonance imaging of the head may be normal or show diffuse cerebral or cerebellar atrophy [59]. Neuropathologic examination reveals perivascular T-cell infiltrates of the leptomeninges and often the brain and spinal cord. The pattern of infiltration and neuronal loss generally reflects the specific constellation of neurological deficits present in the patient antemortum [59,60].

### Treatment

Routine infusions of IVIG have greatly improved the long-term survival of patients with XLA, and are associated with reduced incidence of bacterial infections and enteroviral meningoencephalitis [3,58]. However, some patients acquire enteroviral infection with central nervous system disease despite receiving antibody replacement therapy [63–67]. In addition, treatment of established enteroviral meningoencephalitis with IVIG benefits some, but by no means all, affected patients [60,62,68], and relapses occur [60,68]. Antiviral therapy with pleconaril has been administered to agammaglobulinemic patients with chronic enteroviral infection; however, this agent is no longer available [65–67].

## *Chronic Granulomatous Disease*

### Introduction

Chronic granulomatous disease (CGD) is a disorder of phagocytes associated with frequent pneumonias and abscesses of lymph nodes, soft tissue, or bone. The disease is caused by mutations in the various components of phagocyte oxidase, which result in defective intracellular oxidative killing. Continual recruitment of phagocytes to sites of unresolved infection results in granuloma formation [69].

### Epidemiology

X-linked disease accounts for two thirds of affected patients, but autosomal recessive disease occurs as well [69].

### Clinical Manifestations

Children with CGD typically present with infection in infancy or early childhood. The most commonly isolated infectious agent is *Staphylococcus aureus*, but other catalase-producing bacteria and fungi, particularly *Aspergillus* spp., also cause infection. Gastrointestinal and urologic dysfunction may occur as a result of intramural granuloma formation. Mild forms of CGD may not be recognized until adulthood [69].

### Neurological Manifestations

Chorioretinitis without an obvious infectious etiology [9,10,70] affects approximately one quarter [10] of patients with CGD, most often asymptomatically. Nonprogressive, well-circumscribed retinal scars with central atrophy and peripheral clumping of pigment are found [10,70]. These "punched out" lesions may be multiple and are found adjacent to blood vessels, although the vessels themselves appear normal. In addition, areas of atrophic epithelium containing coarse clumps of pigment may be present. The atrophic lesions may be very large, but generally spare the macula. Sight-threatening chorioretinitis occurs infrequently and is associated with retinal ischemia, neovascularization, and macular edema [70]. Histopathologic examination of chorioretinal lesions shows disturbances of all layers of the retina, with distinct areas of hypertrophy and atrophy of the retinal pigment epithelium, and focal infiltration of pigment-containing macrophages [71].

Meningitis and brain abscess occur infrequently in patients with CGD [10,69]. Fungal and bacterial agents are implicated in both processes [10]. Granulomatous lesions of the central nervous system may be found postmortem [72]. Leptomeningeal infiltration with pigmented, lipid-laden macrophages has been demonstrated in two patients with CGD whose histories suggested the occurrence of a chronic central nervous system process [73,74].

### Treatment

Treatment of CGD includes surgical drainage of abscesses, prolonged antibiotic treatment of infections, and antibacterial and antifungal prophylaxis. In addition, regular administration of gamma-interferon has proven to be beneficial [69].

## *Chédiak–Higashi Syndrome*

### Introduction

Chédiak–Higashi syndrome (CHS) is a rare, autosomal recessive disorder consisting of partial oculocutaneous albinism, recurrent pyogenic infections, and the laboratory finding of giant, cytoplasmic granules in most cell types. The majority of patients eventually experience one or more episodes of an "accelerated phase" of disease in which organ infiltration with lymphohistiocytes occurs. Death caused by sepsis, pneumonia, or hemorrhage often occurs during this phase of disease [6,75].

## Pathogenesis

CHS is caused by mutations in the CHS1 gene which is found on 1q42–43 [76,77] and encodes a protein involved in trafficking of intracellular vesicles [6]. Aberrant migration of melanosomes leads to clumping rather than the normal dispersion of melanin and results in pallor of the iris, retina and skin, and hair [78]. Ocular manifestations of CHS, which include increased red reflex, photophobia, and nystagmus in bright light, presumably result from decreased ocular pigment [79]. Most patients also have some degree of neutropenia, which worsens during the accelerated phase. NK and T-cell cytotoxicity is impaired, whereas B-cell function is normal. A mild bleeding tendency is linked to a platelet storage pool deficiency [6].

## Clinical Manifestations

Children with CHS may experience frequent sinopulmonary and skin infections in early life [75]. The accelerated phase usually develops between a few months and 6 years of age. Viral infection, particularly with Epstein–Barr virus, often precedes the onset of lymphoproliferation [75,80]. Patients in the accelerated phase have fever and hepatosplenomegaly. Lymphadenopathy, bleeding, edema, icterus, and neurological abnormalities (see below) also may be present. Laboratory findings include pancytopenia, transaminasemia, and low serum fibrinogen levels [80]. Bone marrow may have normal or low cellularity, and hemophagocytosis or monocytic infiltrates are sometimes seen [79,80]. During the accelerated phase, sepsis or pneumonia with opportunistic bacteria or fungi may occur. The accelerated phase may remit spontaneously or with treatment, but recurrence is the rule [75].

## Neurological Manifestations

Peripheral and cranial neuropathies, seizures, behavioral disturbances, and loss of deep tendon reflexes have all been reported in patients with CHS, usually coincident with onset of the accelerated phase [79]. Histopathological study of autopsy material reveals lymphohistiocytic infiltrates in virtually all neurological structures [81], as well as most other tissues examined [75]. Resolution of neurological abnormalities with remission of the accelerated phase has been described [79,80].

Two distinct subsets of individuals with CHS reach adulthood, those who never enter the accelerated phase of disease [11], and those who survive after stem cell transplantation [82]. In both groups, progressive cerebellar ataxia, distal sensory and motor deficits, and loss of deep tendon reflexes become apparent at the end of the second decade. Nystagmus, tremor, and dementia are also reported. Head imaging may show diffuse cerebral or cerebellar atrophy. Electrophysiologic studies and muscle and nerve biopsy are consistent with axonal neuropathy [11,82].

Mental retardation has been noted in several children and adults reported with CHS [11,79]. Whether cognitive delay is part of the clinical spectrum of CHS or reflects separate genetic lesions in these patients of consanguineous parentage has not been determined [79].

### Diagnosis

The diagnosis of CHS is established by the finding of characteristic, giant, azurophilic, cytoplasmic granules in the neutrophils of the affected patient [6]. Prenatal diagnosis is possible [83,84].

### Treatment

Treatment of children in the accelerated phase with etoposide, corticosteroids, and intrathecal methotrexate may induce a temporary remission of lymphohistiocytic proliferation, but relapse is usual. Bone marrow transplantation has resulted in sustained resolution of the hematologic and immunologic abnormalities of CHS in a number of patients, greatly prolonging life expectancy. However, bone marrow reconstitution does not halt the neurodegenerative aspects of the syndrome [82].

## *Griscelli Syndrome*

### Introduction

Griscelli syndrome includes several rare, autosomal recessive disorders characterized by pigmentary abnormalities, recurrent bacterial infections, and episodic lymphohistiocytic proliferation [12]. Griscelli syndrome group 1 (GS1) accounts for the majority of affected patients and is associated with mutations of the RAB27A gene, whose product participates in intracellular vesicle transport [13].

### Clinical Manifestations

Uncontrolled lymphohistiocytic proliferation, the "accelerated phase," affects GS1 patients most often in infancy or early childhood [85]. Hepatomegaly, lymphadenopathy, and fever predominate. Neurological complications of lymphohistiocytic infiltration of the nervous system include seizures, spasticity, hypotonia, strabismus, nystagmus, ataxia, and coma.

### Diagnosis

The diagnosis of GS1 may be made by the finding of characteristic histopathology of hair and skin, which is distinct from that of CHS [12]. Genetic diagnosis is also possible [85]. Central nervous system disease is associated with elevated cerebrospinal fluid protein levels. Magnetic resonance imaging of the head reveals white matter lesions [86].

### Treatment

Cytoreductive therapy temporarily ameliorates lymphoproliferation, but only stem cell transplant is curative [84,86]. Unlike patients with CHS, GS1 patients do not have chronic neurodegenerative disease.

## *Purine Phosphorylase Deficiency*

### Introduction

Purine nucleoside phosphorylase (PNP) deficiency is a rare, autosomal recessive disorder characterized by recurrent infection, neurological abnormalities, and autoimmune disease [14]. Immunodeficiency results from the accumulation of the PNP substrate, deoxyguanosine, which is toxic to T cells. Neurological abnormalities are a consequence of deficiency of the PNP product, guanosine triphosphate [87].

### Clinical Manifestations

Affected patients have frequent upper and lower respiratory tract infections, diarrhea, and urinary tract infections, most often beginning in infancy or early childhood. Viral infections are particularly difficult for patients to control, but bacterial and fungal pathogens are problematic as well [14].

### Neurological Manifestations

Autoimmune disease most often manifests as hemolytic anemia, but central nervous system vasculitis [88] and stroke [89] have been reported as well. Neurological abnormalities, primarily motor defects, affect more than half of patients with PNP deficiency, and may be recognized before infectious complications occur. Spastic diplegia, hemiplegia and quadriplegia, hypotonia, motor delay, ataxia, and tremor have all been reported. Cognitive delay occurs in some patients [14].

### Diagnosis

Diagnosis of PNP deficiency is supported by the finding of very low serum uric acid levels and may be confirmed by the detection of abnormally low PNP activity in erythrocytes [14].

Results of computed tomographic scanning and magnetic resonance imaging of the brain are unremarkable, as is electroencephalography [90,91].

### Treatment

Stem cell transplantation restores immunocompetence in PNP-deficient patients. Neurological complications, especially motor deficits, require rehabilitation and physical therapy; whereas cognitive deficits require specialized assessment and educational interventions.

### Prognosis

Neurological complications of the disorder are stabilized but not reversed by bone marrow reconstitution [90–93].

## References


1. Sedgwick RP and Boder E. Ataxia-Telangiectasia. In: de Jong JMBV, ed. *Handbook of Clinical Neurology*, 1st ed., vol.16 New York: Elsevier Science, 1991; 347–423.
2. The International Nijmegen Breakage Syndrome Study Group. Nijmegen breakage syndrome. *Arch Dis Child* 2000; 82:400–406.
3. Ochs HD, Smith CI. X-linked agammaglobulinemia. A clinical and molecular analysis. *Medicine* (Baltimore) 1996; 75:287–299.
4. Perry GS 3rd, Spector BD, Schuman LM, Mandel JS, Anderson VE, McHugh RB, Hanson MR, Fahlstrom SM, Krivit W, Kersey JH. The Wiskott-Aldrich syndrome in the United States and Canada (1892–1979). *J Pediatr* 1980; 97:72–78.
5. Purtilo DT, Grierson HL, Davis JR, Okano M. The X-linked lymphoproliferative disease: from autopsy toward cloning the gene 1975–1990. *Pediatr Pathol* 1991; 11:685–710.
6. Spritz RA. Genetic defects in Chediak-Higashi syndrome and the beige mouse. *J Clin Immunol* 1998; 18:97–105.
7. Walport MJ, Davies KA, Botto M. C1q and systemic lupus erythematosus. *Immunobiology* 1998; 199:265–285.
8. Figueroa JE, Densen P. Infectious diseases associated with complement deficiencies. *Clin Microbiol Rev* 1991; 4:359–395.
9. Winkelstein JA, Marino MC, Johnston RB Jr, Boyle J, Curnutte J, Gallin JI, Malech HL, Holland SM, Ochs H, Quie P, Buckley RH, Foster CB, Chanock SJ, Dickler H. Chronic granulomatous disease. Report on a national registry of 368 patients. *Medicine* (Baltimore) 2000; 79:155–169.
10. Goldblatt D, Butcher J, Thrasher AJ, Russell-Eggitt I. Chorioretinal lesions in patients and carriers of chronic granulomatous disease. *J Pediatr* 1999; 134:780–783.

11. Uyama E, Hirano T, Ito K, Nakashima H, Sugimoto M, Naito M, Uchino M, Ando M. Adult Chediak-Higashi syndrome presenting as parkinsonism and dementia. *Acta Neurol Scand* 1994; 89:175–183.
12. Griscelli C, Durandy A, Guy-Grand D, Daguillard F, Herzog C, Prunieras M. A syndrome associating partial albinism and immunodeficiency. *Am J Med* 1978; 65:691–702.
13. Sanal O, Ersoy F, Tezcan I, Metin A, Yel L, Menasche G, Gurgey A, Berkel I, de Saint Basile G. Griscelli disease: genotype-phenotype correlation in an array of clinical heterogeneity. *J Clin Immunol* 2002; 22:237–243.
14. Markert ML. Purine nucleoside phosphorylase deficiency. *Immunodefic Rev* 1991;3:45–81.
15. Emanuel BS, McDonald-McGinn D, Saitta SC, Zackai EH. The 22q11.2 deletion syndrome. *Adv Pediatr* 2001; 48:39–73.
16. Freeman AF, Collura-Burke CJ, Patronas NJ, Ilcus LS, Darnell D, Davis J, Puck JM, Holland SM. Brain abnormalities in patients with hyperimmunoglobulin E syndrome. *Pediatrics* 2007; 119:e1121–1125.
17. Nowak-Wegrzyn A, Crawford TO, Winkelstein JA, Carson KA, Lederman HM. Immunodeficiency and infections in ataxia-telangiectasia. *J Pediatr* 2004; 144:505–511.
18. Swift M, Morrell D, Cromartie E, Chamberlin AR, Skolnick MH, Bishop DT. The incidence and gene frequency of ataxia-telangiectasia in the United States. *Am J Hum Genet* 1986; 39:573–583.
19. Savitsky K, Bar-Shira A, Gilad S, Rotman G, Ziv Y, Vanagaite L, Tagle DA, Smith S, Uziel T, Sfez S, et al. A single ataxia telangiectasia gene with a product similar to PI-3 kinase. *Science* 1995; 268:1749–1753.
20. McKinnon PJ. ATM and ataxia telangiectasia. *EMBO Rep* 2004; 5:772–776.
21. Hecht F, Koler RD, Rigas DA, Dahnke GS, Case MP, Tisdale V, Miller RW. Leukaemia and lymphocytes in ataxia-telangiectasia. *Lancet* 1966; 2:1193.
22. Higurashi M, Conen PE. In vitro chromosomal radiosensitivity in "chromosomal breakage syndromes". *Cancer* 1973; 32:380–383.
23. Woods CG, Taylor AM. Ataxia telangiectasia in the British Isles: the clinical and laboratory features of 70 affected individuals. *Q J Med* 1992; 82:169–179.
24. Farr AK, Shalev B, Crawford TO, Lederman HM, Winkelstein JA, Repka MX. Ocular manifestations of ataxia-telangiectasia. *Am J Ophthalmol* 2002; 134:891–896.
25. Morrell D, Cromartie E, Swift M. Mortality and cancer incidence in 263 patients with ataxia-telangiectasia. *J Natl Cancer Inst* 1986; 77:89–92.
26. Sandoval C, Swift M. Treatment of lymphoid malignancies in patients with ataxia-telangiectasia. *Med Pediatr Oncol* 1998; 31:491–497.
27. Seidemann K, Henze G, Beck JD, Sauerbrey A, Kuhl J, Mann G, Reiter A. Non-Hodgkin's lymphoma in pediatric patients with chromosomal breakage syndromes (AT and NBS): experience from the BFM trials. *Ann Oncol* 2000; 11 Suppl 1:141–145.
28. Morgan JL, Holcomb TM, Morrissey RW. Radiation reaction in ataxia telangiectasia. *Am J Dis Child* 1968; 116:557–558.
29. Gotoff SP, Amirmokri E, Liebner EJ. Ataxia telangiectasia. Neoplasia, untoward response to x-irradiation, and tuberous sclerosis. *Am J Dis Child* 1967; 114:617–625.
30. Rogers PB, Plowman PN, Harris SJ, Arlett CF. Four radiation hypersensitivity cases and their implications for clinical radiotherapy. *Radiother Oncol* 2000; 57:143–154.
31. Reed WB, Epstein WL, Boder E, Sedgwick R. Cutaneous manifestations of ataxia-telangiectasia. *JAMA* 1966; 195:746–753.
32. Lefton-Greif MA, Crawford TO, Winkelstein JA, Loughlin GM, Koerner CB, Zahurak M, Lederman HM. Oropharyngeal dysphagia and aspiration in patients with ataxia-telangiectasia. *J Pediatr* 2000; 136:225–231.
33. McConville CM, Stankovic T, Byrd PJ, McGuire GM, Yao QY, Lennox GG, Taylor MR. Mutations associated with variant phenotypes in ataxia-telangiectasia. *Am J Hum Genet* 1996; 59:320–330.
34. Sutton IJ, Last JI, Ritchie SJ, Harrington HJ, Byrd PJ, Taylor AM. Adult-onset ataxia telangiectasia due to ATM 5762ins137 mutation homozygosity. *Ann Neurol* 2004; 55:891–895.

35. Tavani F, Zimmerman RA, Berry GT, Sullivan K, Gatti R, Bingham P. Ataxia-telangiectasia: the pattern of cerebellar atrophy on MRI. *Neuroradiology* 2003; 45:315–319.
36. Kwast O, Ignatowicz R. Progressive peripheral neuron degeneration in ataxia-telangiectasia: an electrophysiological study in children. *Dev Med Child Neurol* 1990; 32:800–807.
37. Sridharan R, Mehta BC. Visual evoked potentials in ataxia telangiectasia. *J Neurol* 1985; 232:172–174.
38. Taylor MJ, Chan-Lui WY, Logan WJ. Longitudinal evoked potential studies in hereditary ataxias. *Can J Neurol Sci* 1985; 12:100–105.
39. Barbieri F, Santoro L, Crisci C, Massini R, Russo E, Campanella G. Is the sensory neuropathy in ataxia-telangiectasia distinguishable from that in Friedreich's ataxia? Morphometric and ultrastructural study of the sural nerve in a case of Louis Bar syndrome. *Acta Neuropathol (Berl)* 1986; 69:213–219.
40. Waldmann TA, McIntire KR. Serum-alpha-fetoprotein levels in patients with ataxia-telangiectasia. *Lancet* 1972; 2:1112–1115.
41. Masseyeff R, Gilli J, Krebs B, Calluaud A, Bonet C. Evolution of alpha-fetoprotein serum levels throughout life in humans and rats, and during pregnancy in the rat. *Ann NY Acad Sci* 1975; 22;259:17–28.
42. Spacey SD, Gatti RA, Bebb G. The molecular basis and clinical management of ataxia telangiectasia. *Can J Neurol Sci* 2000; 27:184–191.
43. Sun X, Becker-Catania SG, Chun HH, Hwang MJ, Huo Y, Wang Z, Mitui M, Sanal O, Chessa L, Crandall B, Gatti RA. Early diagnosis of ataxia-telangiectasia using radiosensitivity testing. *J Pediatr* 2002; 140:724–731.
44. Gatti RA, Peterson KL, Novak J, Chen X, Yang-Chen L, Liang T, Lange E, Lange K. Prenatal genotyping of ataxia-telangiectasia. *Lancet* 1993; 342:376.
45. Cabana MD, Crawford TO, Winkelstein JA, Christensen JR, Lederman HM. Consequences of the delayed diagnosis of ataxia-telangiectasia. *Pediatrics* 1998; 102:98–100.
46. [No authors listed] NIH consensus conference. Intravenous immunoglobulin. Prevention and treatment of disease. *JAMA* 1990; 264:3189–3193.
47. Su Y, Swift M. Mortality rates among carriers of ataxia-telangiectasia mutant alleles. *Ann Intern Med* 2000; 133:770–778.
48. FitzGerald MG, Bean JM, Hegde SR, Unsal H, MacDonald DJ, Harkin DP, Finkelstein DM, Isselbacher KJ, Haber DA. Heterozygous ATM mutations do not contribute to early onset of breast cancer. *Nat Genet* 1997; 15:307–310.
49. Matsuura S, Tauchi H, Nakamura A, Kondo N, Sakamoto S, Endo S, Smeets D, Solder B, Belohradsky BH, Der Kaloustian VM, Oshimura M, Isomura M, Nakamura Y, Komatsu K. Positional cloning of the gene for Nijmegen breakage syndrome. *Nat Genet* 1998; 19:179–181.
50. Varon R, Vissinga C, Platzer M, Cerosaletti KM, Chrzanowska KH, Saar K, Beckmann G, Seemanova E, Cooper PR, Nowak NJ, Stumm M, Weemaes CM, Gatti RA, Wilson RK, Digweed M, Rosenthal A, Sperling K, Concannon P, Reis A. Nibrin, a novel DNA double-strand break repair protein, is mutated in Nijmegen breakage syndrome. *Cell* 1998; 93:467–476.
51. Gregorek H, Chrzanowska KH, Michalkiewicz J, Syczewska M, Madalinski K. Heterogeneity of humoral immune abnormalities in children with Nijmegen breakage syndrome: an 8-year follow-up study in a single centre. *Clin Exp Immunol* 2002; 130:319–324.
52. Varon R, Seemanova E, Chrzanowska K, Hnateyko O, Piekutowska-Abramczuk D, Krajewska-Walasek M, Sykut-Cegielska J, Sperling K, Reis A. Clinical ascertainment of Nijmegen breakage syndrome (NBS) and prevalence of the major mutation, 657del5, in three Slav populations. *Eur J Hum Genet* 2000; 8:900–902.
53. Chrzanowska KH, Kleijer WJ, Krajewska-Walasek M, Bialecka M, Gutkowska A, Goryluk-Kozakiewicz B, Michalkiewicz J, Stachowski J, Gregorek H, Lyson-Wojciechowska G, et al. Eleven Polish patients with microcephaly, immunodeficiency, and chromosomal instability: the Nijmegen breakage syndrome. *Am J Med Genet* 1995; 57:462–471.
54. Weemaes CM, Hustinx TW, Scheres JM, van Munster PJ, Bakkeren JA, Taalman RD. A new chromosomal instability disorder: the Nijmegen breakage syndrome. *Acta Paediatr Scand* 1981; 70:557–564.

55. Distel L, Neubauer S, Varon R, Holter W, Grabenbauer G. Fatal toxicity following radio- and chemotherapy of medulloblastoma in a child with unrecognized Nijmegen breakage syndrome. *Med Pediatr Oncol* 2003; 41:44–48.
56. Bekiesinska-Figatowska M, Chrzanowska KH, Sikorska J, Walecki J, Krajewska-Walasek M, Jozwiak S, Kleijer WJ. Cranial MRI in the Nijmegen breakage syndrome. *Neuroradiology* 2000; 42:43–47.
57. Lammens M, Hiel JA, Gabreels FJ, van Engelen BG, van den Heuvel LP, Weemaes CM. Nijmegen breakage syndrome: a neuropathological study. *Neuropediatrics* 2003; 34:189–193.
58. Winkelstein JA, Marino MC, Lederman HM, Jones SM, Sullivan K, Burks AW, Conley ME, Cunningham-Rundles C, Ochs HD. X-linked agammaglobulinemia: report on a United States registry of 201 patients. *Medicine* (Baltimore) 2006; 85:193–202.
59. Rudge P, Webster AD, Revesz T, Warner T, Espanol T, Cunningham-Rundles C, Hyman N. Encephalomyelitis in primary hypogammaglobulinaemia. *Brain* 1996; 119:1–15.
60. McKinney RE Jr, Katz SL, Wilfert CM. Chronic enteroviral meningoencephalitis in agammaglobulinemic patients. *Rev Infect Dis* 1987; 9:334–356.
61. Wyatt HV. Poliomyelitis in hypogammaglobulinemics. *J Infect Dis* 1973; 128:802–806.
62. Rotbart HA, Kinsella JP, Wasserman RL. Persistent enterovirus infection in culture-negative meningoencephalitis: demonstration by enzymatic RNA amplification. *J Infect Dis* 1990; 161:787–791.
63. Webster AD, Rotbart HA, Warner T, Rudge P, Hyman N. Diagnosis of enterovirus brain disease in hypogammaglobulinemic patients by polymerase chain reaction. *Clin Infect Dis* 1993; 17:657–661.
64. Misbah SA, Spickett GP, Ryba PC, Hockaday JM, Kroll JS, Sherwood C, Kurtz JB, Moxon ER, Chapel HM. Chronic enteroviral meningoencephalitis in agammaglobulinemia: case report and literature review. *J Clin Immunol* 1992; 12:266–270.
65. Quartier P, Foray S, Casanova JL, Hau-Rainsard I, Blanche S, Fischer A. Enteroviral meningoencephalitis in X-linked agammaglobulinemia: intensive immunoglobulin therapy and sequential viral detection in cerebrospinal fluid by polymerase chain reaction. *Pediatr Infect Dis J* 2000; 19:1106–1108.
66. Rotbart HA, Webster AD; Pleconaril Treatment Registry Group. Treatment of potentially life-threatening enterovirus infections with pleconaril. *Clin Infect Dis* 2001; 32:228–235.
67. Schmugge M, Lauener R, Bossart W, Seger RA, Gungor T. Chronic enteroviral meningoencephalitis in X-linked agammaglobulinaemia: favourable response to anti-enteroviral treatment. *Eur J Pediatr* 1999; 158:1010–1011.
68. Quartier P, Debre M, De Blic J, de Sauverzac R, Sayegh N, Jabado N, Haddad E, Blanche S, Casanova JL, Smith CI, Le Deist F, de Saint Basile G, Fischer A. Early and prolonged intravenous immunoglobulin replacement therapy in childhood agammaglobulinemia: a retrospective survey of 31 patients. *J Pediatr* 1999; 134:589–596.
69. Dinauer MC, The Phagocytic System and Disorders of Granulopoiesis and Granulocyte Function. In: Nathan DG, Orkin SH, Ginsburg E, Look AT, eds. *Nathan and Oski's Hematology of Infancy and Childhood*, 6th ed., Philadelphia: Saunders, 2003; 977–986.
70. Kim SJ, Kim JG, Yu YS. Chorioretinal lesions in patients with chronic granulomatous disease. *Retina* 2003; 23:360–365.
71. Grossniklaus HE, Frank KE, Jacobs G. Chorioretinal lesions in chronic granulomatous disease of childhood. Clinicopathologic correlations. *Retina* 1988; 8:270–274.
72. Walker DH, Okiye G. Chronic granulomatous disease involving the central nervous system. *Pediatr Pathol* 1983; 1:159–167.
73. Riggs JE, Quaglieri FC, Schochet SS Jr, Dove DJ. Pigmented, lipid-laden histiocytes in the central nervous system in chronic granulomatous disease of childhood. *J Child Neurol* 1989; 4:61–63.
74. Hadfield MG, Ghatak NR, Laine FJ, Myer EC, Massie FS, Kramer WM. Brain lesions in chronic granulomatous disease. *Acta Neuropathol* (Berl) 1991; 81:467–470.

75. Padgett GA. The Chediak-Higashi Syndrome. *Advances in Veterinary Science* 1968; 12: 239–284.
76. Nagle DL, Karim MA, Woolf EA, Holmgren L, Bork P, Misumi DJ, McGrail SH, Dussault BJ Jr, Perou CM, Boissy RE, Duyk GM, Spritz RA, Moore KJ. Identification and mutation analysis of the complete gene for Chediak-Higashi syndrome. *Nat Genet* 1996; 14:307–311.
77. Barbosa MD, Nguyen QA, Tchernev VT, Ashley JA, Detter JC, Blaydes SM, Brandt SJ, Chotai D, Hodgman C, Solari RC, Lovett M, Kingsmore SF. Identification of the homologous beige and Chediak-Higashi syndrome genes. *Nature* 1996; 382:262–265.
78. Windhorst DB, Zelickson AS, Good RA. A human pigmentary dilution based on a heritable subcellular structural defect—the Chediak-Higashi syndrome. *J Invest Dermatol* 1968; 50:9–18.
79. Blume RS, Wolff SM. The Chediak-Higashi syndrome: studies in four patients and a review of the literature. *Medicine* (Baltimore) 1972; 51:247–280.
80. Bejaoui M, Veber F, Girault D, Gaud C, Blanche S, Griscelli C, Fischer A. The accelerated phase of Chediak-Higashi syndrome. *Arch Fr Pediatr* 1989; 46:733–736.
81. Sung JH, Meyers JP, Stadlan EM, Cowen D, Wolf A. Neuropathological changes in Chediak-Higashi disease. *J Neuropathol Exp Neurol* 1969; 28:86–118.
82. Tardieu M, Lacroix C, Neven B, Bordigoni P, de Saint Basile G, Blanche S, Fischer A. Progressive neurologic dysfunctions 20 years after allogeneic bone marrow transplantation for Chediak-Higashi syndrome. *Blood* 2005; 106:40–42.
83. Diukman R, Tanigawara S, Cowan MJ, Golbus MS. Prenatal diagnosis of Chediak-Higashi syndrome. *Prenat Diagn* 1992; 12:877–885.
84. Durandy A, Breton-Gorius J, Guy-Grand D, Dumez C, Griscelli C. Prenatal diagnosis of syndromes associating albinism and immune deficiencies (Chediak-Higashi syndrome and variant). *Prenat Diagn* 1993; 13:13–20.
85. Menasche G, Pastural E, Feldmann J, Certain S, Ersoy F, Dupuis S, Wulffraat N, Bianchi D, Fischer A, Le Deist F, de Saint Basile G. Mutations in RAB27A cause Griscelli syndrome associated with haemophagocytic syndrome. *Nat Genet* 2000; 25:173–176.
86. Arico M, Zecca M, Santoro N, Caselli D, Maccario R, Danesino C, de Saint Basile G, Locatelli F. Successful treatment of Griscelli syndrome with unrelated donor allogeneic hematopoietic stem cell transplantation. *Bone Marrow Transplant* 2002; 29:995–998.
87. Simmonds HA, Fairbanks LD, Morris GS, Morgan G, Watson AR, Timms P, Singh B. Central nervous system dysfunction and erythrocyte guanosine triphosphate depletion in purine nucleoside phosphorylase deficiency. *Arch Dis Child* 1987; 62:385–391.
88. McGinniss MH, Wasniowska K, Zopf DA, Straus SE, Reichert CM. An erythrocyte Pr auto-antibody with sialoglycoprotein specificity in a patient with purine nucleoside phosphorylase deficiency. *Transfusion* 1985; 25:131–136.
89. Tam DA Jr, Leshner RT. Stroke in purine nucleoside phosphorylase deficiency. *Pediatr Neurol* 1995; 12:146–148.
90. Baguette C, Vermylen C, Brichard B, Louis J, Dahan K, Vincent MF, Cornu G. Persistent developmental delay despite successful bone marrow transplantation for purine nucleoside phosphorylase deficiency. *J Pediatr Hematol Oncol* 2002; 24:69–71.
91. Classen CF, Schulz AS, Sigl-Kraetzig M, Hoffmann GF, Simmonds HA, Fairbanks L, Debatin KM, Friedrich W. Successful HLA-identical bone marrow transplantation in a patient with PNP deficiency using busulfan and fludarabine for conditioning. *Bone Marrow Transplant* 2001; 28:93–96.
92. Myers LA, Hershfield MS, Neale WT, Escolar M, Kurtzberg J. Purine nucleoside phosphorylase deficiency (PNP-def) presenting with lymphopenia and developmental delay: successful correction with umbilical cord blood transplantation. *J Pediatr* 2004; 145: 710–712.
93. Carpenter PA, Ziegler JB, Vowels MR. Late diagnosis and correction of purine nucleoside phosphorylase deficiency with allogeneic bone marrow transplantation. *Bone Marrow Transplant* 1996; 17:121–124.

# Section VIII
# Basic Principles of Selective Neurological Treatments

# Chapter 39
# Basic Principles of Selective Neurological Treatments

**Neil R. Friedman, M.B.Ch.B. and Manikum Moodley, M.B.Ch.B.**

## Basic Principles of Selective Neurological Treatments

Clinical monitoring is directed toward early detection and reversal of potentially life-threatening conditions or morbidity.

## Supportive Care

### *Vital signs*

- ◦ Blood pressure and pulse
  - Cushing's triad/response: Elevation in arterial blood pressure associated with falling pulse rate and irregular respirations is suggestive of raised intracranial pressure (ICP), Cushing triad/response.
  - After an acute ischemic stroke, it is not uncommon to see an elevation in blood pressure.
  - Dysautonomia frequently accompanies Guillain-Barré syndrome (GBS). Fluctuation in blood pressure and cardiac arrhythmias may be life threatening.
  - Stimulant medications typically give rise to altered mental status and hypertension.
- ◦ Respiratory rate
  - Alterations in respiratory rate may reflect underlying neurological dysfunction—such as ataxic breathing, which is suggestive of severe brainstem dysfunction.
- ◦ Fever
  - Fever and, in some instances, hypothermia may reflect infection.

MANAGEMENT ISSUES

- If Cushing's response is suspected, measures should be instituted aimed at reducing raised ICP (*vide infra*).

L.L. Barton and N.R. Friedman (eds.), *The Neurological Manifestations of Pediatric Infectious Diseases and Immunodeficiency Syndromes.*

- When hypertension is the result of an acute ischemic stroke, care should be taken to avoid rapid or excessive lowering of blood pressure, which may result in underperfusion of the penumbra region surrounding the stroke core.
- Blood pressure changes associated with GBS dysautonomia may result in marked fluctuations from hypertension to hypotension. Short-acting agents should, therefore, be used to treat the hypertension.
- Fever should be aggressively treated because it predisposes the young patient to seizures and increases the basal metabolic rate of the brain.

## *Neurological vital signs*

- Level of consciousness
  - Awake, alert, fully responsive
  - Lethargic or somnolent
    - Awakens to gentle stimulus, e.g., voice. Repeat stimulus may be required to maintain attention.
  - Obtundation
    - More vigorous stimulation required to arouse or maintain attention, e.g., may require physical stimulus or raised voice.
  - Stupor
    - Deeper degree of unresponsiveness and more severely impaired arousal than obtundation. Usually requires vigorous physical stimulus to elicit any response.
  - Coma
    - Unresponsive even to persistent external obnoxious stimulus.

The Glasgow Coma Scale (GCS) [1], originally developed as a prognostic tool for head injured patients, has become popular as a quick, reproducible estimate of the level of consciousness of a patient.

### Management Issues

- ABCs: With impaired level of consciousness, protection of airway and management of oropharyngeal secretions is important. Cardiopulmonary monitoring is mandatory. Airway safety and patency should be assessed, and, if necessary, an artificial airway or nasal trumpet inserted. Ventilation may be required if there is hypoxemia or impaired gaseous exchange. Rapid assessment and skillful support are essential to the survival of patients presenting in coma.

- Ocular signs
  - Pupillary reaction
    - Size, symmetry, and responsiveness to light should be assessed.

- Asymmetric pupils should raise concern for raised ICP ("blown pupil"). Remember that certain drugs (anticholinergic and atropine-like drugs), when accidentally rubbed topically on the eye, may cause mydriasis and failure of a pupil to respond.
- Small sluggish or absent pupillary response may occur with certain drugs, e.g., morphine, or with brainstem lesions.
- Fixed, dilated pupils are suggestive of impaired brainstem function.

- Eye movements
  - Gaze deviations:
    - Horizontal gaze deviation may be seen in acute stroke (eyes looking "toward the site of the lesion") or with seizures (typically eyes looking "away from the site of the lesion").
    - Dysconjugate gaze or phorias may be seen during sleep or in patients with impaired consciousness and should "correct" when the patient is awake. Vertical skew deviations raise concern for a possible IVth nerve palsy.
    - Roving eye movements and ocular bobbing may be seen in patients with severe visual impairments, brainstem pathology and/or metabolic encephalopathy respectively.
    - "Sunsetting" sign is the forced or sustained downgaze of the eyes seen in the setting of raised ICP or in pretectal or pineal lesions.

**Management Issues**

- Asymmetric pupils or the presence of "sunsetting" eyes should immediately raise concern for the possibility of raised ICP, and in the case of the former, a unilateral structural lesion with hemorrhage or swelling and imminent herniation. If the pupil is asymmetric and the patient is awake and fully conscious, consider inadvertent introduction of an anticholinergic drug topically to the eye, or a physiological anisocoria.
- Management of suspected raised ICP (*vide infra*).

## *General care*

- Deep venous thrombosis prophylaxis

**Management Issues**

- If the patient is immobilized for any significant period of time, preventive therapies aimed at avoiding deep vein thrombosis should be instituted. This includes the use of subcutaneous heparin and pneumatic stockings.

- Avoidance of contractures and pressure sores

  **Management Issues**

  - It is important to prevent decubitus ulcers, therefore, careful positioning and frequent turning of the patient is important. The skin should regularly be inspected for signs of skin break down.
  - Physical therapy should be instituted early for passive range-of-motion exercises. When safe, exercise and ambulation should be encouraged to help maintain and improve strength and function.
  - Ankle foot orthoses (AFOs) should be used as adjunctive therapy if the patient is immobilized for prolonged periods to help prevent ankle contractures.

- Critical illness myopathy (CIM) or critical illness polyneuropathy (CIP)

  **Management Issues**

  - Newly acquired muscle weakness or unexplained difficulty weaning the ventilator in a critically ill child should raise the suspicion of a CIM or CIP. Risk factors include corticosteroids, nondepolarizing neuromuscular-blocking agents, [2] sepsis, and systemic inflammatory response syndrome [3].
  - Differentiating CIM from CIP clinically can be very difficult and usually requires electrodiagnostic studies.
  - Treatment is essentially supportive because no specific therapies are available. A high index of suspicion is necessary to make the diagnosis. Prognosis is variable and recovery is slow and may occur over weeks to months [3].
  - It is best to avoid corticosteroids and neuromuscular blockade, if possible, once a diagnosis of CIM or CIP is made.

- Aspiration precautions

  **Management Issues**

  - If a patient is unable to protect his/her airway, or if there is oropharyngeal weakness or a reduced gag reflex, consideration to intubation and nasogastric placement should be given.

- Urinary retention

  **Management Issues**

  - A Foley catheter may be required if there is urinary retention.

## Seizures [4–12]

Seizures may be generalized or focal/partial in onset with, at times, subsequent generalization. It is important to know whether the onset of the seizure was observed to determine whether there was a focal onset. After a seizure, the post-ictal stage is characterized by confusion, fatigue, and disorientation.

Acute symptomatic seizures are seizures that arise from an acute brain insult (infection, stroke, etc.) or secondary to systemic derangements (such as electrolyte disturbances, hypoglycemia, etc.).

Most seizures are brief and self-limited. However, repetitive seizures without recovery of consciousness or seizures lasting longer than 10 to 12 minutes [7,8] (operational definition) are regarded as status epilepticus (SE) and are a medical emergency. SE should also be suspected in a patient who remains unresponsive after an observed seizure and who is not returning to baseline mentation. Persistence of SE eventually causes hemodynamic changes, cardiac arrhythmias, acidosis, and neuronal cell death. Rhabdomyolysis and renal failure may also ensue.

### Management Issues

Initial general management:

- The initial management of seizures involves the "ABCs." One needs to ensure a safe and adequate airway, as well as adequate oxygenation and gaseous exchange. Intravenous access should be established and nasal oxygen started. With hypotension and cardiovascular collapse, fluid resuscitation and inotropic drug support may be necessary. If there is hypertension, consider the possibility of an acute stroke or Cushing response (*vide supra*) with raised ICP as the cause, in which case, there should be the judicious use of isotonic fluids.
- Establishing the cause of the seizure is crucial. A quick focused history, and general and neurological examinations should be conducted, and finger stick blood glucose level checked. Blood should also be sent for a complete blood count (CBC), electrolytes, glucose, blood urea nitrogen (BUN) and creatinine, calcium, magnesium, hepatic function tests, and toxicology screen. If there is fever or any concern for infection, blood and urine cultures should be obtained. An additional aliquot of blood should be held for serologies. If meningitis or encephalitis is suspected, a lumbar puncture (LP) is necessary, but if the patient is still seizing, or if there is concern for raised ICP, antibiotics should be started immediately and the LP deferred until the patient is stabilized and raised ICP can be excluded with a computed tomographic (CT) brain scan.
- Fever should be aggressively treated with antipyretics and active cooling if necessary.

Specific management:

- Pharmacotherapy depends on whether the patient is still actively seizing or not.
- Status epilepticus (SE).
  - Initial management of SE involves the administration of lorazepam (0.05–0.1 mg/kg). This should ideally be administered intravenously, however, if intravenous access is not available, rectal Valium (Diastat) is an alternative.
  - If there is no response after 5 minutes, a second dose should be administered. Some authorities recommend the institution of a second anticonvulsant at this time, whereas others would wait another 5 minutes to see whether the seizures abort. The most commonly used second-line agent is fosphenytoin administered at a dose of 18 to 20 mg/kg (if the patient has no hepatic or renal impairment). A maintenance dose should then be initiated 12 hours later until further information

is available. Alternative second-line drugs include intravenous phenobarbital (15–20mg/kg), valproic acid (20mg/kg), and levetiracetam (20mg/kg). There is only limited information regarding the use of the latter two drugs in SE.
    - If the seizures are refractory, a further 5 to 10mg/kg of fosphenytoin can be administered, but, if SE persists, induce coma with either barbiturate anesthesia (phenobarbital or sodium pentobarbital), benzodiazepine infusion (such as a midazolam drip), or propofol. At this point, the patient will need intubation and transfer to an intensive care unit for continuous electroencephalography (EEG) to monitor seizure control and level of anesthesia.

- Focal/partial seizures.
    - A number of different anticonvulsant/antiepileptic drugs (AED) are effective for the treatment of partial seizures. These include many of the newer anticonvulsant medications, such as oxcarbazepine, levetiracetam, topiramate, and lamotrigine. Phenobarbital, phenytoin, carbamazepine, and valproic acid are also effective.
    - The duration of anticonvulsant therapy in treating the patient depends on two main factors—whether the seizure is a symptomatic seizure, and the resolution of the inciting event. In the case of an electrolyte imbalance, for example, there is no need for maintenance therapy. In encephalitis, or a structural lesion, such as a brain abscess that can heal with little residual brain scarring/gliosis, treatment with an AED is usually continued for 6 to 12 weeks. There is some debate regarding whether an EEG should be obtained before discontinuing the AED if the patient has remained asymptomatic and seizure free. If the underlying etiology of the seizure has resulted in significant brain injury, such as a stroke with encephalomalacia, the issue of maintenance drug therapy is more complex and controversial. If the EEG shows epileptiform discharges 6 to 12 weeks after the inciting event, and given the underlying structural brain damage, many authorities would continue treatment until the patient is seizure free for 2 years (the "gold standard" for the treatment of idiopathic epilepsy).

- Generalized seizures.
    - A number of different AEDs are effective for the treatment of generalized seizures. These include phenobarbital, phenytoin, valproic acid, lamotrigine, topiramate, and levetiracetam.
    - Decision making regarding the duration of treatment is essentially the same as that for partial seizures (*vide supra*).

## Raised Intracranial Pressure

Raised ICP, also referred to as intracranial hypertension, is a medical emergency and is the result of intracranial mass lesions (tumor, abscess, hemorrhage), hydrocephalus (obstructive, communicating), or cerebral edema from a variety of causes (infection/inflammation, ischemia/stroke, metabolic or toxic). One of the most frightening complications of raised ICP is brain herniation (uncal, tentorial, cerebellar, or subfalcine), which may result in death or significant neurological morbidity. Another contributing factor to neurological morbidity is impairment of the cerebral perfusion pressure (CPP) leading to hypoxic–ischemic brain damage. CPP is the difference between the mean arterial pressure (MAP) and the ICP.

Therapeutic interventions are measures that help to increase the CPP and cerebral blood flow (CBF). The skull is rigid and comprises essentially three components—brain tissue (80%), cerebrospinal fluid (10%), and intracranial blood (10%). Treatment modalities, therefore, try to reduce the intracranial volume while trying to increase the MAP.

The clinical symptoms of raised ICP include progressive decline in level of consciousness, headache, early morning and persistent vomiting, diplopia (from cranial nerve palsies—especially VIth cranial nerve), and excessive fussiness or irritability in a younger child. Signs include altered level of consciousness (see above), papilledema, cranial nerve palsies, and Cushing's response.

### Management Issues [13, 14]

- Initial management involves the ABCs (*vide supra*, under seizure management). Caution needs to be taken with intubation, if necessary, to avoid exacerbating the intracranial hypertension.
- General measures include elevation of the head of the bed to approximately 30 degrees [15,16], avoidance of hypotonic fluids, close blood pressure monitoring, avoidance of hyperthermia, and a neurosurgical consultation. If the patient is agitated, he/she should be sedated, and if necessary, paralyzed [17]. If the patient is to be kept paralyzed, continuous EEG monitoring is necessary for the detection of seizures. Seizures, if present, should be identified and treated appropriately. The patients should be monitored for the development of the syndrome of inappropriate antidiuretic hormone (SIADH) secretion [18]. One should avoid fluid restriction because hypovolemia may, in fact, exacerbate the lowering of the CPP.
- Specific measures include:
  - Monitoring of ICP—the placement of an ICP monitoring device allows for more accurate measurement of ICP and better ability to manage CPP. It is important to ensure that the patient does not have disseminated intravascular coagulation (DIC) or thrombocytopenia.
  - Maintenance of CPP [19–22]—CPP should be maintained at or above 70 mmHg and less than 110 mmHg. This involves maintaining or increasing MAP with the use of inotropes and vasopressor support, and/or attempting to reduce the ICP. In many such patients, sedation is an effective means of controlling ICP.
  - Reduction of ICP [23–29]—a number of measures can be instituted to reduce ICP. These tend to be temporary and should be reserved until absolutely necessary, typically to allow time for surgical intervention, if possible.

- Hyperventilation: normocarbia to mild hypocarbia should be achieved with a $pCO_2$ of approximately 28 to 32 mmHg. Aggressive hyperventilation should be avoided because the vasoconstriction induced may result in a deleterious effect of reduced CBF and worsening ischemia and hypoxia.
- Mannitol is a useful adjunctive therapy in reducing raised ICP because of its osmotic effect of drawing fluid into the intravascular compartment. It is usually administered every 4 hours (0.25–1 g/kg). It is important to calculate the difference between the measured serum osmolarity and the calculated osmolarity to ensure that the administered mannitol is cleared before the next dose, thereby avoiding intravascular hypovolemia.
- Corticosteroids: dexamethasone is useful in reducing brain edema caused by vasogenic edema (as seen in brain tumor, abscess, etc.).
- Hypothermia: as with pharmacological approaches, moderate hypothermia (32–33°C) reduces cerebral metabolic rate and, thus, lowers CBF, cerebral blood volume, and ICP.
- Other therapies with unproven outcomes or results include barbiturate coma (reducing basal energy requirement of the brain) and hemispherectomy.

- Neuroimaging—a head CT scan or brain magnetic resonance imaging (MRI) scan should be performed emergently once the patient is stabilized to see whether there is an underlying process or lesion amenable to surgical intervention, such as shunting of hydrocephalus, evacuation of a mass lesion (hematoma, tumor), or drainage of an abscess.

## References

1. Teasdale G, Jennett B. Assessment of coma and impaired consciousness; a practical scale. *Lancet* 1974; 2(7872):81–84.
2. Bird SJ. Diagnosis and management of critical illness polyneuropathy and critical illness myopathy. *Curr Treat Options Neurol* 2007; 9:85–92.
3. Williams S, Horrocks IA, Ouvrier RA, Gillis J, Ryan MM. Critical illness polyneuropathy and myopathy in pediatric intensive care: A review. *Pediatr Crit Care Med* 2007; 8:18–22.
4. Lothman E. The biochemical basis and pathophysiology of status epilepticus. *Neurology* 1990; 40 (suppl 2):13–23.
5. Dunn DW. Status epilepticus in children: etiology, clinical features and outcome. *J Child Neurol* 1988; 3:167–173.
6. DeLorenzo RJ, Towne AR, Pellock JM, Ko D. Status epilepticus in children, adults, and the elderly. *Epilepsia* 1992; 33(suppl 4):S15–S25.
7. Shinnar S, Berg AT, Moshe SL, Shinnar R. How long do new-onset seizures in children last? *Ann Neurol* 2001; 49:659–664.
8. Lowenstein DH, Bleck T, Macdonald RL. It's time to revise the definition of status epilepticus. *Epilepsia* 1999; 40:120–122.
9. Chen YJ, Fang PC, Chow JC. Clinical characteristics and prognostic factors of postencephalitic epilepsy in children. *J Child Neurol* 2006; 21:1047–1051.
10. Riviello JJ, Ashwal S, Hirtz D, et al. Practice parameter: diagnostic assessment of the child with status epilepticus (an evidence-based review): report of the Quality Standards Subcommittee of the American Academy of Neurology and the Practice Committee of the Child Neurology Society. *Neurology* 2006; 67:1542–1550.

11. Chin RF, Neville BG, Peckham C, et al. Incidence, cause, and short-term outcome of convulsive status epilepticus in childhood: prospective population-based study. *Lancet* 2006; 368:222–229.
12. Riviello JJ, Holmes GL. The treatment of status epilepticus. *Semin Pediatr Neurol* 2004; 11:129–138.
13. Rangel-Castillo L, Robertson CS. Management of intracranial hypertension. *Crit Care Clin* 2007; 22:713–732.
14. Jankowitz BT, Adelson PD. Pediatric traumatic brain injury: past, present and future. *Dev Neurosci* 2006; 28:264–275.
15. Feldman Z, Kanter MJ, Robertson CS, et al. Effect of head elevation on intracranial pressure, cerebral perfusion pressure, and cerebral blood flow in head-injured patients. *J Neurosurg* 1992; 76:207–211.
16. Ng I, Lim J, Wong HB. Effects of head posture on cerebral hemodynamics: Its influence on intracranial pressure, cerebral perfusion pressure, and cerebral oxygenation. *Neurosurgery* 2004; 54:593–598.
17. Hsiang JK, Chestnut RM, Crisp CB, Klauber MR, Blunt BA, Marshall LF. Early, routine paralysis for intracranial pressure control in severe head injury: Is it necessary? *Crit Care Med* 1994; 22:1471–1476.
18. Fichman MP, Kleeman CR, Bethune JE. Inhibition of antidiuretic hormone secretion by Diphenylhydantoin. *Arch Neurol* 1970; 22:45–53.
19. Goitein KJ, Tamir I. Cerebral perfusion pressure in central nervous system infections of infancy and childhood. *J Pediatrics*. 1983; 103:40–43.
20. Juul N, Morris G, Marshall B, Marshall F, et al. Intracranial hypertension and cerebral perfusion pressure: influence on neurological deterioration and outcome in severe head injury. *J Neurosurg* 2000; 92:1–6.
21. Rosner MJ, Rosner SD, Johnson AH. Cerebral perfusion pressure: management protocol and clinical results. *J Neurosurg* 1995; 83:949–962.
22. Huang S-J, Hong W-C, Han Y-Y, Chen Y-S, Wen C-S, Tsai Y-S, Tu Y-K. Clinical outcome of severe head injury using three different ICP and CPP protocol-driven therapies. *J Clin Neurosci* 2006; 13:818–822.
23. Horwitz SJ, Boxerbaum B, O'Bell J. Cerebral herniation in bacterial meningitis in childhood. *Ann Neurol* 1980; 7:524–528.
24. Rebaud P, Berthier JC, Hartemann E, Floret D. Intracranial pressure in childhood central nervous system infections. *Intensive Care Med* 1988; 14:522–525.
25. Luerssen TG. Intracranial pressure: current status in monitoring and management. *Semin Pediatr Neurol* 1997; 4:146–155.
26. Lindvall P, Ahlm C, Ericsson M, Gothefors L, Naredi S, Koskinen L-O. Reducing intracranial pressure may increase survival among patients with bacterial meningitis. *Clin Infect Dis* 2004; 38:384–390.
27. Wahlström MR, Olivecrona M, Koskinen L-O, Rydenhag B, Naredi S. Severe traumatic brain injury in pediatric patients: treatment and outcome using an intracranial pressure targeted therapy—the Lund concept. *Intensive Care Med* 2005; 31:832–839.
28. Steiner LA, Andrews PJD. Monitoring the injured brain: ICP and CBP. *Br J Anaesth* 2006; 97:26–38.
29. Fishman RA. Cerebral edema. *N Engl J Med* 1975; 293:706–711.

# Index